A Comprehensive Guide to Reproductive Health and Infertility Medicine for Nurses

Mausumi Das • Michael H. Dahan
Editors

A Comprehensive Guide to Reproductive Health and Infertility Medicine for Nurses

Springer

Editors
Mausumi Das
Assisted Conception Service, Department of Obstetrics and Gynaecology
Glasgow Royal Infirmary, Glasgow, UK

University of Glasgow, Glasgow, UK

Imperial College, London, UK

Michael H. Dahan
Department of Reproductive Endocrinology and Infertility, McGill University,
Montreal, QC, Canada

ISBN 978-3-032-24371-3   ISBN 978-3-032-24372-0 (eBook)
https://doi.org/10.1007/978-3-032-24372-0

This Springer imprint is published by the registered company Springer Nature Switzerland AG
The registered company address is: Gewerbestrasse 11, 6330 Cham, Switzerland

I wish to dedicate this nursing textbook to all the nurses I have worked with through my career who always made my work environment better, corrected my mistakes, laughed at my jokes, did all the required teaching for my patients that I did not have time to, and taught me a great deal about doing research.

Dr. Michael H. Dahan

Preface

Reproductive health and Fertility care are rapidly evolving areas in modern healthcare, sitting at the crossroads of technological advances and meticulous clinical practice. As fertility treatments become more technologically advanced and multifaceted, the knowledge and responsibilities expected of nurses working in this field have expanded in parallel. Nurses are central to the delivery of safe, effective, and compassionate fertility care. They translate complex protocols and procedures into easily understandable, supportive guidance for patients and their partners. This book is written with those nurses in mind.

This book aims to provide nurses a clear, practical, and clinically grounded guide to fertility and assisted conception. It integrates reproductive physiology, evidence-based fertility treatments, contemporary IVF practice, and laboratory procedures in a user-friendly and easy-to-read format. Many of the topics are written by nurses working in the field of fertility care and we are deeply grateful to them for their contribution. Topics include physiology, patient assessment, treatment protocols, medication management, cycle monitoring, laboratory procedures, ethical and legal considerations, and the psychosocial dimensions of infertility. Throughout, the emphasis is on how scientific principles and evidence-based guidelines translate into day-to-day nursing practice and patient care.

Recognizing the diversity of nursing roles within fertility services, this book is relevant to nurses at different stages of experience—from those new to reproductive medicine to experienced nurse practitioners seeking to consolidate knowledge or support advanced practice. While grounded in current evidence and guidelines, the content acknowledges variation in clinical practice across settings and regions across the globe.

Above all, this book reflects the core values of fertility nursing: professionalism, meticulousness, and empathy. Infertility and its treatment can be emotionally and physically demanding for patients, and nurses play a crucial role in ensuring care is not only technically excellent but also respectful, supportive, and patient-centered.

It was with great joy and trepidation that we undertook to edit a textbook on infertility for nurses. We believe that this is the first ever textbook specifically for nurses on infertility medicine. Infertility is a field of medicine to which we often have minimal or no exposure in training and the care of infertility patients is not self-evident. Nevertheless, nursing care is so vital in infertility medicine, with much of the patients' teaching performed by nurses. The current format to learn infertility medicine for nurses has been an internship mechanism which often requires six or more months of effort to become comfortable with the required knowledge. This expertise can be supplemented by online courses often provided by the major societies in our field and by teaching done by drug company representatives which can be prone to bias. As such, we felt that an academic infertility text for nurses was crucial and would fill an important gap, to provide a reference for the experienced nurse, a source for the new inductee, and a place to go to for questions. It is our hope that this text will be made available in most IVF centers across the world for nurses to consult when necessary.

Infertility is also one of the most rapidly growing areas of medical care. It is estimated that in 2020 five million patients underwent fertility treatment worldwide. In 2025 that number was 15 million patients. By 2035 it will be about 50 million patients, and by 2050, 150 million patients will undergo fertility care worldwide. The reason that fertility care is increasing at an exponential rate is due to many factors, but primarily delayed childbearing, due to the educational and work burden, the difficulty to find a stable partner, and the need to be financially established at the time of childbirth, in a climate of increasing economic pressures. In the mid-1800s most women were married and had their first child as a teenager. Today the average age of first birth is 29 years old in many economically advantaged countries and birth rates are plummeting well below subsistence levels. Even on continents such as Asia and Africa, in countries with developing economies, such trends in age of first birth and birthrates are also being noted. To combat these issues many countries are mandating fertility care, and more are certainly on the way to doing so, all of which will increase demands for trained infertility nurses. As such this text will certainly become an invaluable reference.

We recruited a broad range of world-renowned experts to write these chapters. These experts included nurses, mental health professionals, religious leaders, and physicians with an international representation. The goal of which was to make sure that nuances in infertility care across the globe were represented. Infertility is affected by cultural and religious beliefs. As such, we presented an unbiased view of how different religions understand and accept diverse fertility treatments. Infertility is psychologically taxing for patients, with up to 50% of infertility patients failing to function in their jobs and at daily life. As such, we recruited one of the world's most foremost infertility psychologists to write a chapter. Nurses will often need to counsel patients, who are suffering through care and comfort those who failed to achieve a pregnancy with treatment.

We stated that it was with both joy and trepidation that we undertook to edit this text. That is because we find teaching a true joy, and the love of transmitting knowledge is what drove us to undertake this journey. However, we have previously edited several infertility textbooks, and we are aware of how daunting a task this can be. Nevertheless, the importance of spreading knowledge won out over the difficulties which would be encountered. It is our hope that this book will serve as a trusted reference, a learning resource, and a practical companion for nurses committed to delivering high-quality care in fertility and assisted conception.

Sincerely

London, UK — Mausumi Das, MD FRCOG MPH
Montreal, QC, Canada — Michael H. Dahan, MD FACOG FRCSC

Contents

About the Editors

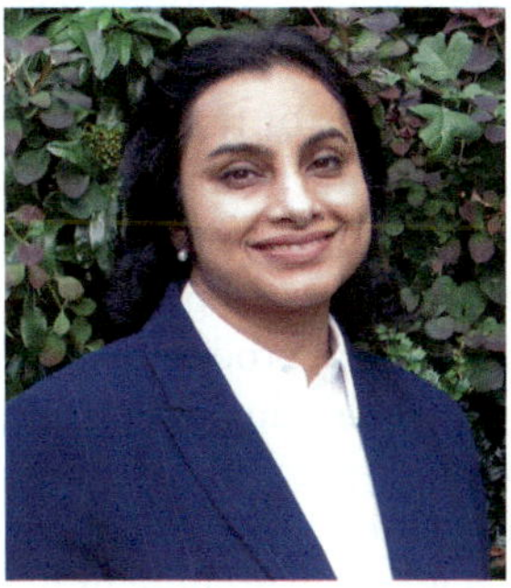

Mausumi Das is a highly accomplished clinician-academic with an established track record of leadership in clinical care, research, education, and strategic service development. She is a Consultant Gynaecologist and Royal College of Obstetricians and Gynaecologists (RCOG) accredited Sub-Specialist in Reproductive Medicine and Surgery. After completing specialist training in Obstetrics and Gynaecology in the United Kingdom, she undertook a prestigious two-year fellowship in Reproductive Endocrinology and Infertility at McGill University in Montreal, Canada, further refining her expertise in the management of complex reproductive disorders and advanced fertility care.

She was awarded a research doctorate by the University of London for her work on the pathogenesis of Polycystic Ovary Syndrome (PCOS) and an MPH degree in Epidemiology by Harvard University, USA. She works as a consultant in Reproductive Medicine at Glasgow Royal Infirmary, Scotland, UK. Alongside her clinical practice, she serves as an Honorary Senior Lecturer at Imperial College, London, and at the University of Glasgow, where her work seamlessly integrates clinical excellence, research innovation, education, and professional leadership.

Deeply committed to education and training, she is the British Fertility Society (BFS) Training Committee lead for Reproductive Endocrinology, an accredited trainer for the specialist certification modules, and an RCOG preceptor for the Subfertility Special Interest Training module. She teaches and supervises PhD, MSc, and BSc students of Reproductive Sciences at Imperial College, London, and is the research theme lead for Optimising Disease Prediction and Prevention for the Women's Health Network, thereby playing a key role in fostering academic excellence and developing the next generation of clinicians and scientists.

Her research has made significant contributions to the field of reproductive medicine, with a strong emphasis on translating scientific evidence into clinical excellence. She is the author of more than 30 peer-reviewed publications and book chapters in the field of reproductive medicine and infertility. She is the editor of the book *Recent Advances in Obstetrics and Gynaecology, volume 28*, and serves on the editorial board of several international journals. An active member of several professional societies, she regularly speaks at national and international conferences. Her work has contributed to advancing knowledge across key areas of reproductive medicine and has informed contemporary clinical practice and ongoing research initiatives.

Her clinical expertise encompasses reproductive endocrinology, fertility care, assisted reproduction and IVF, PCOS, fertility preservation, male infertility, and recurrent implantation failure. Her practice is underpinned by a commitment to delivering compassionate, evidence-based, and personalized care. Throughout her career, she has remained committed to advancing reproductive healthcare through the development and implementation of high-quality, evidence-based clinical guidance, innovative research, clinical excellence, and shared learning, ultimately enhancing reproductive outcomes for patients nationally and internationally.

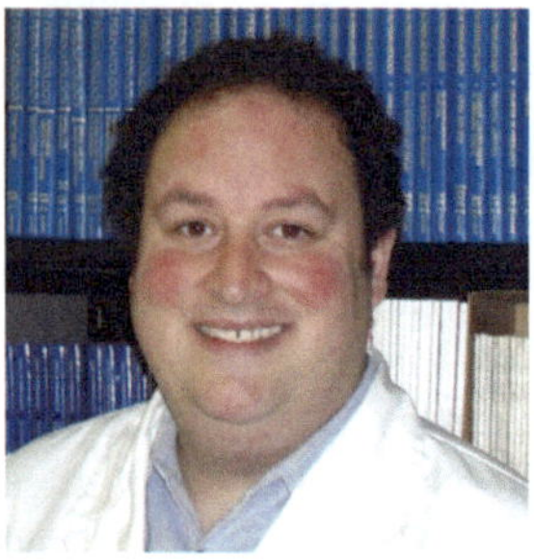

Michael H. Dahan MD, FACOG, FRCSC (of Canada), is an Associate Professor in the Department of Obstetrics and Gynecology at McGill University and a pioneer in IVM, IVF, and Reproductive Endocrinology. He received his medical degree from the State University of New York at Stony Brook in 1996. From 1996 to 2000, he completed a residency in Obstetrics and Gynecology at the Long Island College Hospital of the State University of New York at Down State. In 2003, he completed a fellowship in Reproductive Endocrinology and Infertility with Jeffrey Chang, one of the world's experts in Polycystic Ovary Syndrome, Samuel Yen, the father of Modern Reproductive Endocrinology, and David Meldrum, one of the pioneers of early in vitro fertilization, at the University of California, at San Diego. He was a faculty member at

Washington University in St. Louis, Missouri, and Stanford University in California, where he was a Women's Reproductive Health Research Scholar (WRHR) after finishing his fellowship.

He has more than 25 years of experience in women's health. He has been a member of numerous professional organizations, including the European Society of Human Reproduction, the Society for Reproductive Endocrinology and Infertility, the American Society for Reproductive Medicine, the American College of Obstetrics and Gynecology, the Society for Gynecologic Investigation, the Royal College of Physicians and Surgeons of Canada, the Association of Obstetricians and Gynecologists of Quebec, and the Canadian Fertility and Andrology Society. He is a former Chair of the Associate Committee of the Society for Reproductive Endocrinology and Infertility (SREI).

His research has advanced reproductive health, and he has accomplished many medical firsts. He was the first physician to describe vasospasm-producing pituitary hypofunction and injury, which is known as Dahan's Syndrome. In addition, he facilitated the first pregnancy and live birth resulting from the serial vitrification of embryos gathered through in vitro maturation of oocytes and array-cgh and pgt for fragile x-carrier status in a perimenopausal woman. He developed and first published the protocols for short ovulation delays in women, which are used internationally. He was the first to describe gonadotropin-releasing hormone agonist triggering for IVM. He collected 125 eggs from a single patient undergoing in vitro maturation of human oocytes without gonadotropin stimulation to achieve a world record for egg harvest after developing a new oocyte collection technique. There was no danger of ovarian hyperstimulation syndrome when using this approach. He is considered the international expert on how fertility treatments affect the human placenta, with his research greatly furthering the understanding of this domain.

He is the Editor-in-Chief of the journal *Clinical and Experimental Obstetrics and Gynecology* and has served on the editorial boards of 11 other peer-reviewed journals. He is an in-demand public speaker who has been invited to give over 200 talks nationally and internationally.

He is the author of over 300 peer-reviewed publications and an additional 300 plus meeting abstracts. His articles have been published in some of the most important journals in medicine including titles belonging to the Journal of the American Medical Association (JAMA) and in Human Reproduction Update (the highest impact factor journal in Reproductive Medicine). Over 180 media and newspaper articles have described his research findings worldwide. He has received more than $1.3 million in research grants. The Consumers' Research Council has named Dr. Dahan three times one of America's finest Obstetricians and Gynecologists. He was chosen for inclusion in Who's Who in Medicine. He was awarded the R. Howard Webster Award for Research in 2008. He is a member of the Sigma Xi scientific honors society and received the King Charles Coronation Medal for important contributions in medical research and for bringing an international reputation to Canadian science. He was chosen by Stanford University as one of the top 2% of scientists in the world.

He was the editor of the texts *Handbook of Current and Novel Protocols for the Treatment of Infertility* **published by Elsevier, and** *In-Vitro Maturation of Human Oocytes: The McGill Protocols* **the first edition and the second edition, published by Index of Science Ltd.**

What Is Infertility: Female and Male Reproductive Systems, the Pathophysiology of Reproduction, Definition and Causes of Infertility

1

Ciara Heatherwick, Maha Gumssani, and Mausumi Das

1.1 Introduction

This chapter aims to give an understanding of the physiology of follicular development in the ovary, how oocytes (known as eggs, ovum or gametes) are produced and the ovary's role in preparing the endometrium for implantation. It will include a description of the hypothalamic-pituitary-ovarian (HPO) axis which controls ovarian function and ovulation. This chapter also provides a concise overview of the male reproductive system. It explains how the hypothalamic-pituitary-testis (HPT) axis controls the hormones needed for sperm production and testosterone synthesis. It describes the role of the testes in sperm production, secreting hormones and regulating temperature, and describes how sperm mature and travel through the epididymis, vas deferens and accessory glands. Lastly, an overview of infertility, prevalence and common causes of female and male infertility are discussed.

C. Heatherwick
Department of Nursing, Assisted Conception Service, Glasgow Royal Infirmary, Glasgow, UK
e-mail: Ciara.Heatherwick2@nhs.scot

M. Gumssani
Department of Metabolism, Digestion and Reproduction, Imperial College, London, UK
e-mail: m.gumssani24@imperial.ac.uk

M. Das (✉)
Assisted Conception Service, Department of Obstetrics and Gynaecology, Glasgow Royal Infirmary, Glasgow, UK

University of Glasgow, Glasgow, UK

Imperial College, London, UK
e-mail: Mausumi.das@nhs.scot; mausumi.das@imperial.ac.uk

M. Das, M. H. Dahan (eds.), *A Comprehensive Guide to Reproductive Health and Infertility Medicine for Nurses*, https://doi.org/10.1007/978-3-032-24372-0_1

Throughout the field of fertility and reproduction, different names are used for the same thing. This may confuse people starting to learn about this area of healthcare and can make it seem more daunting than it should be. This chapter will use one standard anatomically correct term for each and other commonly used terms in brackets.

1.2 Ovarian Physiology

Ovaries are normally located in the pelvis, with one on either side of the uterus. Between the uterus (womb) and the ovary are uterine tubes (also known as salpinges, fallopian tubes, oviducts), tubular structures that transport the oocytes (eggs) from the ovary to the uterus. These tubes project from the uterine horns (cornua) at upper outer aspects of the uterus but are not attached to the ovary.

The ovaries are formed as a pair in the very early stages of development of a female foetus. The primordial germ cells originate in the yolk sac around week 3–4 of embryonic development and migrate to the developing ovaries by week 6. Ovaries can be identified as early as the 8th week of gestation (while the baby is part of the maternal pregnancy), and the germ cells which go on to develop into oocytes can be seen as early as the 10th week of gestation [12]. At the 20th week, there will be around 6–8 million of these germ cells present in the ovaries, but by the time of birth, it reduces to 1–2 million and, when a female reaches puberty, that number will have reduced to 300,000–500,000, of which 400–500 will ovulate and release as an oocyte during her lifetime [14]. The other follicles fail to develop an egg and eventually stop developing and die. Menopause is the state when the follicles have been severely depleted, stopping egg development and fertility, and the ovaries cannot produce sufficient oestrogen hormone, causing periods to stop.

In the ovary, an oocyte develops within a structure called a follicle, and in adults, the oocyte and follicle progress through several stages before the oocyte is released during ovulation (see Fig. 1.1). During the first stage of development from primordial to primary follicle, the membrane of the oocyte (the zona pellucida) forms, the granulosa cells start to grow and the oocyte increases in size [14]. The second stage involves

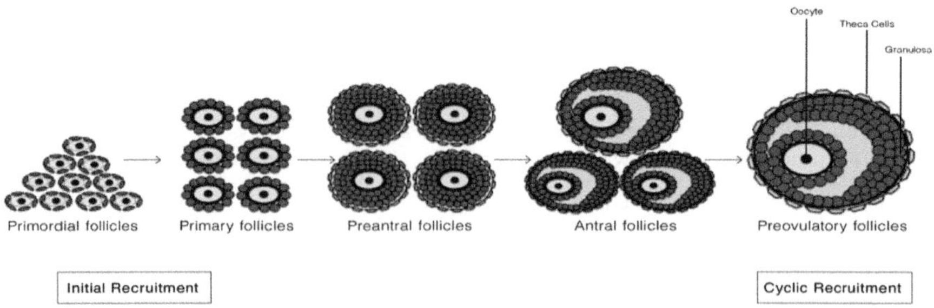

Fig. 1.1 Stage of folliculogenesis. (Diagram by M. McKendrick Adapted from Hannon and Curry (2018) [76])

development to the pre-antral and antral stages when the theca cells start to form. Normally, out of the cohort of follicles which go through the first and second stages every month, one of these follicles will develop on to the pre-ovulatory stage in response to hormonal stimulation. This development from primary follicle to preovulatory follicle lasts around 85 days. The other cohort of follicles which had started to develop will die off in a process called apoptosis [14]. The hormonal stimulation of the follicles in the ovaries is controlled by the brain and will be discussed next.

1.3 Natural Conception

In the human body, for natural conception to occur, two things must happen. An oocyte must be released from one of the ovaries and sperm must be present in the uterine tubes ready to fertilise the oocyte. An oocyte is released during ovulation, a culmination of a series of coordinated signals controlled by the hypothalamus and anterior pituitary in the brain. The hypothalamus will send hormonal signals to the anterior pituitary gland, another part of the brain, which in turn produces hormones which are sent to the ovary, and this makes up the hypothalamic-pituitary-ovarian

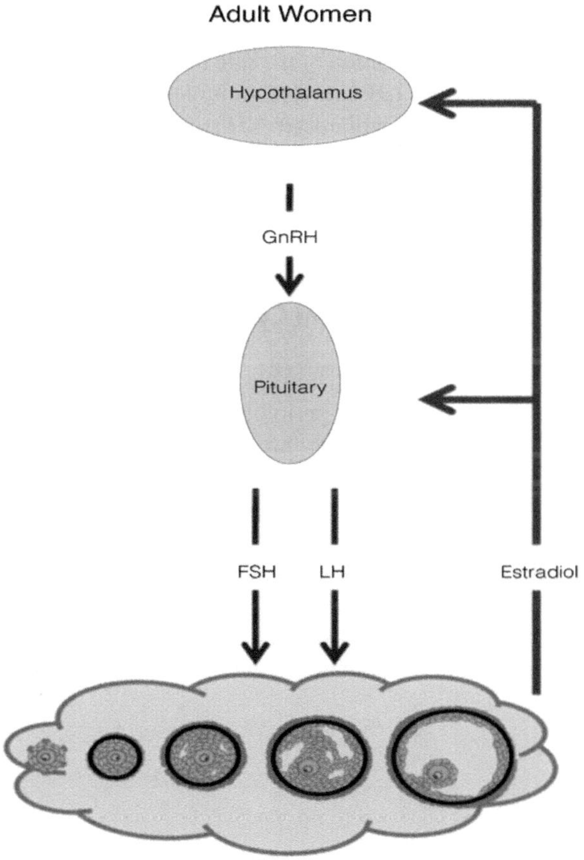

Fig. 1.2 The HPO axis. (Diagram by M. McKendrick Adapted from Hagen et al. (2023) [77])

(HPO) axis (see Fig. 1.2). The HPO axis works on feedback signals being sent between the hypothalamus, the pituitary and the ovary, and is an integral part of the female reproductive system. It is important to have a basic concept of what that involves, to then recognise and understand how a disruption to this pathway can cause ovulatory disorders and lead to infertility.

1.3.1 The Hormones Responsible for Ovulation

The hypothalamus is an area of the brain, located below the thalamus in the centre of the brain, which releases hormones to control many different systems of the body, including ovulation. The hormone that is released as part of the HPO axis is called gonadotropin releasing hormone (GnRH) (see Fig. 1.2). Gonad means ovary (or testicle), and tropin means a hormone released by one gland that stimulates the release of hormones in another gland. So, GnRH is simply a hormone released by the hypothalamus to stimulate the anterior pituitary gland to release hormones to stimulate the ovary (or the testicle).

Two hormones released by the anterior pituitary which have a role in stimulating the ovaries are follicle-stimulating hormone (FSH) and luteinising hormone (LH). The name of FSH makes it clear what the role of that hormone is—to stimulate the follicles in the ovary. LH is less obvious, but the name comes from the Latin name for yellow, an indication of the role it plays in forming the corpus luteum, which has a yellow colour. LH can also stimulate growth of larger follicles once they reach 14 mm or greater in diameter. LH stimulates the theca cells to produce male androgens which are then turned into oestrogens including oestradiol, the main blood marker of ovarian stimulation. LH, through androgens, increases the amount of FSH receptors in the follicle, potentiating the response to FSH.

1.4 The Menstrual Cycle

The length of a menstrual cycle is the number of days from day 1 of a period until the day before the next period. This can vary from person to person, but a regular menstrual cycle can be anything from a 21-day cycle to 35-day cycle, with the average cycle being 28 days long.

Ovarian function in the menstrual cycle is split into two phases: pre- and post-ovulation (see Fig. 1.3). Pre-ovulation, the follicular phase, includes follicular development leading up to ovulation in the ovaries and the menstrual and proliferative phase of endometrial development in the uterus. The post-ovulation stage is known as the luteal phase, when the ruptured follicle is developing into the corpus luteum, and the endometrium enters the secretory phase.

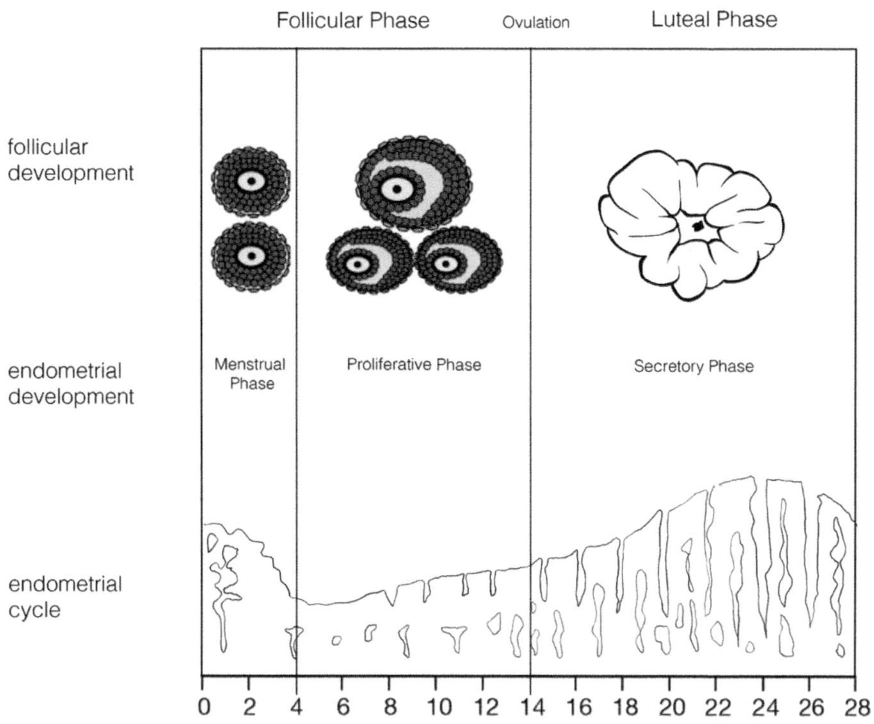

Fig. 1.3 The menstrual cycle. (Diagram by M. McKendrick Adapted from Reed and Carr (2018) [78])

1.4.1 The Follicular Phase

This is the stage from day 1 of the menstrual cycle until ovulation. In an average 28-day cycle, this stage would normally last for around 14 days but can be shorter or longer depending on the length of the cycle. For example, if a woman's menstrual cycle is 21 days long, the follicular phase will be shorter than 14 days. The luteal phase (the second half of the cycle) is usually always 14 days and as such the duration of the follicular phase varies from 7 to 21 days based on cycle length. Cycles less frequent than every 35 days are less likely to be ovulatory or result in the development of an egg.

Throughout the follicular phase, FSH and LH molecules are transmitted from the anterior pituitary gland via the blood to the ovaries, where they attach to specific receptors within the follicles. LH binds to receptors on the theca cells to stimulate them to produce androgens (such as androstenedione) which then diffuse into the granulosa cells. FSH binds to receptors on the granulosa cells and stimulate those cells to convert the androgens produced by the theca cells into oestrogen. This oestrogen is sent back out into the circulatory system and performs two functions in the menstrual cycle. Firstly, it circulates to the uterus to stimulate development of the endometrium (lining of the uterus) in preparation for an embryo to implant.

Secondly, as part of the HPO axis, it feeds back to the brain and if oestrogen levels are low, the brain will produce more FSH and LH to further stimulate follicular growth. This cycle continues until oestrogen levels are high, which will prompt the brain to reduce the amount of FSH and LH released. At this stage, because of the reduction in available FSH and LH, most of the follicles which had begun the development from the primordial to antral stage will die off through apoptosis and only one follicle will graduate to the preovulatory phase.

1.4.2 The Proliferative Phase

The uterus has three layers: the perimetrium, an outer membrane of epithelial cells; the myometrium, a middle layer of smooth muscle which facilitates uterine contractions (such as during labour to help deliver the baby); and the endometrium, an inner layer of cells [6]. The endometrium differentiates into two layers, depending on the stage of the menstrual cycle. The stratum basalis is the base layer which is abundant in oestrogen receptors and does not shed. The stratum functionalis grows from the stratum basalis during the follicular phase. During menstruation at the start of a cycle, the stratum functionalis breaks down and is shed via the cervix and vagina, in what is commonly known as a period. Around the same time, regeneration of the stratus functionalis also begins, with new layer of epithelial and stem cells starting to grow. After around 5–6 days, in response to the rise in oestrogen circulating in the blood from the developing follicles, the endometrium enters its proliferative phase. By day 8–10 of the cycle, the proliferative stage has peaked and each opposing layer of the stratum functionalis has grown from 0.5 mm to 3.5 6 mm in height [14]. This layer now consists of a dense network of glands, blood vessels, endothelial and stromal cells in preparation for fertilisation and a resulting embryo.

In summary, during the follicular phase, the brain will send hormones to the ovaries to stimulate growth of follicles, which will ultimately result in one of these follicles maturing and reaching pre-ovulation. While these follicles are growing in response to hormonal stimulation from the brain, they produce androgens which are then converted into oestrogen within the follicles. This oestrogen is then received by receptors in the base layer of the endometrium which will stimulate development of the functional layers of the endometrium.

1.4.3 The Luteal Phase

This stage begins at ovulation. In a normal 28-day cycle, this is usually at day 14. If the cycle is shorter or longer though, ovulation may occur before or after day 14. It is important to establish how long a woman's normal menstrual cycle is to assess when ovulation is likely to occur.

The dominant pre-ovulatory (Graafian) follicle will continue to produce oestrogen, and this increasing level of circulatory oestrogen will feed back to the brain, resulting in a surge of LH being released. This surge of LH causes the follicle to expand and rupture, resulting in ovulation and the release of a mature oocyte from the follicle. Post–ovulation, the ruptured follicle becomes the corpus luteum, and during the luteal phase it is responsible for the continued production of not only oestrogen, but another hormone called progesterone, both essential in the continued development of the endometrium.

1.4.4 The Secretory Phase

During the luteal phase, endometrial development enters its secretory phase in response to increasing amounts of oestrogen and progesterone from the corpus luteum. For the next 7 days after ovulation, the glands and blood vessels in the stratum functionalis continue to grow and the stromal cells become increasingly oedematous. Various substances are secreted by the endometrium which prepare the environment for an embryo to be able to implant. While this is happening, the released oocyte begins its journey along the uterine tube towards the uterus.

1.5 Fertilisation and Implantation

1.5.1 Fertilisation of the Oocyte

Once ovulation has occurred and a mature oocyte has been released from the ovary, the fimbriae (finger-like protrusions at the ovary end of the uterine tube, also known as the fallopian tube) sweep the oocyte into the uterine tube and move it gently towards the uterus. At this stage, for fertilisation to occur, sperm must have been introduced into the uterus via the cervix, either though ejaculation or insemination. The oocyte will meet the sperm in the uterine tube and one single sperm will enter the oocyte by penetrating its zona pellucida membrane. The nucleus of both the sperm and oocyte must then fuse together to supply the correct number of chromosomes to allow fertilisation. The fertilised oocyte will undergo a series of meiosis and cell division and become an embryo. While continuing to develop and grow, the embryo will continue its journey along the uterine tube until it reaches the endometrium, around 3 days after ovulation. Implantation of the blastocyst stage embryo will begin around 1–3 days after it reaches the endometrium, within the uterine cavity [14]. Rarely, a molar pregnancy can occur, when there is abnormal fertilisation of the egg by the sperm. This type of pregnancy is abnormal. A molar pregnancy cannot develop into a healthy baby. It may end on its own, with a miscarriage, or may be treated with a procedure to remove the pregnancy. After treatment for a molar pregnancy, regular blood and urine tests are needed to check that the hCG hormone level is returning to normal. There is a small risk that the molar cells can become cancerous and can spread to the lungs, liver and brain. If this happens, it will require chemotherapy for treatment.

The embryo reaches the endometrium in the secretory phase of development, around 6 or 7 days after ovulation, when the cells of the endometrium are receptive to an embryo attaching and implanting. The cells of the embryo release a hormone called human chorionic gonadotropin (hCG), signalling to the body a pregnancy has occurred. The corpus luteum in the ovary responds to this signal by continuing to provide progesterone and other important growth factors and hormones to support an ongoing pregnancy [8].

Rarely, a pregnancy may implant in the uterine tube or even the ovary or abdominal cavity. This is known as an ectopic pregnancy and will not lead to the development of a healthy baby. It can rupture causing haemorrhage if left untreated. Treatment involves medicines to cause the pregnancy to stop growing and reabsorb or surgical excision.

If an oocyte does not fertilise and an embryo does not implant, the lack of hCG will signal to the ovary that a pregnancy has not occurred. The corpus luteum will degenerate and levels of oestrogen and progesterone will start to fall. As a result, the endometrium which has been relying on these hormones to maintain its growth will start to break down and shed, resulting in menstruation around day 28 of the cycle, and the follicular phase will begin again.

1.5.2 Implantation of the Embryo

Implantation begins once the embryo has reached the endometrium. Trophoblast cells are the outer layer of cells which make up the embryo and will go on to form the placenta. It is these cells that produce hCG which signals to the ovary that a pregnancy has occurred. They start to extrude from the embryo and attach by 'sticking' to the endothelial cells on the surface of the endometrium and then expand into the stromal cells within, clearing a space for the blastocyst cells to enter. This stage is completed 14 days after ovulation [14].

As the corpus luteum continues to receive hCG, it will keep producing oestrogen and progesterone to maintain the endometrium which is essential for a pregnancy to develop. This means menstruation will not happen at the normal time in a woman's cycle, and this lack of a period will usually be the first indication of pregnancy. At this stage, hCG should be detected by a urine pregnancy test which will confirm the pregnancy. hCG can also be detected with a blood test and normal levels will vary from person to person depending on the stage of pregnancy and number of embryos implanted. If a woman requires serum hCG tracking, the tests should be done 48 h apart and, normally, serum hCG levels should increase by 50–63% every 48 h [17]. If this increase does not occur, it suggests an impending miscarriage or ectopic pregnancy, although rarely such a pregnancy can be normal (about 6–8% of the time).

1.5.3 Early Pregnancy Development

Once the embryo has successfully implanted, the trophoblast cells continue to differentiate into cells which form the circulatory system between the mother and foetus. These cells invade the endometrial stroma and blood supply and go on to form the placenta to facilitate exchange of gases, nutrients and waste between the two.

1.6 What Is Infertility?

It is globally accepted that for infertility to be diagnosed, 12 months of regular, unprotected sexual intercourse must have taken place without pregnancy occurring [4, 18]. Regular intercourse should occur 2–3 times per week. Couples do not need to track ovulation and time intercourse. If a woman's cycles occur less frequently than every 35 days, the couple should seek care after 3–6 month of unprotected intercourse because ovulation is less likely. Older women at least 35 years of age should seek care after 6 months of failure to conceive, to diagnose any issues requiring rapid intervention due to advanced age. However, this does not consider single individuals or same-sex couples who cannot conceive naturally but where their cause of infertility is not defined by the above criteria. Nonetheless, this definition of infertility is widely accepted by health care practitioners when deciding to refer people in heterosexual relationships for fertility investigations and treatment. According to the WHO [19], it is a basic human right to decide how many children to have and when to have them. Infertility takes away this human right and is reported to negatively impact the lives of the people affected, who may experience violence, social stigma, depression and anxiety because of their infertility. A recent systematic review found that females with infertility are 40% more likely to suffer from depression than their fertile counterparts [11]. Depression is also more common in their partners. Approximately, 85% of couples conceive by 1 year of unprotected intercourse. However, a more recent evaluation suggested that 34% of couples conceive the first month of attempted conception and 85% of healthy couples conceive within 6 months of sexual relations without contraception.

A report by the WHO [19] found that infertility prevalence statistics estimated around 17.5% of people globally will experience infertility across their lifetime. Infertility can be caused by disorders of the male or female reproductive and endocrine systems, which may present in many ways. As well as heterosexual couples presenting with the WHO definition of infertility, single people and couples in a same-sex relationship may also choose fertility treatments to enable them to have a child using donor gametes (oocytes or sperm). As part of the initial consultation when a person or couple present to the infertility service, a full reproductive, sexual and medical history should be taken to identify any potential causes of fertility disorders and inform which further investigations are required.

1.7 Female Infertility

Female infertility can be caused by a range of disorders which disrupt the HPO axis, conditions which affect ovarian function, abnormalities of the uterus or uterine tubes such as fibroids or tubal blockages and diseases such as endometriosis. Initial investigations of the female wishing to attempt a pregnancy could include a serum progesterone test in the mid-luteal phase of their menstrual cycle (i.e. day 21 of a 28-day cycle) to assess if they are ovulating. If they report an irregular cycle, FSH, LH and androgen levels as well as thyroid function and prolactin levels should be assessed to identify any endocrine or hypothalamic cause of their irregular cycles. A 3D transvaginal ultrasound scan will examine the uterine shape to identify abnormalities and the morphology of the ovaries. A tubal patency test such as a hysterosalpingo contrast sonography (HyCoSy) or an HSG (hysterosalpingogram) will assess for any blockages or damage to the uterine tubes.

1.7.1 Ovulatory Disorders

Ovulatory disorders are thought to cause fertility problems in around 25% of couples trying to conceive [10]. As described above, ovulation and a regular menstrual cycle rely on the communication and functional relationship between the hypothalamus, anterior pituitary and ovary. It is not surprising then that if any of these glands or organs are dysfunctional, damaged or decline due to age or disease, the ovary's ability to produce a mature follicle and ovulate a healthy oocyte will be affected.

The International Federation of Gynaecology and Obstetrics (FIGO) has produced a system of classification to identify which system of the HPO axis is causing ovulatory dysfunction and then consider what the potential causes for disruption are [9]. They describe type 1 disorders as arising from the hypothalamus, type 2 from the pituitary and type 3 from the ovaries. Described in Table 1.1 are a list of the potential causes, and some examples of how these causes may contribute to ovulatory dysfunction, as explained by Balen et al. [2].

The list of examples given is not exhaustive and there are several different causes of each type of ovulatory dysfunction. The mode of investigation will depend on the likely cause, as will treatment. When categorising the types of ovulatory disorder, Munro et al. [9] considered that polyendocrine metabolic ovarian syndrome (PMOS)

Table 1.1 Categorization of Ovulatory Disorders

Cause	Example	Type
Genetic	Kallman's syndrome when the patient does not produce GnRH due to a failure of the neurones producing GnRH to migrate to the correct anatomic location	1
Autoimmune	Addison's disease is a rare endocrine disorder characterised by insufficient production of cortisol and aldosterone by the adrenal glands	3
Iatrogenic	Radiation	2
Neoplasm	Prolactinoma	2
Functional	Stress/weight related/exercise	1
Infection/ inflammation	Tuberculosis	1,2,3
Trauma	Injury to the gland or ovary	1,2,3
Physiologic	Pregnancy should always be ruled out when a patient misses her period	1
Idiopathic	Premature ovarian insufficiency	3
Endocrine	Hypothyroidism	2

Balen et al. [2]

should be regarded as a type of ovulatory disorder on its own, making it type 4 in their system of classification.

1.7.1.1 Polyendocrine Metabolic Ovarian Syndrome (PMOS)

PMOS is a complex condition which does not always present in the same way in every woman. It involves both the endocrine and reproductive systems, making it difficult for women to get a definitive diagnosis and appropriate treatment. In May 2026, a global expert and patient consensus recommended renaming polycystic ovary syndrome (PCOS) to polyendocrine metabolic ovarian syndrome (PMOS), which better reflects its multisystem endocrine and metabolic nature [79]. Some women may experience irregular cycles, hirsutism, baldness, acne, insulin resistance and obesity. However, other women may only experience irregular cycles and further investigation with serum hormone levels and ultrasound will be required to diagnose PMOS and eliminate other causes of ovulatory dysfunction.

According to the Rotterdam criteria [16], clinical diagnosis of PMOS requires at least two of the following three markers:

1. An ovulatory disorder
2. Clinical evidence of hyperandrogenism (excess androgen production) including increased facial or body hair or acne
3. Ultrasound diagnosis of polycystic ovaries

Investigations include taking a full history of the menstrual cycle, blood tests for androgen levels (testosterone, sex hormone binding globulin to estimate free testosterone and androstenedione) and LH levels and an ultrasound scan of the ovaries.

Hyperandrogenism can cause ovulatory dysfunction by disrupting the hormonal pathways that control the menstrual cycle and ovulation. For example, higher levels of LH will result in higher levels of androstenedione, leading to increased production of oestrogen, reducing the need for the anterior pituitary to release FSH. It is less likely that any of the antral follicles in the ovaries will develop into a mature follicle and ovulate, meaning the progesterone level will not rise and a period will not happen regularly. It is important to note that infertility is not the only clinical manifestation of PMOS and that women with the syndrome are also at increased risk of cardiovascular disease in later life, type 2 diabetes mellitus and of developing endometrial hyperplasia and cancer [7].

Treatments for PMOS vary depending on the individual and the clinical manifestations of the syndrome. If a woman wishes to conceive, then advice around diet for women with insulin resistance, exercise and the benefits of weight loss (if overweight) should be explained. A progesterone-containing medication to induce a withdrawal bleed should also be offered in these cases to prevent the development of uterine cancer.

1.7.2 Uterine Abnormalities

The uterus is normally around 7–8 cm in length and is similar in shape to an upside-down pear. There are four components that make up the whole uterus: the cervix, isthmus, uterine body and fundus. The *cervix* is at the inferior (bottom) and has two openings at either end, the external os and the internal os. The external os opens into the vagina allowing sperm to enter the uterus and menstrual blood to exit. The cervix also produces a thick mucus for most of the month (except around the time of ovulation) to provide protection from infection. The internal os is at the proximal end and opens into the *isthmus*, an area between the cervix and *uterine body*. As previously described, the uterine body consists of the perimetrium, myometrium and endometrium. The *fundus* is located at the superior (top) end of the uterine body.

Development of the uterus normally occurs in the early stages of foetal development when two Mullerian ducts fuse together and is completed by the twelfth gestational week [14]. Congenital uterine abnormalities (CUAs) are a result of the incomplete fusion of the two ducts and can vary in severity from an absence of a uterus to a completely septate uterus, cervix and vagina [1]. It is estimated that around 8% of women presenting with infertility will have CUA and this likelihood increases to 25% in women with a history of infertility and pregnancy loss [5].

CUAs can be diagnosed with a 3D transvaginal ultrasound scan which can assess the shape of the uterus and identify any anomalies. Further imaging with magnetic resonance imaging (MRI) can confirm the severity of the abnormality. Despite the effect a CUA can have on fertility, the only treatment available is a hysteroscopic resection of the septum, if severe. However, evidence to prove the effectiveness of this intervention is limited; therefore, recommendations are that it is only carried out in a research capacity [13].

1.7.3 Tubal Abnormalities

Infertility can be caused by damage to, or absence of, the uterine tubes that act as a conduit from the ovaries to uterus. Damage can be caused by infection or inflammation, leading to tubal scarring, meaning the oocyte/embryo cannot pass through to the uterus. It can also result in fluid accumulation within the tube (hydrosalpinx) causing a complete occlusion. Infection in the uterine tubes can be caused by pelvic inflammatory disease (PID), including sexually transmitted infections (STIs) such as chlamydia, but also because of a ruptured appendix or previous ectopic pregnancy. The uterine tubes can also be damaged by a previous sterilisation, which involves deliberate surgical occlusion of the tubes to prevent pregnancy. Absence of the uterine tubes could be a result of a salpingectomy (surgical removal of the uterine tube) because of an ectopic pregnancy growing in the tube which could rupture, endangering the life of the woman. Endometriosis, a condition where cells similar to the lining of the uterus, or endometrium grow outside the uterus, can also block or damage the fallopian tubes by causing inflammation and scarring.

When assessing if tubal damage could be a cause of infertility, a full surgical, sexual and reproductive history is essential to identify any risk factors including pelvic surgery, STI or previous ectopic pregnancy. If indicated, one way to assess tubal patency is with a hysterosalpingo contrast sonography (HyCoSy) which involves injecting an echo-enhancing solution into the uterus while performing a trans vaginal ultrasound scan and observing tubal flow of the solution through the uterine tubes [3]. Another possible test is the hysterosalpingogram done by radiology, where X-ray images are used to detect tubal passage of a dye.

1.7.4 Unexplained Infertility

It is estimated that in around 15–30% of couples with infertility, a cause will not be found, leading to a diagnosis of unexplained infertility [15]. It is expected that this diagnosis will be reached after a series of investigations which will ultimately exclude any identifiable cause of infertility. However, Romualdi et al. [15] found when developing their evidence-based guideline on management of a couple with unexplained infertility that investigations are not standardised. It could therefore be argued that for many couples the cause of their infertility is not 'unexplained', more that fertility investigation has not been extensive enough to identify a cause. However, according to Romualdi et al. [15], although there are many investigations which have a robust evidence base proving their benefit in the investigation in the infertile couple, such as a 3D TVS and HyCoSy and semen analysis, many others do not have enough evidence to support standardised use and require further research.

1.7.4.1 The Male Reproductive Hormonal Axis

The male reproductive system depends on the hypothalamic-pituitary-testis (HPT) axis, a coordinated hormonal network that controls hormone production and supports sperm development [20].

1.7.4.2 Hypothalamus: The Hormonal Control Centre

Located at the base of the brain, the hypothalamus acts as the command centre for reproductive hormones. It releases gonadotropin-releasing hormone (GnRH) in rhythmic pulses, with cycles occurring every 90–120 min. However, this process is influenced by factors such as seasonal changes and circadian rhythms [20].

1.7.4.3 Pituitary Gland: The Hormone Distributor

The pituitary gland is located just below the hypothalamus. It has two parts:

The posterior lobe (neurohypophysis):

- Controlled by nerve signals from the hypothalamus
- Releases oxytocin and vasopressin

The anterior lobe (adenohypophysis):

- Receives hormone signals from the hypothalamus through a network of blood vessels called the portal system.
- These signals stimulate the release of luteinizing hormone (LH) and follicle-stimulating hormone (FSH). LH stimulates Leydig cells in the testes to produce testosterone, while FSH supports sperm development by acting on Sertoli cells.
- Additionally, the pituitary gland produces prolactin and growth hormone, which contribute to male reproductive health [20].

1.7.4.4 Steroid Feedback Mechanism: Maintaining Hormonal Balance

The body maintains hormone levels through feedback mechanisms.

Testosterone Regulation Mechanism

- *Testosterone's Role*:
  Testosterone plays a key role in regulating hormone levels. It signals the brain and pituitary gland to decrease the release of GnRH, which in turn lowers the production of other hormones like LH and FSH.
- *Conversion to Other Hormones*:
  In the testes and other parts of the body, testosterone is converted into dihydrotestosterone (DHT) and oestradiol. Both hormones help control reproductive functions [20].
- *Effect on FSH*:
  When FSH stimulates Sertoli cells in the testes, they produce a hormone called inhibin. Inhibin helps reduce the amount of FSH released by the pituitary gland [21].

1.7.4.5 Formation of the Male Reproductive System

Key Hormones

During foetal development, hormones like testosterone, DHT and anti-Müllerian hormone (AMH) are crucial for defining male characteristics, including the scrotum and the penis.

Role of AMH

AMH produced by Sertoli cells prevents the development of female reproductive structures including the uterus and the upper two-thirds of the vagina, ensuring a male pattern [22].

Role of Testosterone

Testosterone made by foetal Leydig cells helps forms the Wolffian duct system, which later develops into male reproductive organs like the vas deferens, epididymis and accessory glands [20].

Genetic Control

The early development of the testes begins with the SRY gene on the Y chromosome. This gene *works together* with other transcription factors to start the process of male sex differentiation [23].

Pubertal Development in Males Puberty in boys starts with the growth of the testes. This process is triggered by an increase in GnRH from the hypothalamus, which signals the anterior pituitary gland to release FSH and LH. LH stimulates Leydig cells to produce testosterone, leading to the growth and darkening of the scrotum and penis [24].

Secondary Sexual Characteristics As boys go through puberty, they start to develop facial, underarm, chest, and pubic hair. Their voices become deeper, and they experience growth spurts, getting taller in a short period of time. Another important sign of reproductive maturity is the first ejaculation, which shows that their bodies are now capable of reproduction [24].

Completion of Puberty Puberty is considered complete when the growth plates in the bones close. However, some changes, like muscle development and voice deepening, can continue into the early 20s [24].

1.7.4.6 Male Reproductive Anatomy

The male reproductive system serves two main functions: producing androgens like testosterone to support reproductive function, as well as making and transporting sperm to the female reproductive system for fertilisation [24, 25]. A deep

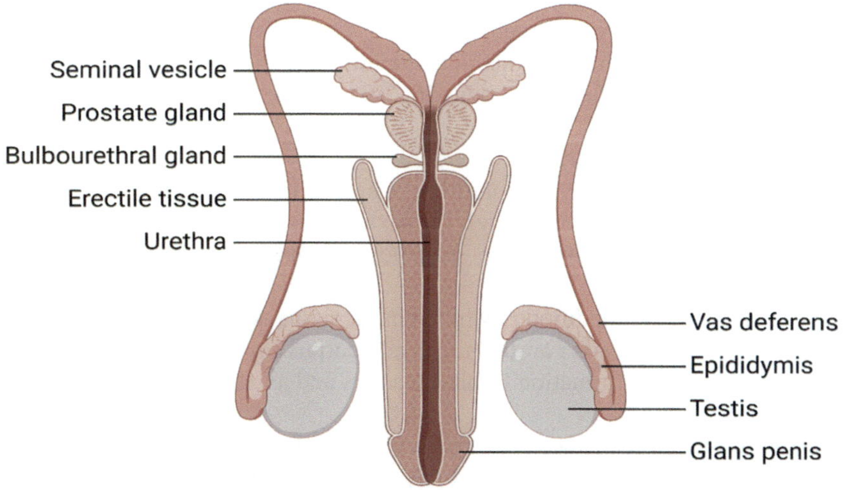

Fig. 1.4 The male reproductive system. The diagram shows the main parts of the male external genitalia and accessory glands. (Image taken from BioRender. Jayasena [31], https://BioRender.com/g26b978) [31]

understanding of male reproductive anatomy and physiology is important for identifying and addressing male infertility [25].

1.7.4.7 External Structures

Penis The penis is an external organ of the male reproductive system (see Fig. 1.4) and plays a vital role in both reproduction and urination [26].

1.7.4.8 Primary Function

- Transfer sperm into the female reproductive tract during sexual intercourse.
- Contains the urethra, which allows for the passage of both urine and semen [27].

1.7.4.9 Structure of the Penis

The penis is structurally divided into three parts:

1. *Root*:

The base of the penis, which is attached to the pelvic region [26].

2. *Body (shaft)*:

The long, cylindrical part of the penis that surrounds the penile urethra (the channel that carries urine and semen) [28]. It consists of three cylindrical erectile tissues and does not contain muscles [26]. These tissues include:

Two corpora cavernosa located on the lateral sides of the shaft [29].

One corpus spongiosum located on the ventral (underside) of the shaft, which surrounds the urethra [26].

3. *Glans (Head)*: The sensitive, rounded tip containing numerous nerve endings that enhance sexual pleasure and facilitate arousal (see Fig. 1.4) [26, 27].

1.7.4.10 Functions of the Penis

Intercourse: Becomes erect for penetration.
Ejaculation: Releases semen through the urethra.
Urination: Expels urine from the body [26, 30].

1.7.4.11 Clinical Relevance

Erectile Dysfunction (ED): A condition where a man struggles to achieve or maintain an erection firm enough for sexual intercourse. It can be caused by many factors such as vascular, neurological, hormonal and psychological factors [32].

Peyronie's Disease: A condition in which fibrous tissue develops in the tunica albuginea (the protective layer around the penile corpus cavernosum). This condition can cause pain, the formation of hard plaques and an abnormal curvature of the penis [33].

Priapism: A condition characterised by an erection that lasts for a long time, often causing pain, and it occurs without any sexual stimulation or persists after the end of sexual stimulation [34].

1.7.4.12 Scrotum Overview

The scrotum is a pouch of skin and muscle located beneath the penis. It holds and supports the testes outside the body to keep them cool [35, 36].

1.7.4.13 Function

Temperature Regulation: The scrotum keeps the testes at the ideal temperature of 32–35 °C, which is essential for spermatogenesis [36]. Hotter temperatures may damage sperm, including that induced by jacuzzi spas and tight underwear.

Muscle Movement: Two muscles, the dartos and cremaster, help manage testicular temperature. They move the testes closer to the body when it is cold and lower them when it is hot [36].

Heat Release: The scrotum helps keep the testes cool by releasing heat through its sweat glands, thin skin and minimal fat, allowing the body get rid of extra heat [37, 38].

Cooling Blood Flow: Blood vessels in the scrotum cool the blood before it reaches the testes [39].

1.7.4.14 Clinical Relevance

Hydrocele Accumulation of fluid in the scrotum, causing swelling [40, 41].

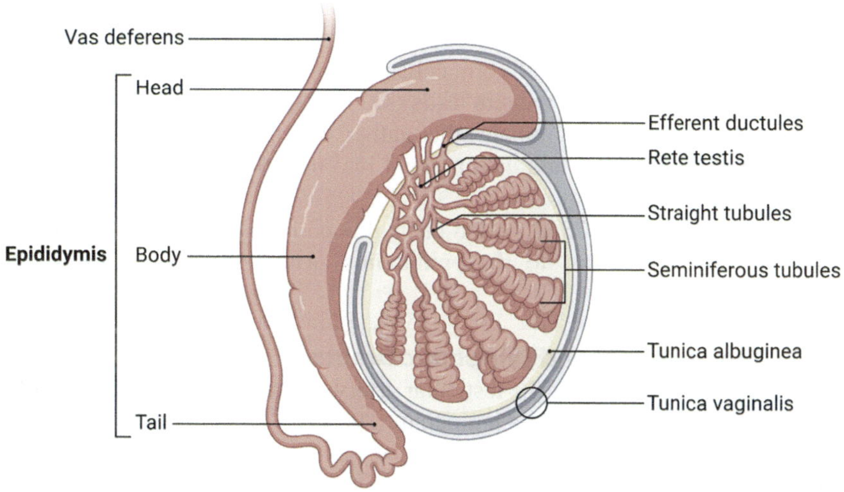

Fig. 1.5 A simple illustration of the human testis and the epididymis. It shows the seminiferous tubules, where sperm is produced; the epididymis, where sperm matures and is stored; and the vas deferens, which acts as the route for sperm to leave the testis (Image taken from BioRender; https://BioRender.com/g26b978 [31])

1.7.4.15 Internal Structures

Testes

The testes are located inside the scrotum and are covered by a thin layer called the tunica vaginalis, except at the back (see Fig. 1.5). At the back of the testis, it is connected to the epididymis, which leads to the vas deferens [42]. The testes are attached to the scrotum by the spermatic cord and cremaster muscles, which help keep them in place and move them when needed [28].

Primary Function Spermatogenesis and testosterone secretion [28, 43].

1.7.4.16 Structure of the Testes

Size: In young men, the average testicular volume is about 15–25 mL, with a length of around 4.5–5.1 cm [44]. Smaller testicles may be associated with testicular failure (partial or complete), due to injury, radiation or genetic causes.

Temperature Regulation: The testes are positioned outside the abdominal cavity to stay 2–4 °C cooler than the body's normal temperature. This cooler environment is essential for normal sperm production [45].

1.7.4.17 Internal Anatomy

Tunica Albuginea: The outer protective layer of the testis, made of strong fibrous tissue (see Fig. 1.5). From this layer, thin walls called septa extend inward and meet a thicker area called the mediastinum. This helps divide the testis into smaller sections called lobules [43].

Lobules: The testis contains around 200–400 lobules, each holding 1–3 seminiferous tubules [28, 46].

Seminiferous Tubules: The site of germ cells (sperm) production, where the tubules form loops and connect to the rete testis (see Fig. 1.5) [20].

Rete testis: A network of tiny tubules that gathers sperm and testicular fluids from the seminiferous tubules and directs them into the efferent ducts (see Fig. 1.5) [20, 42].

Efferent Ducts: A series of fine, coiled ducts that carry sperm and testicular fluids from the rete testis and to the epididymis, where the sperm mature (see Fig. 1.5) [42].

1.7.4.18 Blood Supply and Lymphatic Drainage

The testes receive blood from the testicular artery and are drained by the pampiniform plexus, which helps regulate temperature [47].

1.7.4.19 Cell Types in the Testis

Sertoli Cells

Location Located inside the seminiferous tubules of the testes.

Function

- Support, protect, and nourish developing sperm cells (germ cells). They help guide the sperm as they move toward the lumen of the seminiferous tubules, providing an ideal environment for their growth and maturation [29, 48].
- Form the blood-testis barrier to protect sperm from the immune system [29, 49].
- Sertoli cells also secrete substances like inhibin, anti-Müllerian hormone (AMH) and fluid to help transport sperm to the epididymis [29, 48].
- Facilitates spermiation (the release of mature spermatids into the lumen of the seminiferous tubule) [50].
- During germ cell maturation, the Sertoli cells remove the unnecessary or leftover parts of developing sperm cells through a process called phagocytosis [29].

Leydig Cells

Location Located between the seminiferous tubules in the interstitial tissue [20].

Function

- *Leydig cells* produce male hormones, called androgens, from cholesterol. This process is controlled by luteinizing hormone (LH) [24, 51]. Testosterone is their main product, and its production starts at puberty, when LH signals the Leydig cells to start producing and releasing testosterone [28].
- Convert testosterone to dihydrotestosterone (DHT) in peripheral tissues.

1.7.4.20 Androgens from Leydig Cells

Support male reproductive function and the development of secondary sexual characteristics [52].

Support spermatogenesis [28].

1.7.4.21 Clinical Relevance

Varicocele: Abnormal enlargement of veins in the pampiniform plexus, which disrupt the temperature regulation of the testes and affect sperm production. [53].

Cryptorchidism: A condition where one or both testicles fail to descend into the scrotum before birth, it can affect sperm production and fertility [54]. The higher temperatures of the abdominal cavity may injure the testicle. Therefore, the descent of the testicles (orchidopexy) is done surgically and it is preferable to do this in the first year of life.

Sertoli Cell-Only Syndrome: A condition where the seminiferous tubules contain only Sertoli cells and no spermatogenic cells [55].

Testicular torsion: Testicular torsion occurs when the spermatic cord twists, blocking blood flow to the testicle. This condition is considered a medical emergency and requires immediate surgical intervention [56]. If left untreated, the testicle dies and sperm production may be compromised.

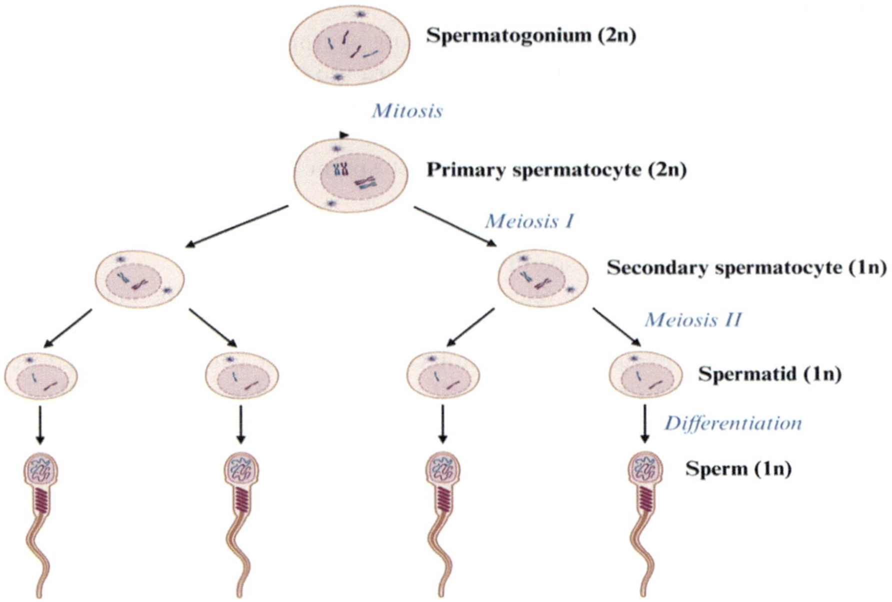

Fig. 1.6 Stages of spermatogenesis. (Image taken from BioRender. Jayasena [31], https://BioRender.com/d55i045) [31]

1.7.4.22 Spermatogenesis

Spermatogenesis is the process by which sperm cells develop in the seminiferous tubules of the testes. It starts with germ cells that undergo a series of stages to mature into fully developed sperm [57].

Sperm production usually takes around 74 days [58]. However, studies in healthy men reported that the entire process of producing mature ejaculated sperm can take between 42 and 76 days [59].

1.7.4.23 Stages of Spermatogenesis

The process occurs in three main phases (see Fig. 1.6):

1. *Proliferation and Differentiation of Spermatogonia (mitosis)*: Mitotic division of spermatogonia (stem cells) to produce primary spermatocytes.
2. *Meiosis (reduction phase)*: Each primary spermatocytes undergoes two meiotic divisions to form haploid spermatids.
3. *Spermiogenesis (maturation phase)*: Spermiogenesis is the process where haploid spermatids develop and transform into fully mature sperm cells (spermatozoa). During this phase, important structures like the acrosome (a cap-like structure that helps sperm penetrate the egg) and the flagellum (tail for motility) are developed [43, 57, 60, 61].

1.7.4.24 Regulation of Spermatogenesis

Spermatogenesis is regulated by hormones, with key roles played by LH, FSH, and androgens.

- *Luteinizing Hormone (LH)*: LH stimulates the Leydig cells in the testes to produce testosterone, which is essential for spermatogenesis [62].
- *Follicle-Stimulating Hormone (FSH)*: FSH stimulates the Sertoli cells, which provide nourishment and support to the developing sperm.
- *Androgens (Testosterone)*: Testosterone is produced in response to LH within the seminiferous tubules, where it plays a vital role in the production of sperm [63].

1.7.4.25 Sperm Transport

Epididymis

The epididymis is long, coiled tube (about 3.8 meters) that runs along the back and side of the testis [64].

Primary Function Sperm maturation, storage, and transport [65].

1.7.4.26 Structure of the Epididymis

The epididymis consists of three main sections (see Fig. 1.5):

1. *Head (Caput Epididymis)*: This part collects sperm from the efferent ducts and begins the maturation process.
2. *Body (Corpus Epididymis)*: Sperm continue to mature in this section.
3. *Tail (Cauda Epididymis)*: Fully matured sperm are stored here until they are ready to travel to the vas deferens [65].

1.7.4.27 Functions of the Epididymis

1. *Sperm Transport*: The epididymis helps transport sperm from the testes to the vas deferens. This journey usually takes about 10–15 days, with muscle contractions driving this process [65].
2. *Sperm Concentration*: It also works to concentrate the sperm by absorbing excess fluid, which is vital for fertility [65].
3. *Sperm Protection*: Protects sperm by neutralising harmful reactive oxygen species and preventing the immune system from attacking them [65].
4. *Sperm Storage*: Mature sperm are stored in the cauda epididymis until ejaculation [65].
5. *Sperm Maturation*: As sperm move through the epididymis, they undergo maturation, gaining the ability to swim and fertilise an egg [65].
6. *Acquisition of Motility*: By the time sperm reach the cauda epididymis, they are fully capable of swimming forward and moving efficiently [65].
7. *Fertilisation Capabilities*: Sperm acquire the necessary factors to bind and penetrate the egg [65].

1.7.4.28 Clinical Relevance

- *Epididymitis*: Inflammation of the epididymis, often causing pain and swelling in the scrotum [66].

1.7.4.29 Duct System

During ejaculation, mature sperm leave the epididymis and travel toward the vas deferens, aided by smooth muscle contractions [29].

1.7.4.30 Vas Deferens

The vas deferens is a muscular tube that carries sperm from the testicles to the urethra, playing a vital role in ejaculation (see Fig. 1.4). It travels through the spermatic cord, pelvis and behind the bladder [29, 43], eventually joining with the seminal vesicle to form the ejaculatory duct [43].

1.7.4.31 Ampulla of the Vas Deferens

The distal end of the vas deferens widens to form the ampulla, where sperm are stored before mixing with seminal fluid for ejaculation [43].

1.7.4.32 Vas Deferens Function

- Carries sperm from the testis and mixes them with fluids from other glands for ejaculation.
- Prevents retrograde ejaculation, where semen flows backwards into the bladder [43].

1.7.4.33 Clinical Application

Bilateral congenital absence of the vas deferens (CAVD): This condition occurs when both vas deferentia are absent, resulting in infertility. However, the exact cause for this condition remains unknown. [67].

Vasectomy: A vasectomy is a minor surgical procedure used for permanent male contraception. It involves blocking or cutting the vas deferens to prevent sperm from being included in the semen during ejaculation [68].

Retrograde Ejaculation A condition where semen moves backwards into the bladder instead of exiting through the urethra during ejaculation [69].

Ejaculatory Duct Obstruction Occurs when there is a blockage in the ejaculatory duct, which prevents semen from entering the urethra [69].

1.7.4.34 Accessory Glands

Semen is produced with the help of three accessory glands in the male reproductive system: the seminal vesicles, prostate and bulbourethral glands [28].

1.7.4.35 Seminal Vesicles

The *seminal vesicles* are glands lined with epithelial cells, when sperm reach the ampulla during ejaculation; they mix with fluid from the seminal vesicles (see Fig. 1.1) [29].

1.7.4.36 Functions of Seminal Vesicles

- They make up about 60% of the total semen volume [29].
- The fluid is rich in sugars, which sperm use to produce ATP, providing them with the energy needed to travel through the female reproductive tract.
- It contains seminogelin proteins, which make the semen thicker and help it coagulate shortly after ejaculation [29].

The mixture of sperm and seminal vesicle fluid moves into the paired ejaculatory ducts, which carry the semen into the prostate gland [29].

1.7.4.37 The Prostate Gland

The prostate is a muscular gland that surrounds the first inch of the prostatic urethra. It is the largest accessory gland in the male reproductive system, roughly the size of a walnut (see Fig. 1.4) [29].

1.7.4.38 Functions of the Prostate

Secretes an alkaline, milky fluid into the semen [29].

During ejaculation, the smooth muscles of the prostate contract, helping to push the semen through the urethra [29].

Adds proteases to the semen, which help in liquefaction and facilitate the release of sperm [29].

1.7.4.39 The Cowper (Bulbourethral) Glands

These are small glands located below the prostate gland [29].

1.7.4.40 Functions

- They release a thick and salty fluid that helps lubricate the urethra, allowing the sperm to move more easily during ejaculation, and cleans out any remaining urine in the urethra.
- It also helps balance the acidity in the vagina, which makes it easier for sperm to swim [29].

1.7.4.41 Male Urethra

- *Structure*: About 20 cm long. It starts at the bladder, passes through the prostate, and travels through glans of the penis (see Fig. 1.4).
- *Function*: Passage for both urine and semen [70].

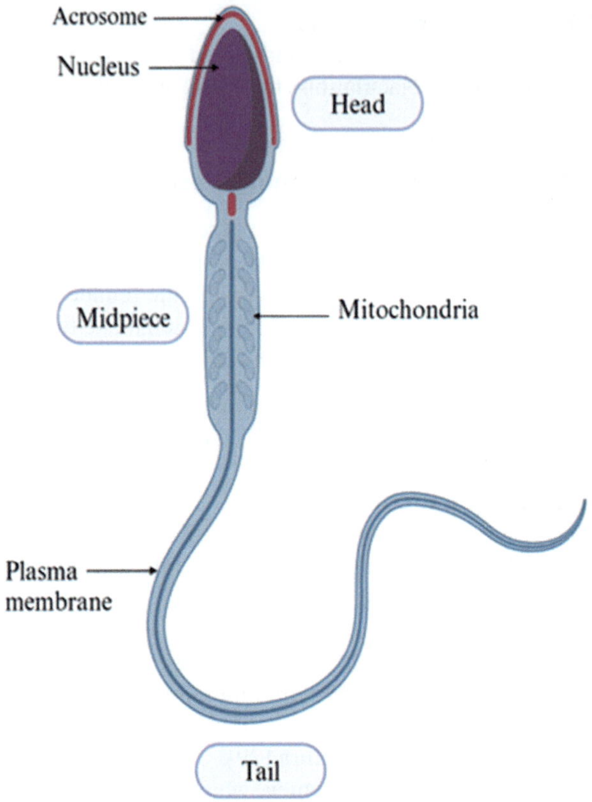

Fig. 1.7 The structure of mature human sperm. The figure highlights the three main parts of sperm: the head, the mid-piece and the tail. (Image created in BioRender. Jayasena [31], https://BioRender.com/d55i045 [31])

1.7.4.42 Mature Sperm Cell (Spermatozoa)

Sperm is a tiny cell designed for movement and can survive for a short period outside the human body. The body produces around 100–300 million sperm every day [71].

A Sperm Has Three Main Parts

- *Head*: The head contains the genetic material (DNA), including 22 autosomes and either an X or Y chromosome. It is capped by the *acrosome* (see Fig. 1.7), which contains enzymes that help the sperm penetrate the egg during fertilisation [71].
- *Mid-piece*: This part contains the mitochondria, which provide the energy needed for the sperm to swim.
- *Tail* (flagellum): The tail helps the sperm move [71].

Table 1.2 WHO 2021 reference values for normal semen parameters

	5th (95% CI)
Semen volume (mL)	1.4 (1.3–1.5)
Total sperm number (per ejaculate 10^6)	39 (35–40)
Sperm concentration (10^6 per mL)	16 (15–18)
Total motility (%)	42 (40–43)
Progressive motility (%)	30 (29–31)
Normal forms (%)	4 (3.9–4)
Vitality (%)	54 (50–56)

The normal range is defined at the fifth percentile with a 95% confidence interval, where values above this threshold are considered normal [72]

1.7.4.43 Semen Analysis: The First Step in Understanding Male Fertility

Semen analysis is the cornerstone of evaluating male fertility. Andrologists evaluate several factors such as semen volume, sperm count, concentration, motility, progressive motility, morphology, and viscosity to identify potential issues affecting a man's ability to conceive.

The World Health Organization (WHO) regularly updates the guidelines for semen analysis, with the latest 6th edition released in 2021. This update includes new reference values to improve diagnostic accuracy. According to WHO, the normal range is defined as the fifth percentile with a 95% confidence interval, meaning that values above this threshold are considered within normal limits (see Table 1.2) [72].

Infertility is defined as the inability of a couple to conceive after 1 year of unprotected intercourse, with male factors contributing to 30–50% of cases [73, 74]. While semen analysis provides valuable insights, it cannot definitively determine fertility unless there are no sperm present or there are severe morphological issues [69].

1.7.4.44 Clinical Relevance

Aspermia: no ejaculation occurs.

Azoospermia is where no sperm are found in the ejaculate, even after centrifugation and microscopic analysis [69]. Fluid is often still present, since it is produced by glands that may continue to function and are located further along the reproductive tract, after the testicles, along the path of ejaculation.

Oligozoospermia occurs when sperm concentration is lower than the WHO reference limit [69].

Asthenozoospermia occurs when the percentage of motile sperm is below the reference limit. In severe cases, known as absolute asthenozoospermia, no motile sperm are present [69].

Teratozoospermia Refers to a condition where the percentage of sperm with normal morphology is lower than the reference limit [69].

Oligoasthenozoospermia is characterised by both low sperm concentration and poor motility [69].

Asthenoteratozoospermia is when sperm exhibit both poor motility and a high percentage of morphological abnormalities [69].

Oligoasthenoteratozoospermia involves low sperm concentration, reduced motility and abnormal morphology, all below the WHO reference limit [69].

Necrozoospermia occurs when the percentage of live sperm is lower than the WHO reference limit, with a high proportion of immotile sperm [69].

Globozoospermia is when sperm cells have little to no acrosomal vesicles [69] and as such have significant difficulty fertilising an oocyte even with ICSI.

Leukocytospermia is when the number of white blood cells (leukocytes) in the semen exceeds one million per milliliter [69].

Cryptozoospermia is a condition where no sperm are found in a fresh semen sample, but some are detected after centrifugation [69].

Hypogonadotropic Hypogonadism is a condition characterised by low levels of testosterone, LH, and FSH, which can lead to oligozoospermia or azoospermia [75].

Retrograde ejaculation: When the ejaculation with the sperm travels backwards into the bladder, instead of out the penis. This often occurs in spinal cord injuries or diabetes mellitus.

1.8 Conclusion

When working in assisted conception and fertility, it is essential to have a basic understanding of normal ovarian and uterine function, and the brain and ovary's role in controlling ovulation and preparing the uterus for pregnancy. This enables further understanding of how a dysfunction of pathways, such as the HPO axis, which control these essential pathways, can lead to infertility. Similarly, an understanding of spermatogenesis and how the HPT axis controls the hormones needed for sperm production and testosterone synthesis is essential for understanding and managing male infertility.

Hopefully this chapter has managed to explain these essential processes in a way that will facilitate further understanding of both normal and abnormal biomechanics of the female and male reproductive systems.

The causes of infertility are extensive and could not be fully explained within the limitations of this chapter. However, the main classifications of female and male infertility have been summarised. Further reading is recommended, particularly around the types of ovulatory dysfunction and disorders of spermatogenesis for healthcare professionals working with women and men presenting with infertility.

References

1. Akhtar MA, Saravelos SH, Li TC, Jayaprakasan K, and the Royal College of Obstetricians, and Gynaecologists. Reproductive implications and Management of Congenital Uterine Anomalies (2024 Second Edition). BJOG Int J Obstet Gynaecol. 2025; https://doi.org/10.1111/1471-0528.18054.

2. Balen AH, Tamblyn J, Skorupskaite K, Munro MG, and for the FIGO Committee on Menstrual Disorders and Related Health Impacts and Reproductive Medicine, Endocrinology and Infertility. A comprehensive review of the new FIGO classification of ovulatory disorders. Hum Reprod Update. 2024;30(3):355–82. https://doi.org/10.1093/humupd/dmae003.
3. Campbell S, Bourne TH, Tan SL, Collins WP. Hysterosalpingo contrast sonography (HyCoSy) and its future role within the investigation of infertility in Europe. Ultrasound Obstet Gynecol. 1994;4(3):245–53. https://doi.org/10.1046/j.1469-0705.1994.04030245.x.
4. Centre for Disease Control. Infertility: frequently asked questions. 2024. Available at: https://www.cdc.gov/reproductive-health/infertility-faq/?CDC_AAref_Val=https://www.cdc.gov/reproductivehealth/infertility/index.htm. Accessed 11 Mar 2025.
5. Chan YY, Jayaprakasan K, Zamora J, Thornton JG, Raine-Fenning N, Coomarasamy A. The prevalence of congenital uterine anomalies in unselected and high-risk populations: a systematic review. Hum Reprod Update. 2011;17(6):761–71. https://doi.org/10.1093/humupd/dmr028.
6. Bastawros H. Human reproduction: a clinical approach. 2023. https://doi.org/10.31274/isudp.2023.148.
7. Teede HJ, Tay CT, Laven J, Dokras A, Moran LJ, Piltonen TT, Costello MF, Boivin JM, Redman LA, Boyle J, Norman RJ, Mousa A Joham, AE. International evidence-based guideline for the assessment and management of polycystic ovary syndrome. 2023. Available at: Accessed 11 Mar 2025.
8. Conrad KP a, Baker VL. Corpus luteal contribution to maternal pregnancy physiology and outcomes in assisted reproductive technologies. Am J Physiol-Regulat Integr Comp Physiol. 2013;304(2) https://doi.org/10.1152/ajpregu.00239.2012.
9. Munro MG, Balen AH, Cho S, Critchley HOD, Díaz I, Ferriani R, Henry L, Mocanu E, van der Spuy ZM, FIGO Committee on Menstrual Disorders and Related Health Impacts, and FIGO Committee on Reproductive Medicine, Endocrinology, and Infertility. The FIGO ovulatory disorders classification system. Int J Gynaecol Obstet. 2022;159(1):1–20. https://doi.org/10.1002/ijgo.14331.
10. National Institute for Health and Care Excellence. What are the causes of infertility? 2023. Available at: https://cks.nice.org.uk/topics/infertility/background-information/causes/#:~:text=Infertility%20is%20a%20disease%20of,(25%25%20of%20couples. Accessed 11 Mar 2025.
11. Nik Hazlina NH, Norhayati MN, Shaiful Bahari I, Nik Muhammad Arif NA. Worldwide prevalence, risk factors and psychological impact of infertility among women: a systematic review and meta-analysis. BMJ Open. 2022;12(3):e057132. https://doi.org/10.1136/bmjopen-2021-057132.
12. Overland MR, Li Y, Derpinghaus A, Aksel S, Cao M, Ladwig N, Cunha GR, Himelreich-Perić M, Baskin LS. Development of the human ovary: fetal through pubertal ovarian morphology, folliculogenesis and expression of cellular differentiation markers. Differentiation. 2023;129:37–59. https://doi.org/10.1016/j.diff.2022.10.005.
13. Regan L, Rai R, Saravelos S, Li T, the Royal College of Obstetricians, and Gynaecologists. Recurrent miscarriage green-top guideline no. 17. BJOG Int J Obstet Gynaecol. 2023;130(12):e9–e39. https://doi.org/10.1111/1471-0528.17515.
14. Taylor HS, Pal L, Seli E. Speroff's clinical gynecologic endocrinology and infertility. 9th ed. Lippincott Williams & Wilkins; 2019.
15. Romualdi D, Ata B, Bhattacharya S, Bosch E, Costello M, Gersak K, Homburg R, Mincheva M, Norman RJ, Piltonen T, Dos Santos-Ribeiro S, Scicluna D, Somers S, Sunkara SK, Verhoeve HR, Le Clef N. Evidence-based guideline: unexplained infertility. Hum Reprod. 2023;38(10):1881–90. https://doi.org/10.1093/humrep/dead150.
16. The Rotterdam ESHRE/ASRM-sponsored PCOS consensus workshop group. Revised 2003 consensus on diagnostic criteria and long-term health risks related to polycystic ovary syndrome (PCOS). Hum Reprod. 2004;19(1):41–7. https://doi.org/10.1093/humrep/deh098.
17. Thompson L, Jewell R. HCG tracking for pregnancy of unknown location. 2023. Available at https://rightdecisions.scot.nhs.uk/media/ypbnbqqt/hcg-tracking-for-pregnancy-of-unknown-location-pul.pdf. Accessed 11 Mar 2025.

18. World Health Organisation. Infertility. 2024. Available at: https://www.who.int/news-room/fact-sheets/detail/infertility. Accessed 11 Mar 2025.
19. World Health Organization. Infertility prevalence estimates, 1990–2021. 2023. Available at: https://www.who.int/publications/i/item/978920068315. Accessed 11 Mar 2025.
20. Goldstein M, Schlegel PN. Anatomy and physiology of the male reproductive system. Cambridge University Press.
21. Hayes FJ, Pitteloud N, DeCruz S, Crowley WF Jr, Boepple PA. Importance of inhibin B in the regulation of FSH secretion in the human male. J Clin Endocrinol Metabol. 2001;86(11):5541–6.
22. Lee MM, Donahoe PK. Mullerian inhibiting substance: a gonadal hormone with multiple functions. Endocr Rev. 1993;14(2):152–64.
23. Sekido R, Lovell-Badge R. Sex determination involves synergistic action of SRY and SF1 on a specific Sox9 enhancer. Nature. 2008;453(7197):930–4.
24. Gurung P, Yetiskul E, Jialal I. Physiology, male reproductive system. In: StatPearls [Internet]. Statpearls Publishing; 2023.
25. Tiwana MS, Leslie SW. Anatomy, abdomen and pelvis: testes. StatPearls Publishing; 2017.
26. Sam P, LaGrange CA. Anatomy, abdomen and pelvis, penis. In: StatPearls [Internet]. StatPearls Publishing; 2023.
27. Lee SH, Ha TJ, Koh KS, Song WC. Ligamentous structures in human glans penis. J Anat. 2019;234(1):83–8.
28. Mohanty SK, Singh R. Overview of the male reproductive system. In: Male infertility: understanding, causes and treatment; 2017. p. 3–12.
29. Goldstein M, Schlegel PN. Surgical and medical management of male infertility. Cambridge University Press; 2013.
30. Tu LH, Spektor M, Ferrante M, Mathur M. MRI of the penis: indications, anatomy, and pathology. Curr Probl Diagn Radiol. 2020;49(1):54–63.
31. Jayasena C. 2025. https://BioRender.com/d55i045
32. Rew KT, Heidelbaugh JJ. Erectile dysfunction. Am Fam Physician. 2016;94(10):820–7.
33. Al-Thakafi S, Al-Hathal N. Peyronie's disease: a literature review on epidemiology, genetics, pathophysiology, diagnosis and work-up. Transl Androl Urol. 2016;5(3):280.
34. Ericson C, Baird B, Broderick GA. Management of priapism: 2021 update. Urol Clin. 2021;48(4):565–76.
35. Garcia RA, Sajjad H. Anatomy, abdomen and pelvis, scrotum. 2019.
36. Durairajanayagam D, Sharma RK, du Plessis SS, Agarwal A. Testicular heat stress and sperm quality. In: Male Infertility: A Complete Guide to Lifestyle and Environmental Factors; 2014. p. 105–25.
37. Waites GM. Thermoregulation of the scrotum and testis: studies in animals and significance for man. In: Temperature and environmental effects on the testis; 1991. p. 9–17.
38. Candas V, Becmeur F, Bothorel B, Hoeft A. Qualitative assessment of thermal and evaporative adjustments of human scrotal skin in response to heat stress. Int J Androl. 1993;16(2):137–42.
39. Sørensen HG, Lambrechtsen J, Einer-Jensen N. Efficiency of the countercurrent transfer of heat and 133Xenon between the pampiniform plexus and testicular artery of the bull under in-vitro conditions. Int J Androl. 1991;14(3):232–40.
40. Cimador M, Castagnetti M, De Grazia E. Management of hydrocele in adolescent patients. Nat Rev Urol. 2010;7(7):379–85.
41. Hoang VT, Van HAT, Hoang TH, Nguyen TTT, Trinh CT. A review of classification, diagnosis, and management of hydrocele. J Ultrasound Med. 2024;43(3):599–607.
42. Bandhauer K, Bartsch G, de Kretser D, Eshkol A, Frick J, Glezerman M, Kerr J, Lunenfeld B, Pöldinger W, Rohr H. Anatomical and functional aspects of the male reproductive organs. In: Disturbances in male fertility; 1982. p. 1–131.
43. O'Donnell L, Stanton P, de Kretser DM. Endocrinology of the male reproductive system and spermatogenesis. 2015.
44. Winter JS, Faiman C. Pituitary-gonadal relations in male children and adolescents. Pediatr Res. 1972;6(2):126–35.

45. Agger P. Scrotal and testicular temperature: its relation to sperm count before and after operation for varicocele. Fertil Steril. 1971;22(5):286–97.
46. Turek PJ. Male reproductive physiology. In: Campbell walsh urology. 11th ed. Philadelphia: Elsevier; 2016. p. 516–37.
47. Dahl EV. A vascular mechanism for maintaining testicular temperature by counter-current exchange. Surg Gynecol Obstet. 1959;108(6):697–705.
48. Li L, Lin W, Wang Z, Huang R, Xia H, Li Z, Deng J, Ye T, Huang Y, Yang Y. Hormone regulation in testicular development and function. Int J Mol Sci. 2024;25(11):5805.
49. Kaur G, Thompson LA, Dufour JM. Sertoli cells–immunological sentinels of spermatogenesis. In: Seminars in cell & developmental biology. Elsevier; 2014.
50. O'Donnell L, Nicholls PK, O'Bryan MK, McLachlan RI, Stanton PG. Spermiation: the process of sperm release. Spermatogenesis. 2011;1(1):14–35.
51. Haider SG. Cell biology of Leydig cells in the testis. Int Rev Cytol. 2004;233(4):181–241.
52. Ye L, Li X, Li L, Chen H, Ge R-S. Insights into the development of the adult Leydig cell lineage from stem Leydig cells. Front Physiol. 2017;8:430.
53. Vanlangenhove P, Dhondt E, Everaert K, Defreyne L. Pathophysiology, diagnosis and treatment of varicoceles: a review. Minerva Urol Nefrol. 2014;66(4):257–82.
54. Cobellis G, Noviello C, Nino F, Romano M, Mariscoli F, Martino A, Parmeggiani P, Papparella A. Spermatogenesis and cryptorchidism. Front Endocrinol. 2014;5:63.
55. Wang X, Liu X, Qu M, Li H. Sertoli cell-only syndrome: advances, challenges, and perspectives in genetics and mechanisms. Cell Mol Life Sci. 2023;80(3):67.
56. Sharp VJ, Kieran K, Arlen AM. Testicular torsion: diagnosis, evaluation, and management. Am Fam Physician. 2013;88(12):835–40.
57. Chu DS, Shakes DC. Spermatogenesis. In: Germ cell development in C elegans; 2013. p. 171–203.
58. Heller CG, Clermont Y. Spermatogenesis in man: an estimate of its duration. Science. 1963;140(3563):184–6.
59. Misell L, Holochwost D, Boban D, Santi N, Shefi S, Hellerstein M, Turek P. A stable isotope-mass spectrometric method for measuring human spermatogenesis kinetics in vivo. J Urol. 2006;175(1):242–6.
60. Griswold MD. Spermatogenesis: the commitment to meiosis. Physiol Rev. 2016;96(1):1–17.
61. Oehninger S, Kruger TF. Sperm morphology and its disorders in the context of infertility. F&S Rev. 2021;2(1):75–92.
62. Smith LB, Walker WH. The regulation of spermatogenesis by androgens. In: Seminars in cell & developmental biology. Elsevier; 2014.
63. Jarow j, Chen h, Rosner w T s, Zirkin b. Assessment of the androgen environment within the human testis: minimally invasive method to obtain intratesticular fluid. J Androl. 2001;22(4):640–5.
64. Jones RE, Lopez KH. Human reproductive biology. Academic; 2013.
65. James ER, Carrell DT, Aston KI, Jenkins TG, Yeste M, Salas-Huetos A. The role of the epididymis and the contribution of epididymosomes to mammalian reproduction. Int J Mol Sci. 2020;21(15):5377.
66. McConaghy JR, Panchal B. Epididymitis: an overview. Am Fam Physician. 2016;94(9):723–6.
67. Patrizio P, Asch RH, Handelin B, Silber SJ. Aetiology of congenital absence of vas deferens: genetic study of three generations. Hum Reprod. 1993;8(2):215–20.
68. Velez D, Pagani R, Mima M, Ohlander S. Vasectomy: a guidelines-based approach to male surgical contraception. Fertil Steril. 2021;115(6):1365–8.
69. Eisenberg ML, Esteves SC, Lamb DJ, Hotaling JM, Giwercman A, Hwang K, Cheng Y-S. Male infertility. Nat Rev Dis Primers. 2023;9(1):49.
70. Stoddard N, Leslie SW. Histology, male urethra. 2019.
71. Clermont Y. Kinetics of spermatogenesis in mammals: seminiferous epithelium cycle and spermatogonial renewal. Physiol Rev. 1972;52(1):198–236.

72. Organization WH. WHO laboratory manual for the examination and processing of human semen. World Health Organization; 2021.
73. Agarwal A, Mulgund A, Hamada A, Chyatte MR. A unique view on male infertility around the globe. Reprod Biol Endocrinol. 2015;13:1–9.
74. Thonneau P, Marchand S, Tallec A, Ferial M-L, Ducot B, Lansac J, Lopes P, Tabaste J-M, Spira A. Incidence and main causes of infertility in a resident population (1 850 000) of three French regions (1988–1989). Hum Reprod. 1991;6(6):811–6.
75. Sharma A, Minhas S, Dhillo WS, Jayasena CN. Male infertility due to testicular disorders. J Clin Endocrinol Metabol. 2021;106(2):e442–e59.
76. Hannon PR, Curry TE. Folliculogenesis. In: Skinner MK, ed. Encyclopedia of Reproduction. 2nd ed. Academic Press; 2018:72–9. https://doi.org/10.1016/B978-0-12-801238-3.64628-7
77. Hagen C, Fischer M, Mola G, Mikkelsen T, Cleemann L, Gravholt C, Viuff M, Juul A, Pedersen A, Main K. AMH and other markers of ovarian function in patients with Turner syndrome: a single center experience of transition from pediatric to gynecological follow-up. Front Endocrinol (Lausanne). 2023;14:1173600. https://doi.org/10.3389/fendo.2023.1173600
78. Reed BG, Carr BR. The normal menstrual cycle and the control of ovulation. In: Feingold KR, Ahmed SF, Anawalt B, et al, eds. Endotext [Internet]. South Dartmouth (MA): MDText.com, Inc.; 2000. Available from: https://www.ncbi.nlm.nih.gov/books/NBK279054
79. Teede HJ, Khomami MB, Morman R, Laven JSE, Joham AE, Costello MF, Patil M, Rees DA, Berry L, Cree MG, Zhao H, Norman RJ, Dokras A, Piltonen T. Global name change consortium. Polyendocrine metabolic ovarian syndrome, the new name for polycystic ovary syndrome: a multistep global consensus process. Lancet. 2026;407(10545):2329–39. https://doi.org/10.1016/S0140-6736(26)00717-8. Epub 2026 May 12. PMID: 42119588.

Role of the Fertility Nurse and the Initial Infertility Workup

2

Shafiqa Awj Allahyar and Nir Kugelman

2.1 Introduction

Infertility is defined as the inability to conceive after 1 year of regular unprotected sexual intercourse. Infertility affects millions of couples worldwide, according to a report published by the WHO. Approximately 17.5% of the adult population—roughly 1 in 6 worldwide—experience infertility, highlighting the urgent need to increase access to affordable, high-quality fertility care for those in need [1].

The etiologies of infertility include tubal factors (14%), ovulatory disorders (21%), and male factors (26%), while approximately 28% remain unexplained after traditional testing [2]. The basic infertility workup includes evaluation of ovarian reserve, tubal patency and uterine anatomy, thyroid and prolactin disorders, confirmation of the diagnosis of polyendocrine metabolic ovarian syndrome (PMOS), assessment of semen parameters, and additional evaluations to ensure that the patient is medically fit and prepared for pregnancy.

The diagnosis and management of infertility are multifaceted, systematic, and sensitive. Fertility nurses are the essential link between patients and healthcare professionals in this journey. Fertility nurses support patients through education, emotional counseling, and clinical guidance to manage the often complex process of infertility evaluation.

S. A. Allahyar (✉)
Fertility Nurse Clinician, McGill University Health Center (MUHC), Reproductive Center, Montreal, Quebec, Canada
e-mail: Shafiqa.Allahyar@MUHC.MCGILL.CA

N. Kugelman
Division of Reproductive Endocrinology and Infertility, Department of Obstetrics and Gynecology, McGill University, Montreal, Quebec, Canada
e-mail: nir.kugelman@mail.mcgill.ca

M. Das, M. H. Dahan (eds.), *A Comprehensive Guide to Reproductive Health and Infertility Medicine for Nurses*, https://doi.org/10.1007/978-3-032-24372-0_2

This chapter discusses the fertility nurses' role in the initial infertility assessment, the interpretation of diagnostic tests, the assessment of female and male partners, and the screening of genetic condition carriers. Fertility nurses are powerful facilitators of early diagnosis and effective interventions through their combination of clinical expertise and patient-centered care.

2.2 Objectives

At the end of this chapter, the reader will be able to:

1. Understand the role of the fertility nurse in the initial infertility workup.
2. Interpret the results and clinical significance of various infertility tests.
3. Understand the assessment of both female and male partners as part of an infertility evaluation.
4. Recognize the importance of carrier screening for genetic conditions in fertility care.

2.3 The Role of the Fertility Nurse

Fertility nurses play a crucial role in connecting patients with the treatment team to ensure the continuity of care, education, and support. This includes the following components of service: [3].

1. *Patient education*
   - *Purpose*: Provide information concerning the nature of infertility, available diagnostic processes, and treatment options.
   - *Key Responsibilities*:
     - Explain the rationale for hormonal tests, imaging studies, and semen testing.
     - Provide counseling on test preparation to ensure accurate results, such as timing hormone tests concerning the menstrual cycle [4].
2. *Emotional Support*
   - *Purpose*: Address the emotional impact of infertility, which may include anxiety, depression, and frustration.
   - *Key Responsibilities*:
     - Provide counseling or refer patients to support groups and mental health professionals.
     - Provide empathy and encouragement to support patients and their partners in coping with disappointment.
3. *Coordination of Care*
   - *Purpose*: Coordinating the logistics required for fertility investigations and treatment.

- *Key Responsibilities*:
  - Arranging appointments and investigations.
  - Liaising between fertility specialists, endocrinologists, urologists, and laboratory services.

4. *Monitoring and Follow-Up*
   - *Purpose*: To monitor patients throughout the investigation process.
   - *Key Responsibilities*:
     - Tracking test outcomes and communicating findings to patients and physicians.
     - Ensuring follow-up visits and changes in treatment occur on a timely basis [5].
5. *Advocacy*
   - *Purpose*: The purpose is to support patients clinically and financially throughout their fertility journey.
   - *Key Responsibilities*:
     - Patient advocacy and navigation through healthcare systems, insurance policies, and financial options for fertility treatments.
     - Empower patients to make informed decisions about their care.

2.4 Initial Infertility Workup

The initial infertility evaluation involves a comprehensive assessment of both partners to identify potential causes of infertility. This process integrates hormonal evaluation, imaging studies, and semen analysis to ensure accurate diagnosis and tailored treatment strategies. Fertility nurses play a key role in coordinating these tests, educating patients about their significance, and facilitating timely diagnosis.

2.4.1 Evaluation of Female Partner

The evaluation of female fertility focuses on ovarian function, hormonal balance, and structural abnormalities in the reproductive system [6]. Understanding hormone levels, their clinical significance, and appropriate units of measurement is essential for accurate interpretation and effective patient care.

2.4.1.1 Hormonal Assessments

Hormonal tests are critical for evaluating ovulatory function, ovarian reserve, and endocrine health. The key hormones assessed incude the following:

- *Follicle-stimulating hormone (FSH)*
  - *Purpose*: To assess ovarian reserve.
  - *Normal* levels: 3–10 mIU/mL (measured on days 2–5 of the menstrual cycle).
  - *Clinical Significance*:
    - Levels >10 mIU/mL suggest diminished ovarian reserve [7].
    - Levels >40 mIU/mL indicate menopause.
    - Levels <3 mIU/mL combined with low estrogen suggest hypothalamic amenorrhea.
- *Luteinizing Hormone (LH)*
  - *Purpose*: Evaluate ovulatory function.
  - *Normal* levels: 1–20 IU/L on day 3 of the cycle
  - *Clinical Significance*:
    - A mid-cycle LH surge (>20 IU/L) triggers ovulation.
    - Excessive fluid intake can dilute urine and lead to false-negative ovulation tests. Urine ovulation tests detect the LH surge, which indicates that ovulation is likely to occur. Therefore, excessive fluid intake may prevent detection of a positive ovulation test.
- *Prolactin*:
  - *Purpose*: To detect hyperprolactinemia, which can interfere with ovulation.
  - *Normal levels*: <25 ng/mL (<600 mIU/L).
  - *Clinical Note*: Elevated prolactin should be retested in the morning, after fasting, and after avoiding sexual activity or nipple stimulation for 48 hours [8]. Levels in women with polyendocrine metabolic ovarian syndrome can reach up to 1.5 times of the upper limit of normal on the assay used and are not considered an issue. Only levels above this should be evaluated in women with polyendocrine metabolic ovarian syndrome.
- *Thyroid function tests*: Thyroid dysfunction significantly impacts fertility. The following parameters are assessed:
  - *Thyroid-stimulating hormone (TSH)*:
    - The normal range is 0.4–4.0 mIU/mL.
    - *Clinical recommendation*: Optimal levels for fertility are <3.0 mIU/mL.
    - *Clinical Significance*:
      - High TSH levels indicate hypothyroidism, which can impair ovulation and increase the risk of miscarriage. Hypothyroidism is typically treated with oral thyroid hormone supplementation to maintain serum TSH levels within the normal range. Thyroid hormones are stable in the body, and once their levels normalize, routine monitoring is only required annually unless there is significant weight gain or loss. However, during pregnancy, thyroid hormone requirements increase, necessitating TSH monitoring at 6–8 weeks of pregnancy and then once per trimester. TSH reflects the brain's regulation of thyroid gland activity. Elevated TSH suggests reduced thyroid function (hypothyroidism) as the brain increases stimulation to compensate. Conversely, low TSH indicates

excessive thyroid activity (hyperthyroidism), reducing the need for brain-derived stimulation. Both hypothyroidism and hyperthyroidism can negatively impact fertility.

  - *Free T4 (thyroxine)*:
    - *Free T4*: normal level: 0.8 to 1.9 ng/dL or 10.3 to 24.5 pmol/L. (T4 is the less active version of the thyroid hormone) [9].
  - *Free T3 (triiodothyronine)*:
    - *Free T3*: 130 to 450 pg/dL, or 2.0 to 7.0 pmol/L. (T3 is the more active version of the thyroid hormone).
    - Low levels of free T3 or free T4 suggest hypothyroidism, while high levels suggest hyperthyroidism.
    - Normal levels of free T3 and free T4 and low or high serum TSH levels suggest subclinical hypo- or hyperthyroidism, respectively, and may be treated or observed on a case-by-case basis.
- *Progesterone*:
  - Progesterone is the hormone associated with the luteal phase following ovulation and is produced by the corpus luteum, the *postovulatory* cyst that forms after the egg is released from the ovary. It serves as a key marker of ovulation, with levels typically ranging from 2 to 25 ng/mL (>30 nmol/L) during the luteal phase of the menstrual cycle.
  - In the follicular phase, serum progesterone levels are lower, typically between 0.1 and 0.7 ng/mL. Values between these two ranges may indicate impending ovulation, as progesterone begins rising 2–3 days before ovulation.
  - During the first trimester of pregnancy, progesterone levels usually range from 10 to 44 ng/mL. Lower levels may suggest the need for additional progesterone supplementation in IVF cycle or could indicate a risk of impending miscarriage or ectopic pregnancy, as unhealthy pregnancies tend to produce less progesterone [10].
- *Estradiol*:
  - *Purpose*: To evaluate ovarian function and the response to stimulation [11].
  - *Normal* levels: 25–75 pg/mL (days 2–5 of the menstrual cycle).

Importance of Units in Hormone Measurements

Accurate interpretation of hormone levels requires attention to units of measurement:

- *mIU/mL or IU/L*: Milli-international units per milliliter (e.g., FSH, LH, TSH, prolactin)
- *ng/mL*: Nanograms per milliliter (e.g., progesterone and prolactin)
- *pg/mL*: Picograms per milliliter (e.g., estradiol and free T3).
- *pmol/L*: Picomoles per liter (alternative metric for thyroid hormones)
- *nmol/L*: Nanomoles per liter (e.g., progesterone, testosterone)

2.4.2 Evaluation of Male Partners

Reproduction is regulated by hormones that function within hypothalamic-pituitary-gonadal (HPG) axis. In males, the maintenance of testicular testosterone (T) production and spermatogenesis is regulated by two pituitary gonadotropins, luteinizing hormone (LH) and follicle-stimulating hormone (FSH). The testicular target cells of LH are the Leydig cells located in the interstitial space whereas the target cells of FSH are the Sertoli cells located in the seminiferous tubules. LH stimulates Leydig cells to produce testosterone, while FSH stimulates Sertoli cells. In synergy with testosterone, Sertoli cells produce regulatory molecules that indirectly support spermatogenesis. Hormonal evaluation, including testosterone, FSH, and LH, provides critical insights into the function of the hypothalamic-pituitary-gonadal (HPG) axis and overall reproductive health [12].

2.4.2.1 Hormonal Assessments

- *Testosterone*: Testosterone is the principal male sex hormone and plays a central role not only in spermatogenesis and libido but also in muscle mass and the development of other secondary sexual traits in males.
  - *Types of Testosterone*:
    - *Total testosterone (TT)*: Total quantity of free and bound testosterone in the blood.
      - Normal range: 300–1000 ng/dL.
      - Most testosterone in the blood is bound to proteins, mainly sex hormone-binding globulin or albumin. It is, therefore, biologically inactive [12].
  - *Free Testosterone (FT)*: It is the biologically active, unbound form of testosterone.
    - Normal range: 5–25 ng/dL. (6–27 nmol/L).
    - Free testosterone is a better marker for the diagnosis of conditions such as infertility or hypogonadism [13].
  - *Clinical insights*: Low total and free testosterone may indicate the following:
    - *Primary testicular failure* (primary hypogonadism). Examples: undescended testes, Klinefelter syndrome, mumps orchitis, and testicular injury (diagnosed by low testosterone and high FSH, LH) [14].
    - Secondary *Hypogonadism*: Malfunction of the hypothalamus or pituitary gland. Examples include pituitary disease, Kallmann syndrome, trauma, and obesity. (diagnosed by low testosterone and normal or low LH).
    - Both types of hypogonadism can cause semen abnormalities and decreased sperm counts. Primary hypogonadism is usually associated with severely impaired sperm motility.
- *FSH (follicle-stimulating hormone)*: FSH produced by the pituitary gland stimulates Sertoli cells in the testes, which are crucial for the development of sperm (spermatogenesis) [14].

- *Normal range*: 1.5–12.4 mIU/mL.
- *Clinical Interpretation*:
  - High FSH: Primary testicular failure. FSH production increases due to reduced negative feedback from impaired testicular function. Examples: Testicular damage (radiation, trauma, or chemotherapy) and Klinefelter syndrome [13].
  - Low FSH: Secondary hypogonadism. Decreased production of FSH due to failure of the hypothalamus or pituitary gland.

- *LH (luteinizing hormone)*: LH plays an important role in sperm production through the stimulation of Leydig cells in the testes [14].
  - *Normal range*: 1.8–8.6 IU/L.
  - *Clinical Interpretation*:
    - *High LH* reflects primary testicular failure since the brain compensates for low testosterone by increasing LH levels.
    - *Low LH* reflects secondary hypogonadism due to pituitary or hypothalamic disease.

The measurements of total testosterone, free testosterone, FSH, and LH are used to distinguish the following:

- *Primary hypogonadism*—testicular failure
- *Secondary hypogonadism*—hypothalamic-pituitary dysfunction [13]

Furthermore, the results of hormonal testing help guide the need for additional investigations, such as karyotyping and genetic testing, as well as appropriate treatment options, including testosterone replacement therapy or assisted reproductive technologies.

2.5 Imaging Tests for Infertility

2.5.1 Imaging Studies for Female Infertility

- *Ultrasound*
  - *Purpose*: Evaluate the endometrial lining, ovaries, and uterus.
  - *Key Assessments*:
    - Antral follicle count (AFC): [2]
      - Timing: Done on cycle days 2–5
      - Follicle Measurement: 2–8 mm in diameter in the ovaries
      - Interpretation:
        - <13 follicles: May indicate decreased ovarian reserve
        - Small ovaries (<2 cm in diameter) may suggest decreased ovarian reserve

- *Hysterosalpingography (HSG)*
  - *Purpose*: X-ray imaging to assess *fallopian tube patency* and detect *uterine abnormalities.*
  - *Normal Results*: Open tubes and a normal uterine cavity.
  - *Clinical Uses*: Identifies:
    - Hydrosalpinx (fluid-filled, blocked tubes).
    - Other tubal obstruction
  - *Additional Considerations*: The use of oil-based contrast during HSG may increase the likelihood of pregnancy, particularly during the first 3 months following the procedure.
  - *Patient Preparation*: Pretreatment with NSAIDs for discomfort reduction. Alternative contrast agents may be considered for patients with iodine allergy.
  - *Clinical Note*: HSG may be painful; patient counseling and preparation are essential.
- *Sonohysterography (Saline Infusion Ultrasound (SIS))*
  - *Purpose*: Enhances visualization of the uterine cavity
  - *Clinical Uses*:
    - Detection of polyps, fibroids, and other uterine abnormalities
    - Assessment of tubal patency (although less accurately than HSG due to possible tubal spasm)
- *HyCoSy (Hysterosalpingo-Contrast Sonography)*
  - *Purpose*: Combines 3D ultrasound with contrast injection to evaluate tubal patency [2]
  - *Clinical Uses*: Identifying blocked fallopian tubes and providing a noninvasive, radiation-free alternative to HSG
  - *Advantages*:
    - Less discomfort than HSG
    - Ideal for patients who cannot tolerate iodine-based contrast

Clinical Imaging Recommendations

- *Hydrosalpinx*: Include an image demonstrating a hydrosalpinx with a blocked fallopian tube on imaging.
- *HSG*: Provides a normal scan to illustrate tubal patency.
- *HyCoSy*: Foam contrast imaging used for clear visualization of the open tubes.

2.5.2 Imaging in Male Reproductive Health

- *Scrotal ultrasonography*:
  Scrotal ultrasound is a noninvasive diagnostic tool for investigating a variety of abnormalities that may result in male infertility [16].

Scrotal Ultrasound Indications:

- *Abnormal physical examination*:
  - Signs and symptoms include a mass, swelling, asymmetry, and painful or uncomfortable states.
  - Varicocele: The problem of enlarged scrotal veins, which may be associated with male infertility in males [17].
- *Suspicion of Varicocele*:
  - Varicoceles may reduce sperm count and motility and increase abnormal morphology
  - Ultrasound provides information on the degree and whether surgery can be conducted [17]
- *Pain or discomfort of the testis*:
  - Provides a diagnosis of testicular pain based on whether infection, trauma, or inflammation is occurring
  - Ultrasound can diagnose hydrocele, epididymitis, or hematomas.
- *History of Infertility*:
  - It enables the evaluation of testicular volume, blood flow, and structural abnormalities that may include obstruction or lesions in the testes that may affect sperm production [17].
- *Hydrocele or epididymal cysts*:
  - Ultrasound can identify fluid collections, including hydrocele and epididymal cysts, which may interfere with sperm transport and potentially affect testicular function.
- *Suspected testicular tumors*:
  - Testicular masses are outlined while separating benign masses from those that could be suspicious, hence requiring further workup.
- *Assessment Post-Trauma*:
  - To assess testicular rupture, hematoma, and impaired vascularity of the testes after trauma.

1. *Indications for the Importance of Scrotal Ultrasound*:

   - Anatomy assessment: details about the anatomy of the testes, epididymides, and scrotal veins.
   - Noninvasive: This is a very safe and painless modality with good accessibility;
   - Scrotal ultrasound is the preferred imaging modality for evaluating varicoceles, hydroceles, and obstructive abnormalities. Accurate imaging is essential for guiding treatment decisions, as some of these conditions may be surgically correctable, potentially improving fertility outcomes.
   - Detection of curable pathology conditions.
   - Guided Treatment Decisions: The results will help in deciding on the need for varicocelectomy, hormonal therapy, or assisted reproductive technology (ART) [17].

2.5.3 Semen Analysis in Male Fertility Evaluation

Semen analysis is the backbone of male fertility evaluation and provides important information about sperm quality and overall fertility. Semen analysis encompasses the volume of the seminal fluid, the motility and concentration of sperm, and morphology to identify possible causes of infertility.

Key Parameters

- *Volume*: normal range: 1.5–5 mL.
  - Low volume (<1.5 mL): Incomplete sample collection, accessory gland hypofunction, and retrograde ejaculation may be suspected [19].
- *pH*: normal: 7.2–8.0.
  - Abnormal pH: May suspect infection or dysfunction of the seminal vesicles.
- *Sperm concentration*: normal: ≥15 million sperm per mL.
  - Clinical significance: A concentration of <10 million/mL should prompt further urologic evaluation to exclude conditions such as testicular malignancy, which occurs in less than 5% of such individuals [19].
- *Sperm motility*: normal: ≥40% motile sperm. Progressive motility: normal: ≥32%.
  - Clinical Insight: Reduced sperm motility (asthenozoospermia) impairs the ability of sperm to move through the female reproductive tract and reach the egg, potentially reducing fertilization potential [19].
- *Sperm morphology*: normal ≥4% normal forms (Kruger strict criteria).
  - Abnormal morphology—teratozoospermia: reduces fertilizing ability. This is generally due to genetic and environmental factors [19].

2.6 Fertility Testing and Screening in Men and Women

2.6.1 Woman Fertility Evaluation

2.6.1.1 Ovarian Reserve Tests

The ovarian reserve is an estimate of a woman's reproductive potential based on the quantity of remaining oocytes. These are the various tests commonly used: [20].

Anti-Müllerian Hormone (AMH)

- The normal range is 1.0–3 ng/mL (7.1–21.4 pmol/l)
- *Clinical Significance*:
  - A concentration of less than 1.0 ng/mL (7.1 pmol/l) indicates an increased risk of poor ovarian response if the patient is undergoing IVF.
  - A concentration above 2.9 ng/mL (20 pmol/l) is associated with an optimal response to ovarian stimulation during IVF.

- *Advantages*: AMH levels can be measured at any point in the menstrual cycle, as they are not cycle-dependent.
- *Considerations*: The results may vary depending on the assay used, requiring careful interpretation in the clinical context [21].

Antral Follicle Count (AFC)

- *Normal range*: 6–10 antral follicles observed via transvaginal ultrasound.
- *Clinical significance*: The AFC provides a direct estimate of the remaining follicle pool and is correlated with the ovarian response during IVF [22].

2.6.1.2 Endometrial Biopsy

Endometrial biopsy is used to evaluate the receptivity of the uterine lining during the luteal phase for implantation.

- *Clinical utility*: Traditionally, it has been used to assess luteal phase defects, although its use has declined due to variability in interpretation.
- *Limitation*: There is considerable variation in the results, depending on the pathologist analyzing the sample [23].

2.6.2 Male Fertility Evaluation

2.6.2.1 Genetic Testing in Male Infertility

Genetic testing reveals the underlying causes of male infertility and, particularly, in individuals presenting with azoospermia. The following are some of the important tests:

Y Chromosome Microdeletions

The Y chromosome contains critical regions responsible for normal spermatogenesis, known as the azoospermia factor (AZF) region [24].

- *Results and Clinical Implications*:
  - *Deletions of AZFa or AZFb*:
    - Poor prognostic value; usually due to non-obstructive azoospermia
    - Sperm retrieval (Micro-TESE): is very unlikely
  - *Deletions in AZFc*
    - Variable phenotypes: some men have sperm production at very low levels.
    - Sperm retrieval for use in IVF/ICSI is often possible.
    - AZFc deletions may be passed on to male offspring, who themselves can be affected by impaired fertility.
- *Recommendation*: Genetic counseling is advised before assisted reproductive technology (ART) because it provides individuals with information about the risks and implications of genetic disorders.

Cystic Fibrosis Transmembrane Conductance Regulator (CFTR) Gene Mutations

Mutations in the CFTR gene have been associated with congenital bilateral absence of the vas deferens, which is a common cause of obstructive azoospermia [25].

- *Results and clinical implications*:
  - Men with congenital bilateral absence of the vas deferens (CBAVD) produce sperm, but due to the absence of the vas deferens, the transport of sperm is impaired.
  - Testicular techniques such as TESA or PESA can be used to obtain sperm.
  - CFTR mutations can be inherited and increase the risk of cystic fibrosis if the female partner is also a carrier.
- *Recommendation*: CFTR carrier screening should be undertaken by both partners to identify genetic risk.

Karyotype Analysis

Karyotyping assesses the structure and number of chromosomes to identify genetic abnormalities that may impact fertility.

- *Common Abnormalities*:
  - Klinefelter syndrome (KS) is the most common chromosomal disorder found in men and is characterized by the typical karyotype of 47,XXY.
    - An extra X chromosome is a major cause of male infertility [26].
    - A potential result is azoospermia or severe oligospermia.
    - Sperm may still be retrieved for IVF/ICSI with micro-TESE.
  - Structural chromosome abnormalities, for example, such as translocations:
    - Robertsonian or reciprocal translocations can result in infertility or recurrent miscarriage.
- *Recommendation*: Genetic counseling, including an understanding of transmission risks and available reproductive options, is important.

2.7 Infectious Disease Screening

Screening for transmissible infections is crucial for ensuring the safety of conception, preventing adverse pregnancy outcomes, and maintaining standards of IVF laboratory safety.

2.7.1 Rubella and Varicella Testing

These tests assess immunity against Rubella and Varicella-Zoster viruses. Which can cause congenital infection during pregnancy if the mother is not immune.

- *Results and Actions*:
  - *Rubella IgG*: A positive result signifies immunity.
    - *If Negative*:
      - Advise MMR (measles, mumps, and rubella) vaccination.
      - Advise avoiding pregnancy for 1-month post-vaccination.
  - *Varicella IgG*: Positive result indicates immunity.
    - *If negative*:
      - Advise Varicella vaccination
      - Advise avoiding pregnancy for 1 month after vaccination
      - Immunity status should be repeated 4–6 weeks post-vaccination, if necessary [27].

2.7.2 HIV, Hepatitis B and C, and Syphilis Testing

The screening of these transmissible infections ensures safety for fertility treatment itself as well as the prevention of maternal-fetal transmission.

- *Results and clinical action*:
  - *HIV*: a negative test indicates no evidence of infection.
  - *Hepatitis B and C*: A negative result indicates no infection.
  - *Syphilis (RPR or VDRL)*: A negative result suggests no evidence of infection.
    - *If positive*:
      - Refer to infectious disease specialists for further management.
      - Adequate treatment before conception is necessary.
      - Appropriate handling and storage of gametes during IVF are required to reduce the risk of cross-contamination [28].

2.7.3 Chlamydia and Gonorrhea Testing

The two most prevalent sexually transmitted infectious agents significantly affect fertility and may further worsen IVF outcomes.

- *Results and clinical action*:
  Negative result: No evidence of current infection.
- If positive:
  - Administration of appropriate antibiotics to both partners.
  - Rescreen post-treatment to confirm clearance.
  - Gametes should be appropriately handled and stored in IVF laboratories to avoid cross-contamination [29].

2.7.3.1 Summary of Actions

Test	Negative result action	Positive result action
Rubella/Varicella	Vaccinate Avoid pregnancy for 1 month	None (immune)
HIV, hepatitis B/C, syphilis	None	Infectious disease referrals; infection treatment
Chlamydia/Gonorrhea	None	Treat both partners; rescreen post-treatment

2.7.3.2 Clinical Significance

- Infectious disease screening can ensure the safety of fertility treatment and reduce the chance of maternal-fetal transmission.
- Vaccination: Congenital infections are prevented, thereby improving the outcome of pregnancy.

2.8 Evaluation of the Female Partner in Recurrent Pregnancy Loss (RPL)

RPL is the condition of experiencing two or more clinical pregnancy losses, as stated by the ASRM and ESHRE. This affects approximately 1–2% of couples [32]. Chromosomal abnormalities, uterine structural abnormalities, infection, immune system dysfunction, and endocrine factors are major risk factors for RPL. However, a significant proportion of RPL cases, approximately 50%, are of unknown etiology and are thus termed unexplained recurrent pregnancy loss. Despite an enormous amount of scholarly work on this topic, the etiology and management of RPL remain poorly understood.

2.8.1 Medical History

Histories play an essential role in the assessment of RPL. The following should be explored:

- *History of the Menstrual Cycle*: Length, regularity, any abnormalities.
- *History of pregnancy*: Past pregnancies, miscarriages, number of living children, and complications.
- *Sexual history*: This history includes the frequency of intercourse, the use of contraception, and sexually transmitted infections.
- *Lifestyle factors*: alcohol intake, smoking, obesity, nutritional habits, exercise.
- *Medical/surgical history*: chronic conditions, surgeries, or medications contributing to infertility [30].

2.8.2 Physical Examination

General physical examination provides insight into the underlying conditions affecting fertility and the outcomes of pregnancy:

1. *General physical examination*
   - Evaluation of general health, including blood pressure, BMI, and the presence of endocrine or systemic diseases.
2. *Pelvic examination*
   - Examines the reproductive system (vagina, cervix, uterus, and ovaries) for abnormalities such as the following:
     (i) Uterine masses (fibroids, polyps)
     (ii) Ovarian cysts
     (iii) Pelvic infections or congenital uterine anomalies.
3. *Pap Smear*
   - Screens for cervical dysplasia or cervical cancer associated with HPV infection.
   - Ensures the health of the cervix in anticipation of pregnancy or fertility treatment.
   - Abnormal results require colposcopy or biopsy before other interventions [31].
4. *Breast examination*
   - *Manual breast examination*: Lumps, tenderness, or abnormalities are detected.
   - *Mammography*: Should be performed for patients ≥40 years of age or those with breast cancer risk factors.

   Why Breast Evaluation Is Important:
     - Pregnancy hormones, such as estrogen and progesterone, cause the growth of breast tissue.
     - Hormone-sensitive breast cancers, such as ER-positive breast cancer, may worsen during pregnancy.
     - Early detection allows timely treatment and protection of maternal and fetal health.
   - *Clinical Note*: The diagnosis of breast cancer before pregnancy allows timely treatment planning and may prevent delays in chemotherapy, radiation, or surgery, which may influence prognosis.

2.8.3 Hormonal Investigations

Hormonal factors have strong implications for RPL, especially in overweight patients. The important tests are as follows:

1. *Serum early follicular FSH and LH (days 2–5 of the cycle)*
    - Follicle-stimulating hormone (FSH)
        - Normal value: 3–10 mIU/mL
        - An FSH level > 10 mIU/mL is suggestive of diminished ovarian reserve
    - Luteinizing hormone (LH)
        - Normal value: 1–20 IU/L
        - Increased LH, which is common in women with PMOS, may impede ovulation and predispose them to miscarriage.
    - *Clinical Insight*: An abnormal FSH/LH ratio may be suggestive of ovarian dysfunction or PMOS [32].
2. *Prolactin*
    - Normal value: <25 ng/mL (<600 mIU/L)
    - Increased prolactin levels impair ovulation and inhibit endometrial development during the luteal phase, preventing implantation.
    - *Clinical Insight*: Overweight patients may have hyperprolactinemia secondary to obesity, medication, or stress. It is preferred to check fasting prolactin levels, avoiding nipple trauma or sexual activity, for 48 hours before testing.
3. *Thyroid function tests (TSH, free T4, and free T3)*
    - TSH: Optimal preconception range: <2.5 mIU/mL
        - High TSH (>4.0 mIU/mL) suggests that hypothyroidism is a known risk factor for miscarriage.
    - Free T4 and free T3:
        - Free T4: 0.8–1.9 ng/dL
        - Free T3: 2.0–7.0 pmol/L
    - *Clinical Insight*: Hypothyroidism is a common factor, especially in overweight patients; it impairs implantation and increases the risk of pregnancy loss [34].
4. *Estradiol (Days 2–5 of Cycle)*
    - Normal range: 25–75 pg/mL
    - High levels of estradiol suppress FSH, masking reduced ovarian reserve.
    - *Clinical Insight*: Overweight patients are often diagnosed with high levels of estradiol because of the peripheral conversion of androgens to estrogens in adipose tissue, which is responsible for abnormalities in the cycle and disorders in endometrial function [35].
5. *Mid-Luteal Serum Progesterone (Days 21–23)*
    - A normal level of >10 ng/mL (>30 nmol/l) confirms adequate ovulation.
    - <10 ng/mL (<30 nmol/l) indicates a defect in the luteal phase that impairs implantation.
    - *Clinical Insight*: Overweight patients very often have insulin resistance, which is sometimes associated with PMOS. These factors are associated with luteal insufficiency. Management of these issues improves pregnancy outcomes [32].

2.8.4 Other Investigations for Overweight Patients with RPL [32]

1. *Coagulation Factors and Thrombophilia Screening*:
   Inherited or acquired thrombophilias may result in placental insufficiency. The following tests are recommended: [33]
   - Lupus anticoagulant (LA)
   - Anticardiolipin antibodies (aCLs)
   - Anti-β2 glycoprotein I antibodies
   - Protein C and protein S deficiency
   - Factor V Leiden mutation
   - Prothrombin gene mutation (G20210A) [33].
2. *Metabolic and insulin resistance testing*
   - Fasting glucose and insulin levels: assessed via the HOMA-IR index.
   - HbA1c: assesses glycemic control.
   - *Clinical Insight*: Insulin resistance in obesity and PMOS promotes inflammation, poor ovulation, and miscarriage [34].
3. *PMOS assessment*:
   Polyendocrine metabolic ovarian syndrome is common in overweight women with irregular cycles. The features include:
   - Increased LH: FSH ratio
   - High androgen–testosterone levels
   - Polycystic ovaries on ultrasound

2.8.5 Lifestyle Modifications and Medical Management

Weight management and lifestyle modification play very important roles in the management of hormonal balance and improvement in fertility outcomes. This includes:

- *Weight loss*: A 5–10% reduction in weight may restore ovulation and improve metabolic health.
- *Dietary and exercise interventions*: Increasing insulin sensitivity and hormonal regulation.
- *Medications*: Metformin is indicated for improving insulin resistance, especially in patients with PMOS [35].

2.8.6 Clinical Recommendations

1. *Hormonal evaluation*: This allows identification of ovulatory dysfunction, thyroid disorders, hyperprolactinemia, and luteal phase defects.

2. *Thrombophilia screening*: Thrombophilia screening is indicated in patients with recurrent miscarriage or risk factors for thrombosis.
3. *Lifestyle therapy*: Weight reduction, exercise, and dietary changes can significantly improve fertility outcomes.
4. *Targeted therapies*: Optimization of hormonal imbalance, metabolic dysfunction, and coagulation disorders to achieve maximum pregnancy success.

2.9 Evaluation of the Male Partner

2.9.1 Medical History

A thorough history is helpful in identifying modifiable risk factors and underlying causes of male infertility. The following are the important points to cover:

1. *Past pregnancies*:
   - Assess past fertility status with current and previous partners.
   - Recurrent pregnancy loss or infertility may indicate genetic, hormonal, or lifestyle-related factors.
2. *Sexual history*:
   - Assess sexual activity patterns, frequency, and concerns such as erectile dysfunction, ejaculatory issues, or STIs.
   - STIs such as chlamydia and gonorrhea cause reproductive tract obstruction and affect sperm quality [36].
3. *Lifestyle factors*:
   - Smoking, alcohol, drugs, diet, weight, stress, and physical activity have direct impacts on fertility.
   - Smoking and alcohol reduce the quality of sperm.
   - Obesity and malnutrition affect hormone levels and sperm production.
   - High stress may reduce testosterone levels sperm motility.
4. *Past medical history*:
   - Chronic diseases such as diabetes and hypertension can lead to erectile dysfunction or hormonal imbalances.
   - History of infection, surgeries, or trauma to the testes gives clues about fertility issues.
5. *History of Surgery*:
   - Groin, testicular, or pelvic surgery may lead to adhesion formation and damage to the reproductive tract.
   - Groin, testicular, and pelvic surgical procedures, such as vasectomy, hernia, and correction of undescended testis, interferes directly with fertility [36].

2.9.2 Physical Examination

The examination is generalized and includes the following:

- *General examination*: assessment of the patient's general health, BMI, and evidence of systemic disease.
- *Examination of the Genitalia*: This assesses the testes, epididymis, and vas deferens for masses, asymmetry, or swelling. It is also a screen for conditions such as varicocele, hydrocele, and testicular atrophy [16].

2.9.3 Laboratory Investigations

2.9.3.1 Hormonal Assessments

Hormonal assessment is indicated when abnormalities are detected on semen analysis. The important hormones to be estimated include the following:

- Serum-free and total testosterone
- Thyroid-stimulating hormone (TSH)
- Prolactin
- Follicle-stimulating hormone (FSH)
- Luteinizing hormone (LH) [16]

2.9.4 Semen Analysis

- Semen analysis—a key in male infertility
- Semen volume and pH
- Sperm concentration
- Sperm motility
- Sperm morphology [16]

2.9.5 Additional Diagnostic Investigations

In some cases, other investigations are needed:

- *Genetic testing*: Chromosomal abnormalities, Y chromosome microdeletions, and cystic fibrosis mutations.
- *Advanced hormonal profiles*: To further investigate the endocrinological causes of infertility.
- *Serology tests*: For HIV, hepatitis, syphilis, Chlamydia, and gonorrhea [12].

2.9.6 Summary

The assessment of male infertility is performed in a stepwise approach, including history taking, physical examination, and imaging studies, such as ultrasound of the scrotum and laboratory tests. Imaging modalities such as ultrasound play an important role in identifying structural and vascular abnormalities, whereas hormonal and semen analyses reveal functional abnormalities. A full assessment will lead to an appropriate diagnosis and permit personalized treatment options that can help achieve the best fertility outcome possible [12].

2.10 Carrier Screening for Genetic Issues

2.10.1 Importance of Carrier Screening

Carrier screening helps in the early identification of couples who are at risk of passing on genetic disorders to their offspring. It is significant in cases of autosomal recessive diseases, X-linked conditions, and individuals with a strong family history of inherited disorders. Early diagnosis allows for options in reproductive choices, early intervention, and methods of risk mitigation [37].

2.10.1.1 Why Carrier Screening Matters

- *Identifies risk*: It estimates the chances of passing on serious genetic conditions.
- *Enables informed decisions*: Couples can proactively make reproductive choices.
- *Facilitates early interventions*: The early diagnosis of genetic disorders can optimize treatment outcomes for affected offspring [37].

2.10.1.2 Common Genetic Tests in Carrier Screening

1. *Cystic Fibrosis (CF)*
   - *Inheritance*: autosomal recessive.
   - *Effect*: Caused by mutations in the CFTR gene, CF primarily affects the respiratory and digestive systems; it may also affect the reproductive system. In males, it can lead to CBAVD, resulting in obstructive azoospermia (absence of sperm in the ejaculate) [38].
   - *Why Test?* Testing for carriers helps evaluate the risk of passing the disease to offspring.
2. *Fragile X Syndrome*
   - *Inheritance*: X-linked disorder.
   - *Impact*: Fragile X syndrome is caused by the expansion of the FMR1 gene and is the most common cause of inherited intellectual disabilities, behavioral problems, and developmental delays. Female carriers are at risk for fragile X-associated primary ovarian insufficiency.
   - Screening is especially useful if there is a family history of unexplained intellectual disabilities or developmental delays.

3. *Spinal Muscular Atrophy (SMA)*
   - *Inheritance*: autosomal recessive.
   - *Effect*: SMA is caused by mutations in the SMN1 gene and leads to progressive degeneration of motor neurons, causes the production of abnormal hemoglobin (HbS).
   - *Why Test?* Screening for carriers is very important, as SMA is one of the most common causes of neuromuscular disorders in childhood.
4. *Thalassemia and Sickle Cell Anemia*
   - *Inheritance*: autosomal recessive hemoglobinopathies.
   - *Effect*:
     - Thalassemia: Anemia and its complications due to mutations that affect hemoglobin production.
     - Sickle cell anemia: A mutation in the HBB gene causes the production of abnormal hemoglobin (HbS), which distort red blood cells, leading to anemia, pain crises, and organ damage [39].
   - *Why Test?* Testing reveals carriers and allows for prenatal or preimplantation genetic testing.
5. *Congenital Adrenal Hyperplasia (CAH)*
   - *Inheritance*: autosomal recessive.
   - *Effect*: This mutation is caused by mutations in the CYP21A2 gene, affecting the production of adrenal hormones:
     - Females: Ambiguous genitalia may arise at birth because of virilization.
     - In males: Severe forms may present with salt-wasting crises and precocious puberty.
   - *Why Test?* Carrier screening permits prenatal intervention, thus minimizing the chances of a catastrophic neonatal outcome [40].

2.10.1.3 Summary of Genetic Tests

These genetic tests detect carriers of some of the most common inherited disorders. They help couples decide on family planning and assess the risk of a particular disorder. Screening is of utmost importance in individuals with the following:

- Family history of some genetic disorders
- Ethnic predisposition to certain disorders
- Unexplained infertility or recurrent pregnancy loss

2.11 Nurse's Role in Genetic Screening

A nurse's role is to educate the patient about the reasons for genetic testing, prepare the patient for testing and follow-up appointments, and reassure the patient emotionally through the process to ensure that the patient understands the results and can make appropriate decisions related to their health and family planning based on their genetic information.

This would also include identifying those most at risk to benefit from genetic screening based on family history, potential risks, and benefits associated with genetic testing and discussion of any concerns the patient might have [41].

The key aspects of a nurse's role in genetic screening include the following:

- *Patient education*: Explain the concept of genetic screening in clear, understandable language, including the purpose and potential implications of testing. A patient's family history should be assessed to identify individuals at high risk for genetic conditions, and the benefits of genetic testing in such situations should be discussed. Tailor information according to the patient's cultural background and health literacy level.
  - Advantages, such as early detection and prevention, as well as the disadvantages and ethical issues of genetic testing.
- *Ordering testing*:
  - Appropriate samples, such as blood and saliva, are collected for genetic testing.
  - Correctly fill out all necessary forms and consent documents and obtain patient consent.
  - Contact and coordinate with genetic testing laboratories for test processing and results follow-up.
- *Counseling following testing*:
  - Explain the genetic test results to the patient in a sensitive manner, describing what the implications are.
  - Addressing on emotional issues that may arise in association with the results, including anxiety or issues with decision-making related to outcomes;
  - Describe follow-up steps depending on the findings: any future genetic counseling, medical monitoring, or reproductive planning options.
- *Referral to genetic counselors*:
  - Mention the conditions under which the patient should be referred to a professional specialist for genetic counseling.
  - Facilitate referral to genetic counselors in complicated cases—when either patient needs detailed discussions about the implications of their genetic findings.

2.11.1 Keywords to Remember

- Ethical Issues: Nurses should be aware of ethical issues associated with genetic testing, privacy, and potential discrimination against individuals due to their genetic background.
- Access to community resources, support groups, and educational materials.
- Continuing Education: Nurses should show interest in continuous education since genetics is evolving daily. This helps them maintain competency in practices related to genetic counseling and testing.
- Genetic disorder carrier screening.
- Importance of carrier screening.

References

1. World Health Organization. 1 in 6 people globally is affected by infertility. 2023. https://www.who.int/news/item/04-04-2023-1-in-6-people-globally-affected-by-infertility.
2. Kondagari L, Kahn J, Singh M. Sonography gynecology infertility assessment, protocols, and interpretation. In: StatPearls [Internet]. Treasure Island (FL): StatPearls Publishing; 2023. Available at https://www.ncbi.nlm.nih.gov/sites/books/NBK572093/.
3. Sagheb Ray Shirazi M, Salarkarimi F, Moghadasi F, Mahmoudikohani F, Tajik F, Bastani Nejad Z. Infertility prevention and health promotion: the role of nurses in public health initiatives. Galen Med J. 2024;13:1–12. https://doi.org/10.31661/gmj.v13i.3534.
4. de Angelis C, Nardone A, Garifalos F, Pivonello C, Sansone A, Conforti A, et al. Smoke, alcohol, and drug addiction and female fertility. Reprod Biol Endocrinol. 2020;18(1):21. https://doi.org/10.1186/s12958-020-0567-7.
5. Gaskins A, Chavarro JE. Role of nurses in reproductive health: strategies and outcomes. Fertil Steril. 2018;110(4):772–9. https://doi.org/10.1016/j.fertnstert.2018.05.026.
6. Dishman M. Female fertility labs explained (PDF). 2016. https://drmeaghandishman.com/wp-content/uploads/2016/08/Dr.-Dishman-Female-Fertility-Labs-Explained.pdf.
7. Deadmond A, Koch CA, Parry JP. Ovarian reserve testing. In: Snyder LJ, Petitti BG, editors. StatPearls. StatPearls Publishing; 2019. https://www.ncbi.nlm.nih.gov/books/NBK279058/.
8. UCSF Health. Prolactin blood test. n.d.; Retrieved January 19, 2025, from https://www.ucsf-health.org/medical-tests/prolactin-blood-.
9. UCSF Health. Free T4 test. n.d.; Retrieved January 19, 2025, from https://www.ucsfhealth.org/medical-tests/free-t4-test.
10. American Society for Reproductive Medicine. The clinical relevance of luteal phase deficiency: a committee opinion. 2015. Retrieved from https://www.asrm.org/globalassets/_asrm/practice-guidance/practice-guidelines/pdf/clinical-relevance-of-luteal-phase-deficiency.pdf.
11. Smotrich DB, Widra EA, Gindoff PR, Levy MJ, Hall JL, Stillman RJ. Prognostic value of day 3 estradiol on in vitro fertilization outcome. Fertil Steril. 1995;64(6):1136–40. [PubMed]
12. UCSF Health. Infertility in men. n.d.; Retrieved January 19, 2025, from https://www.ucsfhealth.org/conditions/infertility-in-men#:~:text=Semen%20Evaluation%20The%20evaluation%20assesses,the%20sperm's%20ability%20to%20fertilize
13. Sizar O, Leslie SW, Schwartz J. Male hypogonadism. In: StatPearls [Internet]. Treasure Island (FL): StatPearls Publishing; 2024; Available at https://www.ncbi.nlm.nih.gov/books/NBK532933/.
14. Santi D, Crépieux P, Reiter E, Spaggiari G, Brigante G, Casarini L, Rochira V, Simoni M. Follicle-stimulating hormone (FSH) action on spermatogenesis: a focus on physiological and therapeutic roles. J Clin Med. 2020;9(4):1014. https://doi.org/10.3390/jcm9041014.
15. Kerr DM, Middleton WD. Ultrasound of normal and abnormal vas deferens. Ultrasound Q (2017). 33: 153–156. J Ultrasound Med. 2022;40:1085–90.
16. Ammar T, Sidhu PS, Wilkins CJ. Male infertility: the role of imaging in diagnosis and management. Br J Radiol. 2012;85(Spec 1):S59–68. https://doi.org/10.1259/bjr/31818161.
17. Azziz R, Norman RJ. Ultrasound in male reproductive Health. Cambridge University Press; 2015.
18. World Health Organization. Laboratory manual for the examination and processing of human semen. 5th ed. World Health Organization; 2010.
19. Wald G, Punjani N, Hayden R, Feliciano M, Dudley V, Goldstein M. Assessing the clinical value of the Kruger strict morphology criteria over the World Health Organization fourth edition criteria. Fertil Sci Rep. 2021;2(2):176–80. https://doi.org/10.1016/j.xfre.2021.04.003.
20. Hansen KR, Craig LB, Zavy MT, Klein NA, Soules MR. Ovarian primordial and nongrowing follicle counts according to the Stages of Reproductive Aging Workshop (STRAW) staging system. Menopause. 2012;19:164–71.

21. Broer SL, Broekmans FJ, Laven JS, Fauser BC. Anti-Müllerian hormone: ovarian reserve testing and its potential clinical implications. Hum Reprod Update. 2014;20(5):688–701. https://doi.org/10.1093/humupd/dmu020.
22. Frattarelli JL, Levi AJ, Miller BT, Segars JH. A prospective assessment of the predictive value of basal antral follicles in in vitro fertilization cycles. Fertil Steril. 2003;80:350–5.
23. Blanco-Breindel MF, Singh M, Kahn J. Endometrial receptivity. In: StatPearls [Internet]. Treasure Island (FL): StatPearls Publishing; 2023; Available from https://www.ncbi.nlm.nih.gov/books/NBK587449/.
24. Yu XW, Wei ZT, Jiang YT, Zhang SL. Y chromosome azoospermia factor region microdeletions and transmission characteristics in azoospermic and severe oligozoospermic patients. Int J Clin Exp Med. 2015;8(9):14634–46.
25. Bieniek JM, Lapin CD, Jarvi KA. Genetics of CFTR and male infertility. Transl Androl Urol. 2021;10(3):1391–400. https://doi.org/10.21037/tau.2020.04.05.
26. Zitzmann M, Aksglaede L, Corona G, et al. European academy of andrology guidelines on Klinefelter syndrome: endorsing organization: European Society of Endocrinology. Andrology. 2020;9(1):145–67. https://doi.org/10.1111/andr.12909.
27. Foley E, Breit S, Marsh C, Ault K, Lydic M. Attitudes toward rubella and varicella vaccination during preconception care. Kansas J Med. 2021;14:215–9. https://doi.org/10.17161/kjm.vol1415205.
28. World Health Organization Regional Office for the Western Pacific. Triple elimination of mother-to-child transmission of HIV, hepatitis B, and syphilis: Provisional agenda item 12. In: The Sixty-eighth session of the WHO Regional Committee for the Western Pacific, Brisbane, Australia, 9–13 October 2017. WHO Regional Office for the Western Pacific: Manila; 2017. Retrieved from http://www.wpro.who.int/about/regional_committee/68/documents/wpr_rc68_7_hiv_hepa_syphilis.pdf.
29. American College of Obstetricians and Gynecologists. Copyright by the American College of Obstetricians and Gynecologists. 2025.
30. American Society for Reproductive Medicine. Evaluation and treatment of recurrent pregnancy loss: a committee opinion. American Society for Reproductive Medicine; n.d.. https://www.asrm.org/practice-guidance/practice-committee-documents/evaluation-and-treatment-of-recurrent-pregnancy-loss-a-committee-opinion.
31. Christiansen OB, Andersen A-MN, Bosch E, Daya S, Delves PJ, et al. Evidence-based investigations and treatments of recurrent pregnancy loss. Fertil Steril. 2005;83(4):821–39. https://doi.org/10.1016/j.fertnstert.2004.10.021.
32. Wang RQ, Deng ZM, Chen GT, et al. Obesity and recurrent spontaneous abortion: the crucial role of weight management in pregnancy. Reprod Biol Endocrinol. 2025;23(1):10. https://doi.org/10.1186/s12958-024-01326-3.
33. Abu-Heija A. Thrombophilia and recurrent pregnancy loss: is heparin still the drug of choice? Sultan Qaboos Univ Med J. 2014;14(1):e26–36. https://doi.org/10.12816/0003333.
34. Amisi CA. Markers of insulin resistance in polycystic ovary syndrome women: an update. World J Diabetes. 2022;13(3):129–49. https://doi.org/10.4239/wjd.v13.i3.129.
35. Rasquin LI, Anastasopoulou C, Mayrin JV. Polycystic ovarian disease. In: StatPearls [Internet]. StatPearls Publishing; 2022. https://www.ncbi.nlm.nih.gov/books/NBK459251/.
36. Leslie SW, Soon-Sutton TL, Khan MAB. Male infertility. In: StatPearls [Internet]. StatPearls Publishing; 2024. https://www.ncbi.nlm.nih.gov/books/NBK562258/.
37. Gregg AR, Aarabi M, Klugman S, Leach NT, Bashford MT, Goldwaser T, Chen E, Sparks TN, Reddi HV, Rajkovic A, Dungan JS, ACMG Professional Practice and Guidelines Committee. Screening for autosomal recessive and X-linked conditions during pregnancy and preconception: a practice resource of the American College of Medical Genetics and Genomics (ACMG). Genet Med. 2021;23(10):1793–806. https://doi.org/10.1038/s41436-021-01203-z.
38. Cai Z, Li H. Congenital bilateral absence of the vas deferens. Front Genet. 2022;13:775123. https://doi.org/10.3389/fgene.2022.775123.

39. Ashley-Koch A, Yang Q, Olney RS. Sickle hemoglobin (HbS) allele and sickle cell disease: a HuGE review. Am J Epidemiol. 2000;151(9):839–45. https://doi.org/10.1093/oxfordjournals.aje.a010288.
40. Momodu II, Lee B, Singh G. Congenital adrenal hyperplasia. In: StatPearls [Internet]. StatPearls Publishing; 2023. https://www.ncbi.nlm.nih.gov/books/NBK448098/.
41. Schaa KL. Assessing patients with a genetic "eye": family history and physical assessment. In: Kasper CE, Schneidereith TA, Lashley FR, editors. Lashley's essentials of clinical genetics in nursing practice. 2nd ed. Springer Publishing Company; 2016. p. 191–214.

[illegible]

3 Causes of Infertility

Abby Mango

3.1 Objectives

1. To understand the underlying causes of female and male infertility
2. To discuss the nursing and medical management of infertility
3. To encourage a holistic approach

3.2 Introduction

Infertility is a disease with multifaceted causes affecting both females and males. It affects about one in seven heterosexual couples that have been having unprotected intercourse over a 12-month period trying to achieve a clinical pregnancy [52, 112]. This chapter will explore the various causes of infertility in females and males and also discuss unexplained infertility. Moreover, key contributors to female infertility such as tubal, ovulatory and congenital factors will be discussed as well as male infertility contributors such as sperm production, hormonal imbalances and structural anomalies. Some aspects of treatment will be covered to give a full scope of infertility.

A. Mango (✉)
Wolfson Fertility Centre, Imperial College Healthcare NHS Trust, London, UK
e-mail: a.mango@nhs.net

M. Das, M. H. Dahan (eds.), *A Comprehensive Guide to Reproductive Health and Infertility Medicine for Nurses*, https://doi.org/10.1007/978-3-032-24372-0_3

3.3 Female Infertility

3.3.1 Knowledge Gap as an Infertility Cause

Fertility knowledge gaps can result in infertility, for example, when a couple incorrectly times intercourse, leading them to miss the ovulation window [95]. According to the National Health Service [97], in some instances, the couple may be having intercourse a few times instead of the recommended 2–3 times a week. Ojah and Pradhan [98] found that poor fertility knowledge gaps need to be addressed, especially for ovulation and the fertile window. Therefore, assessing the patient's knowledge and educating them becomes an integral part of the nurse's role if fertility knowledge gaps are to be reduced.

Furthermore, knowledge gaps or ignorance often prevents couples from accessing health services. In the UK, some ethnic minority patients such as Black and Chinese individuals, tend to access services later than other ethnic groups, which affects treatment outcomes [27]. The Human Fertilisation and Embryology Authority (HFEA) found out that this may be due to cost of private treatment if they do not meet the NHS (National Health Service) funding criteria, or a lack of donors of matching ethnicity. Additionally, it may be due to religious reasons, the need to seek other solutions first, a previous experience with a culturally incompetent professional or mistrust of the services. Historically, there has been a mistrust between the ethnic minorities and the healthcare services [85]. Even though this is still an issue, nurses have the opportunity to step in and bring change by providing individualised care, showing understanding of challenges and cultural differences that patients bring when accessing care.

The age at which an individual starts treatment greatly impacts pregnancy and live birth outcomes. It should be noted that Black, mixed and other ethnic minorities are accessing fertility services later, than Caucasians.

3.3.2 Tubal Factors

Research suggests that about 30% of all infertility cases are due to female infertility [5]. Of all the female infertility causes, 25–35% are attributed to tubal disorders [84]. Fallopian tubes or oviducts are essential for the transportation of a mature ovum from the ovary to the uterus to meet with spermatozoa for fertilisation to occur and the transportation of the embryo to the uterus for implantation [111]. Any disruption to this process due to damage, scarring, partial or total blockage of one or both fallopian tubes could make fertilisation impossible and contribute to infertility [15, 92]. This underscores the profound impact of tubal related infertility as an important area of fertility concern.

Typically, tubal factors are identified through hysterosalpingogram (HSG), hysterosalpingo contrast sonography (HyCosy), or laparoscopy to check for any uterine defects and tubal patency. For women with proximal tubal obstruction, selective salpingography and tubal catheterisation or hysteroscopic tubal cannulation may be treatment options because they improve the chances of pregnancy [77]. Thus, early access to healthcare services could mean improved clinical pregnancy outcomes for patients with tubal factors, especially those resulting from Sexually Transmitted Infections (STIs) and endometriosis.

3.3.3 Other Attributing Factors to Tubal Factor Infertility

3.3.3.1 Sexually Transmitted Infections (STIs)

Sexually transmitted infections are a major causative factor for blocked tubes due to untreated infections, particularly *Chlamydia trachomatis* and *Neisseria gonorrhoeae* that ascend into the fallopian tubes [103]. These infections are known to be asymptomatic sometimes but can result in extensive damage to the fallopian tubes if untreated. Also, it may lead to spermatozoa DNA fragmentation and low motility, thereby impacting pregnancy outcomes [57]. Chlamydia can also increase the risk of miscarriages or ectopic pregnancies. Even though this may be outside of a fertility nurse's day-to-day role, providing sexual health promotion is crucial to help the patient understand the impact on their reproductive health.

Research suggests that about 15% of untreated chlamydia infections will result in Pelvic Inflammatory Disease (PID), which is a cause of infertility [86]. In the UK, nurses must follow the guidance provided by the Human Fertilisation and Embryology Authority (HFEA) on infectious disease screening tests for patients. HFEA also requires fertility clinics to regularly audit their practices, including infectious disease screening [82]. Therefore, nurses must ensure all patients are screened for *Chlamydia trachomatis* and *Neisseria gonorrhoeae* and offered treatment as well as contact tracing if found to have the infection before assisted reproductive technologies (ART) commence [47]. Untreated STIs are known to also lead to hydrosalpinx by affecting the cilia's motion and fimbriae resulting in blocked tubes [90].

3.3.3.2 Hydrosalpinx

Hydrosalpinx is a fluid-filled fallopian tube that results from a previous infection, surgery on the tube, inflammation, adhesions or endometriosis [105]. The fluid hinders the ovum from travelling from the ovary to meet the spermatozoa. Where fertilisation has occurred, the fluid could also cause an ectopic pregnancy, which can be life-threatening [100]. Hydrosalpinx is associated with reduced pregnancy or live birth outcomes, especially for patients undergoing ART [84]. NICE guidelines state that anyone with hydrosalpinx should be offered to have a salpingectomy (the affected fallopian tube removed) to improve the chances of success [47]. Conversely, a hydrosalpinx can be clipped (salpingostomy) or aspirated [6].

3.3.3.3 Adhesions/Asherman's Syndrome

Adhesions can have a significant effect on fertility, resulting in tubal blockage that could lead to hydrosalpinx [93]. Zegers-Hochschild et al. [115] defines adhesions as bands of fibrous scar tissue that may bind to the abdominal and pelvic organs, including the intestines and peritoneum. Abbott and Deans [81] estimate the prevalence of adhesions to be between 1.5% and 21.5% as an incidental finding when performing a hysterosalpingogram (HSG) on women with a history of post-partum uterine curettage.

According to Smikle et al. [107] adhesions could be due to endometriosis, uterine lining infection or previous surgery in the pelvic region, such as appendicectomy, dilation and curettage, or caesarean section leading to damage of the uterine lining. The damage to the lining results in light menstrual periods, no periods, recurrent miscarriage and infertility [96]. Adhesions are treated by performing a hysteroscopic adhesiolysis to separate them. However, this procedure does not guarantee they will not be a recurrence, but it can improve pregnancy rates [114].

3.3.3.4 Endometriosis

According to El-Kharoubi [15, 92] endometriosis can bring about scarring and adhesions in and around the pelvic region. If endometrial-like cells attach to the fallopian tubes, this might lead to partial or complete tubal blockage. Endometriosis is when tissue similar to the uterine lining is found elsewhere in the body. It is a chronic inflammatory condition that affects about 10% of women of reproductive age [48]. Its symptoms vary from having no apparent symptoms to chronic pelvic pain, dyschezia, dysuria, dyspareunia, dysmenorrhoea that affects a person's quality of life and infertility [63, 65]. It does not have a known cause or cure, but a theory by Chauhan [88] attributes it to retrograde menstruation. The gold standard test for endometriosis is laparoscopy [35].

When dealing with women with endometriosis, it is key to understand their fertility needs before offering them treatment options. Most patients that suffer with endometriosis present after a delayed diagnosis and possibly late referral for fertility treatment due to misdiagnosis or lack of knowledge by the professionals [102]. Hence, nurses need to be empathetic [54].

Fallopian tubes are essential in the fertilisation process, and any damage or blockage disrupts the ovum moving from the ovary even though ovulation may have occurred. Similarly, the transportation of spermatozoa to meet the ovum is also hindered, thereby preventing natural conception to occur. There have been several theories suggesting that tubal damage can lead to hormonal imbalance, with nothing being conclusive, leaving room for more studies to be conducted in this area [104].

3.3.4 Ovulatory Disorders

The hypothalamus regulates the female reproductive system together with the pituitary gland. However, any form of stress to the hypothalamus could disturb the menstrual cycle and ovulation [68]. Infertility related to ovulatory disorders represents 25–30% of female infertility [64]. Conditions such as polycystic ovarian syndrome (PCOS), diabetes, hypo- or hyperthyroidism, obesity and hyperprolactinemia all disrupt the menstrual cycle and ovulation process [24]. Furthermore, various hormones facilitate ovulation by communicating between the hypothalamus, the anterior pituitary and the ovary [69, 70].

3.3.4.1 Polyendocrine metabolic ovarian syndrome (PMOS)

In May 2026, a global expert and patient consensus recommended renaming polycystic ovary syndrome (PCOS) to polyendocrine metabolic ovarian syndrome (PMOS), which better reflects its multisystem endocrine and metabolic nature [116]. This chapter uses PMOS in line with current terminology. Both terms describe the same condition, and diagnostic criteria and treatment remain unchanged.

PMOS is a common reproductive, metabolic and endocrine disorder that falls under hypothalamic-pituitary dysfunction [9]. According to the World Health Organisation, PMOS is a hormonal condition that affects approximately 8–13% women of childbearing age by preventing the ovulation process. Louwers and Laven [39] state that it is characterised by hyperandrogenism and anovulation with the following clinical features (see Fig. 3.1):

- irregular or absent periods/amenorrhoea or oligomenorrhoea
- acne
- hirsutism
- multiple cysts around the ovaries
- insulin resistance
- obesity and weight gain (there are some cases of lean PCOS)

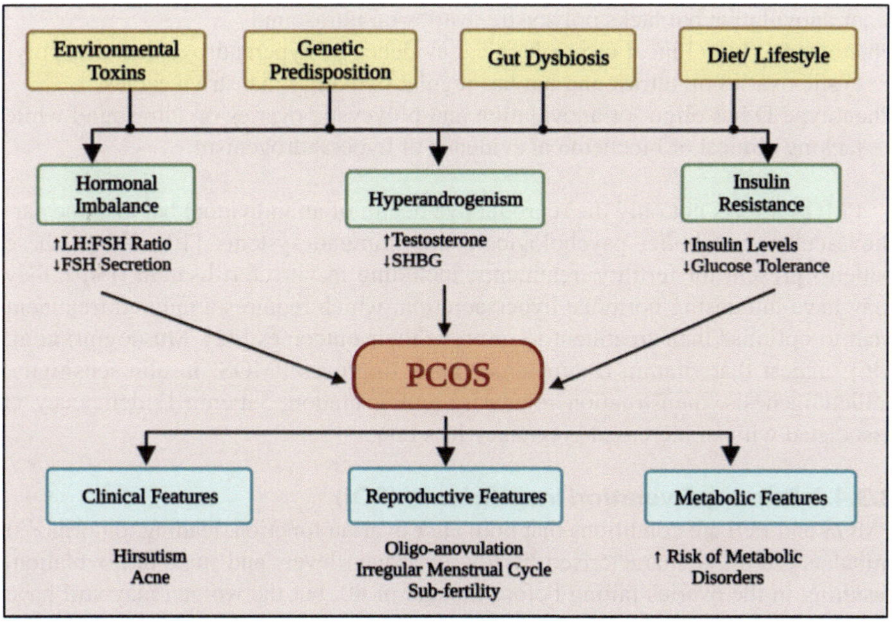

Fig. 3.1 Relationship between PMOS and different elements. (Source: https://www.mdpi.com/2077-0383/12/4/1454. Permission for reproduction: https://www.mdpi.com/openaccess under an open access Creative Commons CC BY 4.0 license)

Being overweight has been noted to increase an individual's risk of or exacerbate PMOS [69, 70]. PMOS patients are often required to lose weight before starting ART, and that can add more stress. Therefore, nurses could create or refer patients to weight loss programmes and offer emotional support, including regular motivational check-ins. Obesity on its own may result in an altered metabolic body state, which can affect ovulation [22].

When diagnosing PMOS, it is vital that all other androgen excess disorders, such as thyroid disorder, premature ovarian failure, adrenal and ovarian androgen-secreting tumours, are ruled out using a tool like the Rotterdam criteria [74]. The Rotterdam Criteria (2003) requires the presence of two out of three of the following features:

- oligo-or anovulation
- biochemical or clinical hyperandrogenism
- presence of polycystic ovaries on ultrasound scan

According to the Rotterdam Criteria, PCOS (PMOS) women can be divided into four phenotypes:

Phenotype A has clinical or biochemical evidence of hyperandrogenism, oligo- or anovulation and polycystic ovaries on ultrasound

Phenotype B has clinical or biochemical evidence of hyperandrogenism, and oligo- or anovulation but lacks polycystic ovaries on ultrasound

Phenotype C has clinical or biochemical evidence of hyperandrogenism and polycystic ovaries on ultrasound but has regular ovulatory menstrual cycles

Phenotype D has oligo- or anovulation and polycystic ovaries on ultrasound while lacking clinical or biochemical evidence of hyperandrogenism.

PMOS affects not only the reproductive health of an individual but also the cardiovascular, metabolic, psychological, and immune systems [10]. When these patients present for fertility treatments, including in-vitro fertilisation (IVF), they may have luteinising hormone hypersecretion, which requires a tailored treatment plan to optimise their treatment to improve their outcomes [42]. Muscogiuri et al. [46] suggest that vitamin D supplementation improves PMOS' insulin sensitivity, folliculogenesis, menstruation regularity and ovulation. Vitamin D deficiency is associated with an increased pregnancy loss rate.

3.3.4.2 Primary Ovulation Insufficiency (POI)

PMOS and POI are conditions that both alter ovarian function, leading to hormonal imbalance. POI is characterised by low oestrogen levels and impaired ovulation, resulting in the ovaries failing before the age of 40, but the woman may still have irregular periods [16]. It is sometimes referred to as premature ovarian failure. POI can be due to idiopathic or iatrogenic causes such as bilateral oophorectomy, chemotherapy, radiation treatments or genetic abnormalities, e.g., Turner syndrome or menopausal hereditary tendencies [43]. POI negatively impacts the individual's physical health, fertility desire and their sexual and mental well-being [17]. POI can be devastating to an individual, especially if they had not considered starting a family. To this end, an offer of oocyte cryopreservation before fertility-impairing treatments such as chemotherapy must be made.

3.3.4.3 Smoking

Smoking has been associated with early menopause and could be a factor for POI [34]. Dhage et al. [11] agree that smoking affects the reproductive system by lowering oestrogen and progesterone levels whilst increasing androgen hormones. Also, smoking brings about poor-quality oocytes, reduced endometrial receptivity, increased risk of ectopics and reduced pregnancy outcomes. NHS IVF eligibility criteria include no smoking for both partners; therefore, individuals coming for ART must be encouraged to stop smoking before treatment can be offered [51].

3.3.4.4 Fibroids

Fibroids are non-cancerous uterine growths known as leiomyomas or myomas, ranging in size from a small grain to a melon [73]. Fibroids affect an estimated 20–50% women of reproductive age but are more prevalent in Black women, which could be attributed to higher oestrogen levels [31]. Fibroids are sensitive to the steroid hormones called oestrogen and progesterone, which aid their growth [23]. They cause heavy or prolonged menstrual periods, iron deficiency anaemia, enlarged abdomen, pelvic pressure, lower back pain, urine frequency, urine retention, and gastrointestinal symptoms. However, some women remain asymptomatic [73]. Vitamin D, tranexamic acid, combined oral contraceptive pills, and GnRH analogue medications help alleviate the symptoms [76]. Some causative factors are obesity, family history, exposure to endocrine-disrupting chemicals and vitamin D deficiency [44].

Fibroids are classed based on their uterine location: intramural (wall of the uterus), submucosal (inside the lining of the uterus), and subserosal (outside of the lining of the uterus) [20]. Surgical intervention remains the standard treatment for fibroids. Myomectomy and uterine artery embolisation (UAE) are usually offered as fertility-preserving solutions.

Some patients suffer painful intercourse (dyspareunia) depending on where the fibroid is located, and some procedures, like transvaginal scans may be uncomfortable. Therefore, it is a nurse's role to advocate for the patient when they find it difficult to express themselves. It is imperative to be their voices.

3.3.4.5 Coital Disorders

Coital disorders can occur as a result of physical or psychosocial problems. Leeners et al. [37] state that they can affect both female and male individuals by impacting their psychological well-being and can also cause infertility. With an infertility diagnosis, sexual desire may diminish in one or both partners, further reducing the chances of pregnancy. The following are coital disorders that affect females:

- Dyspareunia—painful sexual intercourse is estimated to affect about 7.5% of UK women, and it is classed together with vaginismus as a genito-pelvic pain or penetration disorder [36].

- Vaginismus—is a penetration disorder where vaginal muscles go into involuntary spasms, making penetration difficult or impossible. It causes distress to both partners and can result in difficulty conceiving [61].
- Vulvodynia—an idiopathic chronic vulva pain. It is often linked with dyspareunia. Perineal massage could be offered to relieve symptoms of vulvodynia and vaginismus [67].

Coital disorders affect women with Mayer-Rokitansky-Küster-Hauser (MRKH) as well, due to a shortened vagina requiring the use of vaginal dilators [26]. Providing counselling and emotional support may improve coital disorders and confidence to engage in regular intercourse.

3.3.4.6 Female Congenital Disorders

Female congenital disorders are anomalies of the reproductive system affecting the uterus, ovaries, fallopian tubes, cervix and vagina [91]. Below a few are discussed.

- (MRKH) is when a woman with a normal karyotype is born with a shortened vagina, absent cervix and absent or undeveloped uterus [26].
- Turner's syndrome is when a woman is born with one X chromosome, is shorter than average and has underdeveloped ovaries, resulting in primary amenorrhoea, delayed puberty and infertility [33].
- Other congenital uterine anomalies include unicornuate, bicornuate/bicorporeal, uterus didelphys, septate, arcuate and dysmorphic uteri, which result from abnormal Müllerian duct development [65].

In some communities, if a biomedical cause of infertility is not found, some may start to consider other causes, such as witchcraft or that it is God's will for their lives or previous use of contraception [12]. It is therefore recommended that more fertility education programmes be offered to these communities to increase their knowledge of fertility services whilst reducing the myths they hold [21]. Writing patient information leaflets can be beneficial for the patient, which is also part of the HFEA requirement [30]. A nurse's role includes an understanding of these and other causes of infertility outside of the biomedical causes. Having this understanding will encourage a holistic approach to care as well as opportunities for nurses to educate or raise awareness in the communities.

For nurse practitioners or prescribers, this knowledge becomes relevant in how to conduct the patient's consultation or what treatment to prescribe. At every point of encounter, patients must be offered counselling and emotional support, as the diagnosis of infertility could cause stress and depression [30].

3.4 Male Infertility

Male infertility is defined as the inability of a man of reproductive age to impregnate a fertile female despite regular intercourse [112]. Studies show that 20–30% of infertility issues are ascribed solely to the male [108]. Compared to female infertility, male infertility has not received much attention, yet it is clear that there is a decline in sperm quality, with 1 in 20 men affected by infertility [62]. This decline poses severe implications on reproductive health as well as on social and economic statuses of societies.

In a Global Burden of Disease Study 2019, conducted by the Institute for Health Metrics & Evaluation on male infertility, the study showed a gradual global prevalence increase of 76.9% compared to the period 1990–2019 [29]. It is worth noting that the prevalence of infertility generally differs between different countries.

3.5 Diagnosis

Since the last three decades, the WHO has strived to standardize the technique for male andrology by issuing five successive editions of laboratory manuals [4]. Semen analysis remains the cornerstone of male fertility; it gives the clinician a picture and direction into the diagnosis. There has also been special attention to quality assurance and quality control [56]. It is essential for nurses to have a solid grasp of semen analysis to provide accurate information, support and care to the patients.

3.6 Semen Analysis

Sperm is examined microscopically and macroscopically.

1. *Microscopic Examination*
   According to the WHO 2021 (6th edition) criteria for a normal semen analysis:
   - *Sperm count*
   The total sperm count must be ≥16 million per millilitre, or 39 million per ejaculate, to be considered normal.
   - *Motility*
   Normal criteria are total motility (progressive and non-progressive motility) ≥42% and progressive motility (sperm that can "swim" forward) of ≥30%. According to WHO [112], it is important to assess rapidly progressive spermatozoa. Motility is categorised into four groups: rapid progressive, slow progressive, non-progressive, and immotile sperm.
   - *Vitality*
   This measures the amount of live sperm in the ejaculate. The percentage of live sperm must be 54% and above.
   - *Morphology*
   Normal sperm morphology must be at least 4%. Human sperm may have varying sperm morphologies. Sperm abnormalities may be in the head, neck/midpiece and tail.
- *Leukocytospermia*
  This is the presence of white blood cells, and if these are more than one million/ml, it is indicative of an infection [7, 87].

2. *Macroscopic Evaluation*

   These are values and characteristics that one can see with the naked eye; it normally precedes the microscopic examination.

   - *Volume*

   The normal volume of the sample must be 1.5 millilitres or more. Accurate volume is important, as it provides information on the secretory functions of the accessory sex glands in the male reproductive system, which are the prostate gland, seminal vesicles and bulbourethral glands.

   - *Liquefaction*

   Initially the sperm is in a semi-solid mass, and it takes about 20 min for the sample to be liquefied before it is analysed.

   - *Colour*

   The colour of semen is yellowish to greyish. If the sample is pinkish, it may be indicative of the presence of red blood cells; if the sample is too transparent, it may be indicative of the presence of white blood cells.

   - *Viscosity*

   After liquefaction, the normal viscosity is measured by allowing the sample to drop by gravity using a pipette, and it forms small individual drops. Abnormal viscosity will form a thread of more than 2 centimetres long.

- *pH*

  The normal pH ranges should be $\geq$ 7.2 [112].

3.7 Causes

The decline in sperm count and quality worldwide is undeniable, and in several publications, defects in spermatozoa, poor motility, and abnormal morphology remain the leading causes of male infertility worldwide [55].

While there is a variety of seminal problems contributing to male infertility, there are other factors that have been found to contribute to the decline in male fertility.

Male factors can be classified into categories:

1. *Pre-Testicular*

   These are factors that originate outside the testicles but still impact male fertility. Hypogonadotropic hypogonadism, where the body does not produce enough testosterone and spermatogenesis is impaired. This can be a result of a problem in the pituitary gland or hypothalamus, and is estimated to be in 2–5% of cases [71].
2. *Testicular*

   These are factors that are related to the testicles and their function. These factors can affect sperm production, quality and the overall function of the male reproductive health [108].
3. *Post Testicular*

   These are obstructions of the ducts such that the transportation of sperm is impaired, causing low motility rates [83].

3.7.1 Hormonal

- Primary (hypergonadotropic hypogonadism)—Characterized by low serum testosterone level and oligo or azoospermia. Gonadotropin levels also seem to be elevated in these cases. Some of the causes are Klinefelter syndrome, chemotherapy, radiation therapy, gonadectomy, anorchism and cryptorchidism, gonadal dysgenesis, LH resistance [78].
- Secondary (Hypogonadotropic Hypogonadism)—Low testosterone level and sperm count with low or normal follicle-stimulating hormone (FSH) and (LH) luteinising hormone. Testes fail to respond to FSH or LH, which results in impaired testosterone production by the Leydig cells. Some of the causes are high doses and long-term use of anabolic steroids, stress and nutritional imbalance [72].

3.7.2 Varicocele

- This is the enlargement of the scrotal veins which can lead to poor sperm production and quality because of poor thermoregulation. Varicoceles are common and, in many cases, are reversible [45]. Increased scrotal temperature is largely associated with poor sperm quality, also in the case of occupational heat exposure and tight-fitting underwear, though the issue of underwear remains unclear, but there are strong suggestions that it has a negative impact on the quality of sperm [14].

3.7.3 Testicular Tumours or Cancers

- This is where treatments such as chemotherapy or radiation can cause damage to the testicles, thereby impairing sperm production [13]. In some instances, if orchiectomy is done, this leads to infertility. Cancer of the testis is also associated with increased inflammatory markers, and this reduces spermatogenesis. About 22% of men with a history of testicular cancer will need assisted reproductive therapy [58].

3.7.4 Undescended Testicles (Cryptorchidism)

- It is a condition where one or both testes do not descend from the abdomen into the scrotum during foetal development, causing impaired sperm production and spermatogenesis leading to infertility. However, sometimes they can descend within the first 6 months of birth. This condition is usually corrected through orchidopexy between 6 and 18 months of age [106]. Undescended testicles are associated with malignancy in later life [8].

3.7.5 Hypospadias

- It is a male congenital anomaly where the opening of the urethra is located on the underside instead of the tip of the penis, resulting in semen being deposited outside of the vagina. It affects about 1 in 200 male children and can be fixed using surgery [75]. This condition can make sexual intercourse difficult or impossible due to erectile dysfunction or penile curvature. It causes psychological stress from feelings of being different to other males, and urination will also be different—needing to sit instead of standing [53].

3.7.6 Testicular Trauma

- Results from sports injuries, accidents, torsion of the testis could also result in testicular atrophy. About 30–40% of men who had injury to the testicles have abnormal semen parameters. Also, 11% of men with a history of testicular torsion have anti-sperm antibodies present during or after an episode [3].

3.7.7 Retrograde Ejaculation (RE)

- It occurs during an orgasm when the urethral sphincter does not close, causing semen to flow backwards into the bladder instead of coming out through the urethra. It can be partial or complete, which is called dry ejaculate [25]. It accounts for about 0.3–2% of male infertility [59]. Conditions such as spinal cord injury, diabetes neuropathies, colorectal surgeries, transurethral bladder neck incisions, prostatectomies, and multiple sclerosis can lead to RE [2]. Treatment offered includes medical management with anticholinergics and sympathomimetics. When a male with RE comes for ART, he will be required to give a urine sample after ejaculation for sperm retrieval, but this requires a prior arrangement with the embryology team. Techniques such as urine alkalisation and advanced sperm processing methods can be used to improve chances of successful fertilisation [32].

3.7.8 Coital Disorders

- Erectile dysfunction—though it is not a direct causative factor of infertility, it contributes by making intercourse difficult or impossible. Sexual dysfunction may be a result of high blood pressure, diabetes, heart disease, vascular problems, some antidepressants, antipsychotic medications, psychological and hormonal factors [18].

3.7.9 Sexually Transmitted or Urinary Tract Infections

- These can lead to epididymitis, urethritis, prostatitis, seminal vesiculitis or orchitis, causing inflammation and can destroy testicular tissue, resulting in reduced sperm production, but they can be curable [19].

3.7.10 Immunological Factors

- Some studies show that bacterial and viral infections invoke inflammatory system processes, and this increases the polymorphonuclear leukocytes and granulocytes, leading to oxidative stress [1]. Ultimately, the increase in oxidative stress may cause a change in the immune cells of the testis, bringing about irreversible damage to the testis and affecting normal spermatogenesis. Another factor is the presence of anti-sperm antibodies, which ensues in sperm agglutination; this impairs sperm mobility. Not only does it result in male infertility, but it also affects early implantation and pregnancy [40].

3.7.10.1 Unexplained Infertility

Unexplained infertility accounts for about 1 in 4 cases in the UK [50]. Unexplained or idiopathic infertility refers to when there is no known or obvious cause of infertility found after the couple has had all recommended tests. However, according to Sadeghi [66], this depends on the quantity, quality and nature of diagnostic tests done. The NICE guidelines recommend that couples who find themselves with unexplained infertility problems and have not conceived after 2 years of regular unprotected sex, must be offered IVF treatment [52]. It is important to note that the time it takes to conceive naturally does vary from one couple to another.

ESHRE believes that there may be other factors that contribute to unexplained infertility, for example,

- Cervical mucus: cervical mucus supports the sperm to travel up to the egg during ovulation. However, when the mucus is thick, the sperm might not be able to swim through the cervix and vagina and get to the uterus [49].
- Oocyte quality: there is no test available that measures oocyte quality. The current available tests measure the ovarian reserve, or how many oocytes the woman has through anti-mullerian hormone and ultrasound scan. However, these diagnostic tests do not reveal oocyte quality. Oocyte quality can be noted after egg collection [28].
- Endometrial receptivity: There are theories that imply that the endometrium has a window of implantation that is the best time for an embryo to implant successfully, therefore increasing pregnancy and live birth outcomes. However, conducted studies show that there may be no improvement to clinical pregnancy outcome [109].
- Sperm quality: similarly to egg quality, semen analysis only reveals problems with sperm. Apart from the issues identified at semen analysis testing, there may

be other issues with the sperm contributing to infertility that may not be identifiable using semen analysis [38].

3.8 Conclusion

In conclusion, infertility is a diverse condition with numerous causes that impact a wide range of individuals (Table 3.1). Both females and males can account for the causes separately or together. Knowledge gaps around infertility, sexually transmitted infections and coital disorders affect both females and males. It is crucial to emphasise tubal disorders and ovulatory disorders, as they significantly impact female infertility. Additionally, pretesticular, testicular and post-testicular disorders effect men similarly. For nurses to provide the best management for infertility, it is crucial to have an understanding of the different causes. When these factors are addressed, it contributes to provision of effective nursing care. A nurses' role extends beyond the clinical interventions to the provision of education, raising awareness and providing emotional support. This chapter has discussed causes of infertility, along with diagnostic and treatment options, and highlighted the need for personalised care to enhance reproductive outcomes [7, 52, 55, 87, 112].

Table 3.1 Summary of male infertility causes

Cause/investigation	Obstructive (post-testicular)	Non-obstructive (testicular)	Non-obstructive (hypothalamic–pituitary)
Congenital causes	Vasal aplasia Cystic fibrosis Müllerian cysts	Genetic Cryptorchidism Anorchia	Kallman's syndrome Isolated FSH deficiency
Acquired causes	Gonorrhoea Chlamydia Tuberculosis Prostatitis Vasectomy	Radiotherapy Chemotherapy Orchitis Trauma Torsion	Craniopharyngioma Pituitary tumour Pituitary ablation Anabolic steroids
Testicular size	Normal	Small, atrophic	Small, prepubertal
FSH investigation	Normal	Elevated	Low
Testosterone investigation	Normal	Low	Low

References

1. Asadi N, Bahmani M, Kheradmand A, Rafieian-Kopaei M. The impact of oxidative stress on testicular function and the role of antioxidants in improving it: a review. J Clin Diagn Res. 2017;11(5):1–5. https://doi.org/10.7860/JCDR/2017/23927.9886.
2. Belladelli F, Pozzi E, Fallara G, Capogrosso P, Salonia A. Orgasm and ejaculation disorders. In: Practical clinical andrology; 2023. p. 75–87. https://doi.org/10.1007/978-3-031-11701-5_7.
3. Bhardwaj R, Chakravarthy S, Misra S. Testicular torsion: successful management of a late-diagnosed case. Cureus. 2021;13(8):1–4. https://doi.org/10.7759/cureus.16845.
4. Boitrelle F, Shah R, Saleh R, et al. The Sixth Edition of the WHO Manual for Human Semen Analysis: A Critical Review and SWOT Analysis. Life (Basel). 2021;11(12):1368. https://doi.org/10.3390/life11121368NHS.
5. British Fertility Society. What is infertility? » British Fertility Society. 2025.Available at: https://www.britishfertilitysociety.org.uk/fei/what-is-infertility/. Accessed 11 Nov 2024.
6. Capmas P, Suarthana E, Tulandi T. Management of Hydrosalpinx in the era of assisted reproductive technology: A systematic review and meta-analysis. J Minim Invasive Gynecol. 2021;28(3):418–41. https://doi.org/10.1016/j.jmig.2020.08.017.
7. Catena ME, Gomez MB, Cayetano SR, Fernande S Sperm test results explained Interpretation & normal values. 2024a. Available at: https://www.invitra.com/en/results-of-the-sperm-analysis/. Accessed 14 Oct 2024.
8. Cho A, Thomas J, Perera R, Cherian A. Undescended testis. BMJ. 2019;364:l9–26. https://doi.org/10.1136/bmj.l926.
9. Christ JP, Cedars MI. Current guidelines for diagnosing PCOS. Diagnostics (Basel). 2023;13(6):1–11. https://doi.org/10.3390/diagnostics13061113.
10. Deswal R, Narwal V, Dang A, Pundir CS. The prevalence of polycystic ovary syndrome: a brief systematic review. J Human Reprod Sci. 2020;13(4):261–71. https://doi.org/10.4103/jhrs.JHRS_95_18.
11. Dhage VD, Nagtode N, Kumar D, Bhagat A. K. A narrative review on the impact of smoking on female fertility. Cureus. 2024;16(4):1–6. https://doi.org/10.7759/cureus.58389.
12. Dierickx S, Balen J, Longman C, Rahbari L, Clarke E, Jarju B, Coene G. We are always desperate and will try anything to conceive': the convoluted and dynamic process of health seeking among women with infertility in the West Coast Region of The Gambia. PLoS One. 2019;14(1):1–20. https://doi.org/10.1371/journal.pone.0211634.
13. Dimitriadis F. Impact of testicular cancer on male fertility. In: Current and future advances in male infertility; 2024. p. 67–85. https://doi.org/10.1007/978-3-031-62648-7_4.
14. Durairajanayagam D, Sharma RK, Du Plessis S, Agarwal A. Testicular heat stress and sperm quality. In: Male infertility a complete guide to lifestyle and environmental factors, vol. 30; 2014. p. 105–25. https://doi.org/10.1007/978-1-4939-1040-3_8.
15. El-Kharoubi AF. Tubal pathologies and fertility outcomes: a review. Cureus. 2023a;15(5):1–8. https://doi.org/10.7759/cureus.38881.
16. Endocrine Society. Primary Ovarian Insufficiency. 2022. Available at: https://www.endocrine.org/patient-engagement/endocrine-library/primary-ovarian-insuffiency. Accessed 2 Jan 2025.
17. Federici S, Rossetti R, Moleri S, Munari EV, Frixou M, Bonomi M, Persani L. Primary ovarian insufficiency: update on clinical and genetic findings. Front Endocrinol. 2024;15:1–33. https://doi.org/10.3389/fendo.2024.1464803.
18. Fiala L, Lenz J, Sajdlova R. Effect of increased prolactin and psychosocial stress on erectile function. Andrologia. 2021;53(4) https://doi.org/10.1111/and.14009.
19. Fijak M, et al. Infectious, inflammatory and "autoimmune" male factor infertility: how do rodent models inform clinical practice? Hum Reprod Update. 2018;24(4):416–41. https://doi.org/10.1093/humupd/dmy009.

20. Freytag D, Günther V, Maass N, Alkatout I. Uterine fibroids and infertility. Diagnostics (Basel). 2021;11(8):1–13. https://doi.org/10.3390/diagnostics11081455.
21. Gameiro S, El Refaie E, de Guevara BB, Payson A. Women from diverse minority ethnic or religious backgrounds desire more infertility education and more culturally and personally sensitive fertility care. Hum Reprod. 2019;34(9):1735–45. https://doi.org/10.1093/humrep/dez156.
22. Gautam D, et al. The challenges of obesity for fertility: a FIGO literature review. Int J Gynecol Obstet. 2023;160(1):50–5. https://doi.org/10.1002/ijgo.14538.
23. George JW. The burden of uterine fibroids: an overview. J Histotechnol. 2023;46(4):153–5. https://doi.org/10.1080/01478885.2023.2265185.
24. Gordon CM. Functional hypothalamic amenorrhea: an endocrine society clinical practice guideline. J Clin Endocrinol Metabol. 2017;102(5):1413–39. https://doi.org/10.1210/jc.2017-00131.
25. Gupta S, et al. A comprehensive guide to sperm recovery in infertile men with retrograde ejaculation. World J Men's Health. 2022;40(2):208–16. https://doi.org/10.5534/wjmh.210069.
26. Herlin MK, Petersen MB, Brännström M. Mayer-Rokitansky-Küster-Hauser (MRKH) syndrome: a comprehensive update. Orphanet J Rare Dis. 2020;15(1):1–16. https://doi.org/10.1186/s13023-020-01491-9.
27. HFEA. Ethnic diversity in fertility treatment. 2021. Available at: https://www.hfea.gov.uk/about-us/publications/research-and-data/ethnic-diversity-in-fertility-treatment-2021/. Accessed 12 Jan 2025.
28. Homer H. A. The role of oocyte quality in explaining "unexplained" infertility. Semin Reprod Med. 2020;38(1):21–8. https://doi.org/10.1055/s-0040-1721377.
29. Huang B, Wang Z, Kong Y, Jin M, Ma J. Global, regional and national burden of male infertility in 204 countries and territories between 1990 and 2019: an analysis of global burden of disease study. BMC Public Health. 2023;23(1):1–12. https://doi.org/10.1186/s12889-023-16793-3.
30. Human Fertilisation and Embryology Authority. Code of practice. Version 9.4. London: HFEA; 2024. Available from: https://portal.hfea.gov.uk/media/yrkn55xa/2024-10-01-hfea-code-of-practice-v9-4.pdf.
31. Jefferies K, et al. Uterine fibroids and black people of African descent globally: a scoping review protocol. BMJ Open. 2024;14(8):1–6. https://doi.org/10.1136/bmjopen-2024-085622.
32. Jefferys A, Siassakos D, Wardle P. The management of retrograde ejaculation: a systematic review and update. Fertil Steril. 2012;97(2):306–12. https://doi.org/10.1016/j.fertnstert.2011.11.019.
33. Kikkeri NS, Nagalli S. Turner syndrome. 2023. Available at: https://www.ncbi.nlm.nih.gov/books/NBK554621/. Accessed 12 Jan 2025.
34. Kundu S, Acharya SS. Exploring the triggers of premature and early menopause in India: a comprehensive analysis based on National Family Health Survey, 2019–2021. Sci Rep. 2024;14(1):1–15. https://doi.org/10.1038/s41598-024-53536-9.
35. Lee D, Kim SK, Lee JR, Jee B. Management of endometriosis-related infertility: considerations and treatment options. Clin Exp Reprod Med. 2020;47(1):1–11. https://doi.org/10.5653/cerm.2019.02971.
36. Lee NMW, Jakes AD, Lloyd J, Frodsham LCG. Dyspareunia. BMJ, (Clini Res Ed.). 2018;36(1):23–41. https://doi.org/10.1136/bmj.k2341.
37. Leeners B, Tschudin S, Wischmann T, Kalaitzopoulos DR. Sexual dysfunction and disorders as a consequence of infertility: a systematic review and meta-analysis. Hum Reprod Update. 2023;29(1):95–125. https://doi.org/10.1093/humupd/dmac030.
38. Levine H, Jørgensen N, Martino-Andrade AJ, et al. Temporal trends in sperm count: a systematic review and meta-regression analysis. In: Human Reproduction Update; 2017. p. 646–59.
39. Louwers YV, Laven JSE. Characteristics of polycystic ovary syndrome throughout life. Ther Adv Reprod Health. 2020;14:1–9. https://doi.org/10.1177/2633494120911038.

40. Mannucci A, Argento FR, Fini E, Coccia ME, Taddei N, Becatti M, Fiorillo C. The impact of oxidative stress in male infertility. Front Mol Biosci. 2022;5(8):1–9. https://doi.org/10.3389/fmolb.2021.799294.
41. Mariano M, Balen AH. Treatment update for anovulation and subfertility in polycystic ovary syndrome. Curr Opin Endocr Metab Res. 2020;12:53–8. https://doi.org/10.1016/j.coemr.2020.03.003.
42. Mikhael S, Punjala-Patel A, Gavrilova-Jordan L. Hypothalamic-pituitary-ovarian axis disorders impacting female fertility. Biomedicine. 2019;7(1):1–9. https://doi.org/10.3390/biomedicines7010005.
43. Mishra GD, et al. Optimising health after early menopause. Lancet. 2024;403(10430):958–68. https://doi.org/10.1016/S0140-6736(23)02800-3.
44. Mohammadi R, et al. Correlation of low serum vitamin D with uterine leiomyoma: a systematic review and meta-analysis. Reprod Biol Endocrinol. 2020;18(1):1–8. https://doi.org/10.1186/s12958-020-00644-6.
45. Munoz-Lopez C, Wong A, Lewis K, Bole R, Vij SC, Lundy SD. The evolving landscape of male Varicocele pathophysiology in the era of multi-omics: a narrative review of the current literature. Biology. 2024;13(2):1–14. https://doi.org/10.3390/biology13020080.
46. Muscogiuri G, et al. Shedding new light on female fertility: the role of vitamin D. Rev Endocr Metab Disord. 2017;18(3):273–83. https://doi.org/10.1007/s11154-017-9407-2.
47. National Institute for Clinical Excellence. Fertility: assessment and treatment for people with fertility problems. In: Clinical guideline CG11. London: National Institute for Clinical Excellence; 2004.
48. National Institute for Health and Care Excellence. Fertility problems: assessment and treatment. In: NICE guideline NG257. London: National Institute for Health and Care Excellence; 2026. Available from: https://www.nice.org.uk/guidance/ng257.
49. Najmabadi S, Schliep KC, Simonsen SE, Porucznik CA, Egger MJ, Stanford JB. Cervical mucus patterns and the fertile window in women without known subfertility: a pooled analysis of three cohorts. Hum Reprod. 2021;36(7):1784–795.
50. National Health Service (NHS) Causes of infertility. 2023. Available at: https://www.nhs.uk/conditions/infertility/causes/.
51. NHS. IVF. 2021. Available at: https://www.nhs.uk/conditions/ivf/availability/#:~:text=ICBs%20may%20have%20additional%20criteria,not%20smoking. Accessed 20 Nov 2024.
52. NICE. Fertility problems: assessment and treatment. 2017. Available at: https://www.nice.org.uk/guidance/cg156/chapter/recommendations. Accessed 14 Dec 2024.
53. Nordenvall AS, Chen Q, Norrby C, Lundholm C, Frisén L, Nordenström A, Almqvist C, Nordenskjöld A. Fertility in adult men born with hypospadias: a nationwide register-based cohort study on birthrates, the use of assisted reproductive technologies and infertility. Andrology. 2019;8(2):372–80. https://doi.org/10.1111/andr.12723.
54. Norton W, Holloway D. Understanding the nice guidance on endometriosis. Pract Nurs. 2020;31(1):8–16. https://doi.org/10.12968/pnur.2020.31.1.8.
55. Okonofua FE, Ntoimo LFC, Omonkhua A, Ayodeji O, Olafusi C, Unuabonah E, Ohenhen V. Causes and risk factors for male infertility: a scoping review of published studies. Int J General Med. 2022;15:5985–97. https://doi.org/10.2147/IJGM.S363959.
56. Pacey AA. Are sperm counts declining? or did we just change our spectacles? Asian J Androl. 2013;15(2):187–90. https://doi.org/10.1038/aja.2012.165.
57. Padubidri VG, Daftary SN. Shaw's textbook of gynecology. In: 16th ed. New Delhi: Elsevier India; 2014. p. 1–596.
58. Parekh NV, Lundy SD, Vij SC. Fertility considerations in men with testicular cancer. Transl Androl Urol. 2020;9(1):14–23. https://doi.org/10.21037/tau.2019.08.08. PMID 32055481, https://pmc.ncbi.nim.nih.gov/articles/PMC6995852.
59. Parnham A, Serefoglu EC. Retrograde ejaculation, painful ejaculation and hematospermia. Transl Androl Urol. 2016;5(4):592–601. https://doi.org/10.21037/tau.2016.06.05.

60. Pfeifer SM, et al. ASRM müllerian anomalies classification 2021. Fertil Steril. 2021;116(5):1238–52.
61. Raveendran AV, Rajini P. Vaginismus: diagnostic challenges and proposed diagnostic criteria. Balkan Med J. 2024;41(1):80–2. https://doi.org/10.4274/balkanmedj.galenos.2023.2022-9-62.
62. Ravitsky V, Kimmins S. The forgotten men: rising rates of male infertility urgently require new approaches for its prevention, diagnosis and treatment. In: Biology of Reproduction; 2019. p. 872–74.
63. RCOG. Reproductive implications and management of congenital uterine anomalies. BJOG. 2023;127(5):1–13. https://doi.org/10.1111/1471-0528.15968.
64. Rebar RW. Ovulatory dysfunction. 2024. Available at: https://www.msdmanuals.com/professional/gynecology-and-obstetrics/infertility-and-recurrent-pregnancy-loss/ovulatory-dysfunction#Diagnosis_v1068828. Accessed 12 Jan 2025.
65. Royal College of Obstetricians and Gynaecologists. Management of subfertility. In: Royal College of Obstetricians and Gynaecologists. Reproductive implications and management of congenital uterine anomalies. Scientific Impact Paper No. 62. London: RCOG; 2019.
66. Sadeghi RM. Unexplained infertility, the controversial matter in management of infertile couples. J Reprod Infant Psychol. 2015;16(1):1–2.
67. Schlaeger JM, Glayzer JE, Villegas-Downs M, Li H, Glayzer EJ, He Y, Takayama M, Yajima H, Takakura N, Kobak WH, McFarlin BL. Evaluation and treatment of vulvodynia: state of the science. J Midwifery Womens Health. 2023;68(1):9–34. https://doi.org/10.1111/jmwh.13456.
68. Shufelt CL, Torbati T, Dutra E. Hypothalamic amenorrhea and the long-term health consequences. Semin Reprod Med. 2017;35(3):256–62. https://doi.org/10.1055/s-0037-1603581.
69. Silvestris E, de Pergola G, Rosania R, Loverro G. Obesity as disruptor of the female fertility. Reprod Biol Endocrinol. 2018a;16(1):1–13. https://doi.org/10.1186/s12958-018-0336-z.
70. Silvestris E, de Pergola G, Rosania R, Loverro G. Obesity as disruptor of the female fertility. Reprod Biol Endocrinol. 2018b;16(1):1–13. https://doi.org/10.1186/s12958-018-0336-z.
71. Sizar O, Leslie SW, Schwartz J. Male hypogonadism. 2024. Available at: https://www.ncbi.nlm.nih.gov/books/NBK532933/. Accessed 16 Nov 2024.
72. Spaziani M, Carlomagno F, Tarantino C, Angelini F, Vincenzi L, Gianfrilli D. New perspectives in functional hypogonadotropic hypogonadism: beyond late onset hypogonadism. Front Endocrinol. 2023;14(11):1–9. https://doi.org/10.3389/fendo.2023.1184530.
73. Stewart EA, Laughlin-Tommaso SK, Catherino WH, Lalitkumar S, Gupta D, Vollenhoven B. Uterine fibroids. Nat Rev Dis Primers. 2016;16043(2) https://doi.org/10.1038/nrdp.2016.43.
74. Unfer V. When one size does not fit all: reconsidering PCOS etiology, diagnosis, clinical subgroups, and subgroup-specific treatments. Endocrine and Metabolic Science. 2024;14:100159.
75. Van der Horst HJ, de Wall LL. Hypospadias, all there is to know. Eur J Pediatr. 2017;176(4):435–41. https://doi.org/10.1007/s00431-017-2864-5.
76. Vilos GA, Allaire C, Laberge P, Leyland N. The management of uterine leiomyomas. J Obstet Gynaecol Can. 2015;37(2):157–78. https://doi.org/10.1016/S1701-2163(15)30338-8.
77. Vitale SG. Tubal factor infertility: which is the possible role of tubal microbiota? A fresh look to a busy corner focusing on the potential role of hysteroscopy. 2022;3(2):88–93. https://doi.org/10.53260/grem.22302034.
78. Vogiatzi MG. Hypogonadism treatment & management: approach considerations, medical care, surgical care. 2024. Available at: https://emedicine.medscape.com/article/922038-treatment?form=fpf. Accessed 12 Jan 2025.
79. Zayed AA, El-Hadidy MA. Sexual satisfaction and self-esteem in women with primary infertility. Middle East Fertil Soc. 2020a;25(13):2–5. https://doi.org/10.1186/s43043-020-00024-5.
80. Anon. What is infertility? British Fertility Society. n.d..; Available at: https://www.britishfertilitysociety.org.uk/fei/what-is-infertility/.

81. Abbott J, Deans R. Accelerating the science after 125 years of treating intrauterine adhesions. J Minim Invasive Gynecol. 2021;28(2):151–2. https://doi.org/10.1016/j.jmig.2020.12.028.
82. Akande V, Turner C, Horner P, Horne A, Pacey A, British Fertility Society. Impact of chlamydia trachomatis in the reproductive setting: British fertility society guidelines for practice. Hum Fertil (Camb). 2010;13(3):115–25. https://doi.org/10.3109/14647273.2010.513893.
83. American Society for Reproductive Medicine (ASRM); American Urological Association. Diagnosis and treatment of infertility in men: AUA/ASRM guideline (Part I). 2020. Available from: https://www.asrm.org/practice-guidance/practicecommittee-documents/diagnosis-and-treatment-of-infertility-in-men-auaasrm-guideline-part-i-2020/
84. ASRM. Role of tubal surgery in the era of assisted reproductive technology: a committee opinion (2021) [online]. 2021. Available at: https://www.asrm.org/practice-guidance/practice-committee-documents/role-of-tubal-surgery-in-the-era-of-assisted-reproductive-technology-a-committee-opinion-2021/.
85. Bazargan M, Cobb S, Assari S. Discrimination and medical mistrust in a racially and ethnically diverse sample of California adults. Ann Fam Med. 2021;19(1):4–15. https://doi.org/10.1370/afm.2632. PMID: 33431385; PMCID: PMC7800756.
86. Brunham RC, Gottlieb SL, Paavonen J. Pelvic inflammatory disease. N Engl J Med. 2015;372(21):2039–48. https://doi.org/10.1056/nejmra1411426.
87. Catena ME, Gómez MB, Cayetano SR, Fernández S. Sperm test results explained: interpretation and normal values. Invitra; 2024. Available from: https://www.invitra.com/en/results-of-the-sperm-analysis/
88. Chauhan S, More A, Chauhan V, Kathane A. Endometriosis: a review of clinical diagnosis, treatment, and pathogenesis. Cureus. 2022;14(9):e28864. https://doi.org/10.7759/cureus.28864.
89. Chen J, Chen J, Fang Y, Shen Q, Zhao K, Liu C, Zhang H. Microbiology and immune mechanisms associated with male infertility. Front Immunol. 2023;14:1139450. https://pmc.ncbi.nlm.nih.gov/articles/PMC9989213. PMID 36895560.
90. Dinu M-D, Hamoud BH, Amza M, Sima R-M, Conea I-M, Gorecki G-P, Pleş L. Is chronic pelvic inflammatory disease an exclusively medical gynecological disease, or it may be a surgical challenge? Surg Tech Dev. 2024;13(3):301–12. https://doi.org/10.3390/std13030023.
91. Dahiphale SM, Potdar J, Acharya N, Jyotsna G, Saloni, Desale R. Congenital anomalies of the female genital tract: a comprehensive review. Cureus. 2024;16(3):e56753. https://doi.org/10.7759/cureus.56753.
92. El-Kharoubi AF. Tubal pathologies and fertility outcomes: a review. Cureus. 2023b;15(5):e38881. https://doi.org/10.7759/cureus.38881.
93. Gebeh AK, Metwally M. Surgical management of tubal disease and infertility. Obstet Gynaecol Reprod Med. 2019;29(5):123–8.
94. Hamad Zubi ZB, Hamad Alfarisi HA. Hyperlipidemia and male infertility. Egypt J Basic Appl Sci. 2021;8(1):385–96. https://doi.org/10.1080/2314808X.2021.1977080.
95. Hoffman JR, Delaney MA, Valdes CT, et al. Disparities in fertility knowledge among women from low and high resource settings presenting for fertility care in two United States metropolitan centers. Fertil Res Pract. 2020;6:15. https://doi.org/10.1186/s40738-020-00084-1.
96. Hooker AB, de Leeuw RA, Emanuel MH, Mijatovic V, Brolmann HAM, Huirne JAF. The link between intrauterine adhesions and impaired reproductive performance: a systematic review of the literature. BMC Pregnancy Childbirth. 2022;22(1):837. https://doi.org/10.1186/s12884-022-05164-2. PMID: 36376829; PMCID: PMC9664654.
97. NHS. Trying to get pregnant. [online] nhs.uk. 2020. Available at: https://www.nhs.uk/pregnancy/trying-for-a-baby/trying-to-get-pregnant/.
98. Ojah P, Pradhan MR. Can a lack of knowledge of the ovulatory cycle result in primary infertility? Evidence from selected South Asian countries. Hum Fertil. 2024;28(1):2441832. https://doi.org/10.1080/14647273.2024.2441832.

99. NICE. Overview: endometriosis: diagnosis and management: guidance. n.d..; Available at: https://www.nice.org.uk/guidance/ng73. Accessed 12 Jan 2025.
100. Palagiano A, Cozzolino M, Ubaldi FM, Palagiano C a, Coccia ME. Effects of Hydrosalpinx on endometrial implantation failures: evaluating salpingectomy in women undergoing in vitro fertilization. Revista Brasileira de Ginecologia e Obstetrícia/RBGO Gynecol Obstetrics. 2021;43(04):304–10. https://doi.org/10.1055/s-0040-1722155.
101. HFEA. Patient support pathway. n.d.-a. Available at: https://portal.hfea.gov.uk/knowledge-base/emotional-support-for-patients-resources/patient-support-pathway/. Accessed 12 Jan 2025.
102. Requadt E, Náhlik A, Jacobsen AL, Ross WT. Patient experiences of endometriosis diagnosis: A mixed methods approach. BJOG: Int J Obstetrics Gynaecol. 2023; https://doi.org/10.1111/1471-0528.17719.
103. Tsevat DG, et al. Sexually transmitted diseases and infertility. Am J Obstet Gynecol. 2017;216(1):1–9.
104. Shao R, Feng Y, Zou S, Weijdegård B, Wu G, Brännström M, Billig H. The role of estrogen in the pathophysiology of tubal ectopic pregnancy. Am J Transl Res. 2012;4(3):269–78. Epub 2012 Jul 20. PMID: 22937205; PMCID: PMC3426394.
105. Sharif K, Coomarasamy A, editors. Assisted reproduction techniques: challenges and management options. Newark: Wiley, Incorporated; 2021. Available from: ProQuest Ebook Central. [24 December 2024].
106. Sharma A, Minhas S, Dhillo WS, Jayasena CN. Male infertility due to testicular disorders. J Clin Endocrinol Metab. 2020;106(2):e442–59. PMID33295608
107. Smikle C, Yarrarapu SNS, Khetarpal S. Asherman Syndrome. [Updated 2023 Jul 24]. In: StatPearls [Internet]. Treasure Island (FL): StatPearls Publishing; 2024. Available from: https://www.ncbi.nlm.nih.gov/books/NBK448088/.
108. Stephen W, Taylor L, Sutton S, Khan MAB. Male infertility. In: StatPearls [Internet]. Treasure Island (FL): StatPearls Publishing; 2024.
109. Sun B, Yeh J. Non-invasive and mechanism-based molecular assessment of endometrial receptivity during the window of implantation: current concepts and future prospective testing directions. Front Reprod Health. 2022;4:863173. https://doi.org/10.3389/frph.2022.863173.
110. HFEA. The code of practice version 9.4 is now available. n.d.-b.; Available at: https://www.hfea.gov.uk/about-us/news-and-press-releases/2023/the-code-of-practice-version-94-is-now-available/. Accessed 12 Jan 2025.
111. Ward SM. AB277. SPR-04 Myosalpinx contractions are essential for egg/embryo transport in the oviduct. Transl Androl Urol. 2016;5(Suppl 2):AB277. https://doi.org/10.21037/tau.2016.s277. PMCID: PMC5143247.
112. World Health Organization. Infertility. World Health Organization; 2024. Available at: https://www.who.int/news-room/fact-sheets/detail/infertility.
113. NICE. Treatments for women | Information for the public | Fertility problems: assessment and treatment | Guidance |. n.d..; Available at: https://www.nice.org.uk/guidance/cg156/ifp/chapter/treatments-for-women#if-your-fallopian-tubes-are-blocked, www.nice.org.uk.
114. Yang J, et al. The influence of the location and extent of intrauterine adhesions on recurrence after Hysteroscopic adhesiolysis. BJOG: Int J Obstet Gynaecol. 2015;123(4):618–23. https://doi.org/10.1111/1471-0528.13353.
115. Zegers-Hochschild F, et al. The international glossary on infertility and fertility care, 2017. Hum Reprod. 2017;32(9):1786–801. https://doi.org/10.1093/humrep/dex234.
116. Teede HJ, Khomami MB, Morman R, Laven JSE, Joham AE, Costello MF, Patil M, Rees DA, Berry L, Cree MG, Zhao H, Norman RJ, Dokras A, Piltonen T. Global Name Change Consortium. Polyendocrine metabolic ovarian syndrome, the new name for polycystic ovary syndrome: a multistep global consensus process. Lancet. 2026;407(10545):2329–39. https://doi.org/10.1016/S0140-6736(26)00717-8. Epub 2026 May 12. PMID: 42119588.

4 Preparing a Patient for Treatment

Francesca Steyn

4.1 Introduction

Preparing a patient for fertility treatment is an in-depth process that encompasses clinical preparation, emotional well-being, and informed decision-making. Fertility nurses are well placed to support in this area of care as they are often the first and most consistent point of contact, guiding patients through diagnostic assessments, lifestyle modifications, and consent processes. This chapter provides a structured approach to patient preparation, incorporating professional standards and clinical guidelines.

4.2 The Role of the Fertility Nurse

Fertility nurses play an essential role in coordinating and delivering pre-treatment care. The nurse acts as an advocate, educator, and facilitator, ensuring continuity across the patient journey.

Key responsibilities include:

- Conducting baseline assessments
- Supporting informed consent and provision of information
- Coordinating investigations and multidisciplinary input
- Delivering education on treatment options and procedures
- Promoting emotional well-being and managing expectations

F. Steyn (✉)
Department of Obstetrics and Gynecology, Wales Fertility Institute, Port Talbot, UK
e-mail: Francesca.steyn@wales.nhs.uk

M. Das, M. H. Dahan (eds.), *A Comprehensive Guide to Reproductive Health and Infertility Medicine for Nurses*, https://doi.org/10.1007/978-3-032-24372-0_4

4.3 Initial Assessment and Referral Pathways

The standard for fertility assessments for individuals and couples include the following referral criteria [1]:

- Inability to conceive after 12 months of regular unprotected intercourse or assessment after 6 months in a woman at least 35 years of age
- Known clinical causes of infertility (e.g. anovulation, severe male factor, age-related decline, bilateral tubal blockage)
- Same-sex couples and individuals seeking donor conception

Baseline investigations should be completed prior to treatment planning and should include:

- Hormonal profiling—follicle-stimulating hormone (FSH), luteinising hormone (LH), and oestradiol (E2) usually performed on days 2–5 of the menstruation and anti-Müllerian hormone (AMH) performed any time
- Ultrasound scanning (antral follicle count, uterine assessment, and ovarian diameter measurement)
- Semen analysis and if indicated examination of the male reproductive organs as per WHO guidelines [2]
- Screening for infectious diseases
- Lifestyle and psychological well-being assessments

Fertility nurses are well placed to lead this part of the patient journey and can provide timely coordination of investigations, interpret results in collaboration with the medical team, and provide patient education and information throughout.

4.4 Optimising Patient Outcomes

4.4.1 Physical and Lifestyle Preparation

Optimising general health enhances fertility treatment outcomes [1]. Nurses should assess and support the following:

- *Body mass index (BMI)*: Aim for a BMI of 19–30 kg/m^2 before treatment. Recommend weight reduction if time is permitting and BMI is elevated.
- *Smoking cessation*: Strongly advised due to reduced efficacy and increased miscarriage risk.
- *Alcohol reduction*: Complete abstinence during treatment and pregnancy attempts is recommended for both members of the couple.
- *Folic acid supplementation*: 400–1000 mcg daily (or 5 mg (5000 mcg) if high risk).

Fertility nurses may refer patients to specialist services such as dietitians, smoking cessation clinics, or counselling where appropriate.

4.4.2 Preconception Care

Preconception care is an integral component of fertility treatment preparation. It aims to identify and modify clinical, behavioural, and social risks to the individual's health or pregnancy outcome through prevention and management. The importance of preconception care to improve fertility outcomes is that it reduces risks of miscarriage and congenital abnormalities and promotes maternal well-being [3].

Key elements of preconception care include:

- *Medication review*: Identifying and adjusting medications that may impair fertility or pose teratogenic risks (e.g. retinoids, ACE inhibitors, and NSAIDs). This includes a review of any substance misuse and anabolic steroid use.
- *Immunisation status*: Reviewing and updating vaccinations, especially for rubella, varicella, and hepatitis B.
- *Infection screening*: Ensuring screening for blood-borne viruses (HIV, Hepatitis B/C), syphilis, chlamydia, and other sexually transmitted infections.
- *Management of long-term conditions*: Supporting optimisation of chronic conditions such as diabetes, thyroid disorders, and epilepsy before conception.
- *Genetic risk assessment*: Identifying any familial or ethnic risks that may necessitate carrier screening or referral to clinical genetics.
- *Review of any supplements or OTC (over the counter medications)*: Some supplements and medications that can be purchased OTC can influence potential outcomes and well-being so it's critical to ensure all information is captured.

Fertility nurses have a pivotal role in delivering preconception education and promoting a proactive approach to health optimisation. The integration of preconception counselling into all new patient consultations, particularly for those with comorbidities, recurrent pregnancy loss, or complex treatment histories, is always indicated [3, 4].

4.4.3 Psychological Well-Being

Treatment can be emotionally demanding. There is an importance of early psychosocial screening and access to counselling [3]. Nurses should:

- Explore patient expectations and understanding
- Identify previous reproductive trauma or anxiety
- Encourage use of in-house or external counselling services
- Promote coping strategies and peer support

4.5 Informed Consent and Legal Considerations

Nurses play a critical role in supporting patients to:

- Understand treatment options and associated risks
- Review the success rates and limitations
- Complete consents (including embryo storage, donation, and legal parenthood)
- Make autonomous, informed decisions

Consent is a continuous process, not a one-time event. Nurses should revisit consent regularly and ensure access to appropriate information in multiple formats, including digital platforms. It is also important to ensure that patients are also informed about withdrawing their consent and the procedure for doing this [3–5].

4.6 Patient Education and Treatment Planning

Education is central to patient autonomy and compliance. Nurses are well placed to provide evidence-based information on:

- Treatment protocols (e.g. IVF, ICSI, IUI, ovulation induction)
- Medication administration and side effects
- Monitoring and follow-up schedules
- Self-care during stimulation and early pregnancy

Innovative platforms such as e-consent systems and patient applications can enhance accessibility. Visual aids, written materials, and recorded sessions to support learning are often used and encouraged [6].

4.7 Coordination and Multidisciplinary Collaboration

Preparing a patient involves working closely with:

- Fertility specialists
- Embryologists
- Andrologists
- Counsellors
- Pharmacists
- Administrative teams

The fertility nurse acts as a coordinator and patient advocate when preparing the treatment cycle, ensuring information sharing and alignment across teams. Multidisciplinary team (MDT) meetings provide an opportunity to discuss complex cases and tailor treatment plans accordingly [7].

4.8 Ethical and Cultural Considerations

Patients may present with diverse backgrounds and values. Nurses must provide non-judgemental, culturally sensitive care. Ethical dilemmas can include:

- Use of donor gametes or surrogacy
- Fertility preservation in transgender or oncology patients
- Disparities in treatment access
- Discarding of gametes and embryos

Nurses should remain informed, seek supervision, and involve the ethics committee where needed.

4.9 Preparing for Specific Treatment Pathways

Each fertility treatment has unique preparatory needs. Examples include:

- *Ovulation induction*: Baseline scan, hormone levels, patient instruction on timing and intercourse
- *IUI*: Cycle monitoring, partner semen preparation, synchronisation with ovulation, and co-ordination of the availability of donor sperm
- *IVF/ICSI*: Understand and teach the diverse protocols, stimulation start date, trigger, egg collection, embryo transfer
- *Oncological fertility preservation*: Urgent counselling, rapid stimulation protocols, oncology liaison

Ensuring that the protocol has been tailored to the patients' medical history and diagnostic results will enhance safety and success.

4.10 Conclusion

Patient preparation is a cornerstone of safe and effective fertility treatment. The fertility nurse plays an indispensable role in clinical assessment, education, and emotional support. By following national and international recommendations and best practice, nurses ensure that patients are empowered, informed, and ready for the journey ahead.

References

1. National Institute for Health and Care Excellence (NICE). Fertility problems: assessment and treatment. NICE guideline [CG156]; 2017.
2. World Health Organization. WHO laboratory manual for the examination and processing of human semen. 6th ed. Geneva: WHO; 2021.

3. British Infertility Counselling Association. Guidelines for good practice in fertility counselling. 4th ed. BICA; 2019. Retrieved from https://www.bica.net/item/1/BICA/Guidelines-for-Good-Practice-in-Infertility-Counselling.html.
4. Royal College of Nursing (RCN). Career and competence framework for fertility nursing. London: RCN Publishing; 2023.
5. Human Fertilisation and Embryology Authority (HFEA). Code of practice [internet]. London: HFEA; 2025; [cited 2025 May 21]. Available from: https://www.hfea.gov.uk.
6. Steyn FM, Tyler SN, Stevenson E, Perry S. Innovations in fertility nursing: the impact of COVID-19 on the delivery of patient care. Fertil Steril. 2021;116(3):e31. https://doi.org/10.1016/j.fertnstert.2021.07.092.
7. Human Fertilisation and Embryology Act 1990, as amended by the Human Fertilisation and Embryology Act 2008.

5 Procedures and Scanning

Ayse Seyhan

5.1 Imaging in Reproductive Health

Ultrasound-based examinations have become an increasingly vital component in the field of gynecology due to their noninvasive nature, efficiency, and growing adaptability. Over the past few decades, the frequency and scope of ultrasound use in diagnosing a multitude of gynecological conditions have significantly expanded.

Ultrasound-based examinations have become a cornerstone in the evaluation and management of infertility. Baseline ultrasound offers an essential reference for assessing reproductive health and identifying underlying issues. Saline infusion sonography is pivotal in assessing the uterine environment and detecting any abnormalities that might impair implantation. Additionally, tubal imaging modalities, which include techniques like HyCoSy and HyFoSy, aid in assessing the patency and overall health of the fallopian tubes, a critical aspect of comprehensive infertility evaluations.

Monitoring ovulation induction through ultrasound enables precise, real-time tracking of follicular development, which is crucial for timely medical intervention in ovulation triggering. During controlled ovarian stimulation, ultrasound provides detailed visualizations of the ovarian response, helping to optimize treatment protocols for individuals undergoing fertility treatments.

Early pregnancy ultrasound also plays a vital role in confirming intrauterine pregnancy, evaluating fetal development, and identifying any complications that may require intervention.

A. Seyhan (✉)
Atlas University, Istanbul, Türkiye

American Hospital Women's Health Clinic, Istanbul, Türkiye
e-mail: ayseseyhan@amerikanhastanesi.org

M. Das, M. H. Dahan (eds.), *A Comprehensive Guide to Reproductive Health and Infertility Medicine for Nurses*, https://doi.org/10.1007/978-3-032-24372-0_5

In the following sections, we will explore each of these ultrasound applications in detail, highlighting their contributions to modern gynecological practice and their impact on fertility treatment outcomes.

5.2 Baseline Ultrasound

Baseline scanning is the foremost among imaging modalities for evaluating and managing a patient's reproductive health. This procedure provides a crucial reference point that allows for the comprehensive evaluation of ovarian reserve and pelvic anatomy, offering insights into underlying issues that may affect fertility.

5.3 Ovarian Reserve

Female infants are born with approximately 500,000 to 1 million oocytes [1]. As they age, this initial reserve declines through natural processes such as follicular atresia and ovulation, ultimately leading to menopause when the ovarian reserve is exhausted and no oocytes are left [2].

Ovarian reserve refers to the number of oocytes remaining in the ovaries [3]. Understanding a woman's ovarian reserve is of great value, particularly for those considering fertility treatments. While it's common knowledge that ovarian reserve decreases as women age, it's crucial to recognize the significant individual variation in ovarian reserve among women of the same chronological age [2].

Directly measuring ovarian reserve by counting primordial follicles is not feasible, as it would require the removal of ovarian tissue. Therefore, indirect methods have been developed. These noninvasive tests include biochemical tests (Follicle Stimulating Hormone (FSH), AntiMullerian Hormaone (AMH)) and imaging to provide estimates of ovarian reserve [3]. Antral follicle count (AFC) is a transvaginal ultrasound test that measures the number of visible small follicles in the ovaries [4].

AFC typically encompasses follicles with a mean diameter ranging from 2 to 10 mm and represents the total number of antral follicles in both ovaries [5] (Fig. 5.1). It is generally recommended to perform follicle counting during the early follicular phase of the menstrual cycle [5]. This timing reduces the likelihood of encountering an ovarian cyst or corpus luteum, which could obscure some antral follicles. However, assessing AFC can be conducted at any stage of the menstrual cycle. This flexibility helps reduce the logistical burden on patients and decreases the number of clinic visits required.

AFC has proven to be a reliable predictor of ovarian reserve and potential responsiveness to exogenous gonadotropins. A lower AFC suggests a reduced ovarian reserve and may predict suboptimal response, characterized by the retrieval of fewer oocytes [3]. This scenario increases the likelihood of cycle cancellation due to insufficient follicular development or not obtaining good embryo quality available for transfer. Conversely, a high AFC is indicative of a robust ovarian reserve,

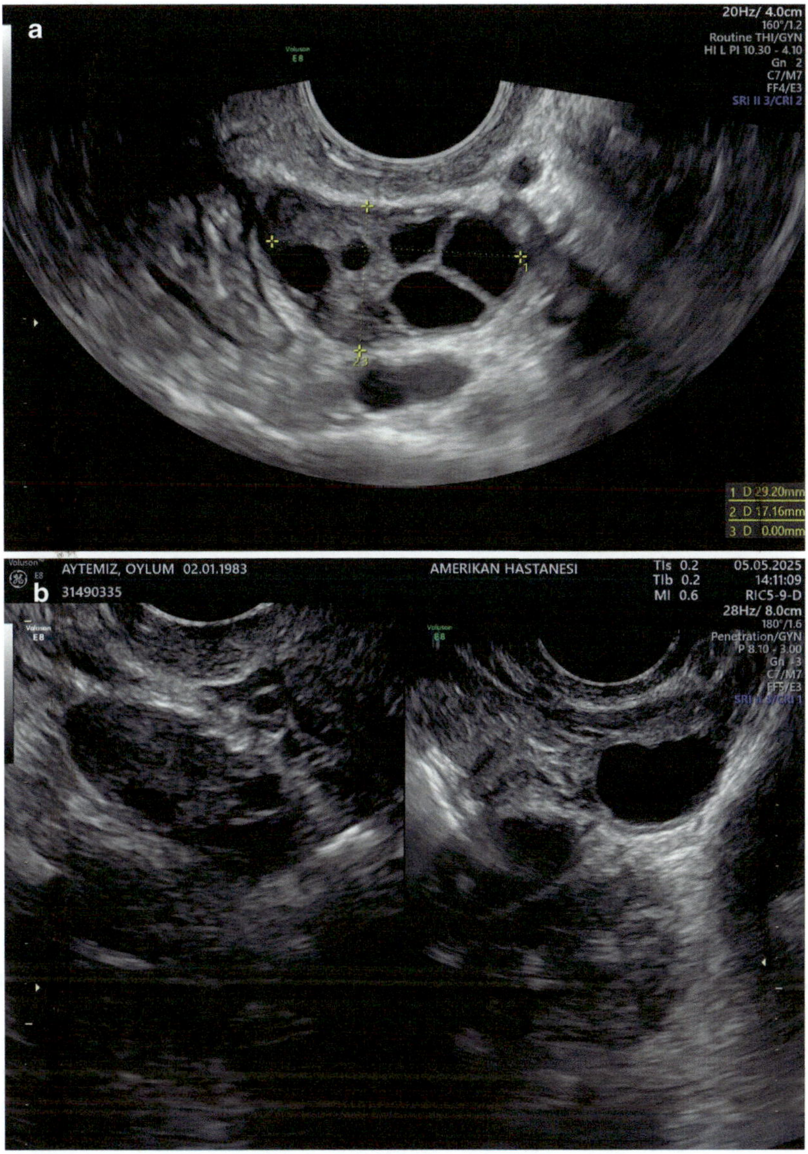

Fig. 5.1 Ovaries visualized with 2D Transvaginal US. (**a**) Antral follicle count of 5 observed in the left ovary. (**b**) Total antral follicle count: 3 follicles identified—2 in the right ovary and 1 in the left ovary

suggesting a risk of exaggerated ovarian response and a higher risk of ovarian hyperstimulation syndrome (OHSS), which is associated with significant morbidity and even mortality [6].

In an effort to define the patients with predicted poor ovarian response (POR), the European Society of Human Reproduction and Embryology (ESHRE) published the Bologna criteria in 2011. AFC was identified as one of three indicators of POR, and cutoff values were established as AFC <5–7 [7] although more recently an AFC of 12 or less was associated with a suboptimal ovarian response per the POSEIDON criteria. An AFC ≥ 24 has been shown to be associated with higher risk of OHSS [8]. Determining which patients are at risk for developing OHSS is essential for selecting the appropriate dosage of gonadotropins and choosing the right final trigger agent for oocyte maturation. This proactive strategy is intended to reduce and potentially eliminate the incidence of OHSS.

When considering the role of AFC, it is important to recognize that while AFC provides valuable insights into ovarian reserve, it does not assess oocyte quality—a crucial factor in predicting live birth rates. Female age is the single most important predictor of fecundity and IVF outcome [3].

As such, caution is advised when using AFC to predict IVF outcomes due to its limited ability to forecast live birth success. Understanding that ovarian reserve (oocyte quantity) is different from oocyte quality is essential for accurately consulting a couple undergoing fertility treatment.

5.4 Ovarian Cysts and Hydrosalpinx

Ultrasound offers valuable insights into the physiological changes that occur throughout the ovarian cycle. It enables accurate and reproducible measurements of follicular size and growth. The corpus luteum, which serves as an indicator of ovulation, typically appears as a unilocular cyst with a reticular pattern, fine, thin intersecting lines that represent fibrin strands, and may contain a retractile clot [9] (Fig. 5.2). The corpus luteum is a physiological cyst, and it is important to differentiate these cysts from other commonly seen benign ovarian cysts such as dermoid cysts and endometriomas.

Endometriomas are often identified on ultrasound as unilocular cysts with homogeneous low-level echogenicity, sometimes described as having a "ground glass" appearance [9] (Fig. 5.3). It's important to recognize that isolated endometriomas are relatively rare; in fact, studies show that about 85% of patients with endometriomas also exhibit other signs of pelvic endometriosis or adenomyosis detectable through transvaginal ultrasound (TVS) [10]. When both ovaries contain endometriomas and are located very close to each other, often adhering together behind the uterus in the pouch of Douglas (a condition known as 'kissing ovaries'), 89% of patients are found to have severe pelvic endometriosis [11]. Therefore, evaluating the entire pelvis is crucial to detect any additional endometriotic lesions in patients with endometrioma.

Typical dermoid cysts demonstrate one or more of the following ultrasound feature(s): diffuse or regional hyperechoic component(s) with shadowing, hyperechoic lines and dots, and floating echogenic spherical structures [9] (Fig. 5.4). The

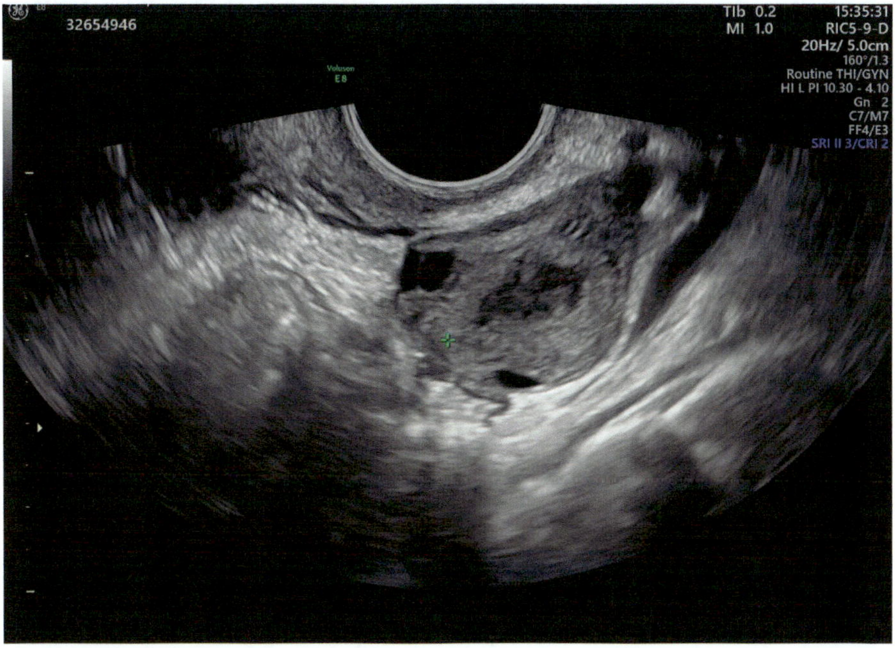

Fig. 5.2 Corpus luteum cyst exhibiting a retraced clot at the center of the lesion

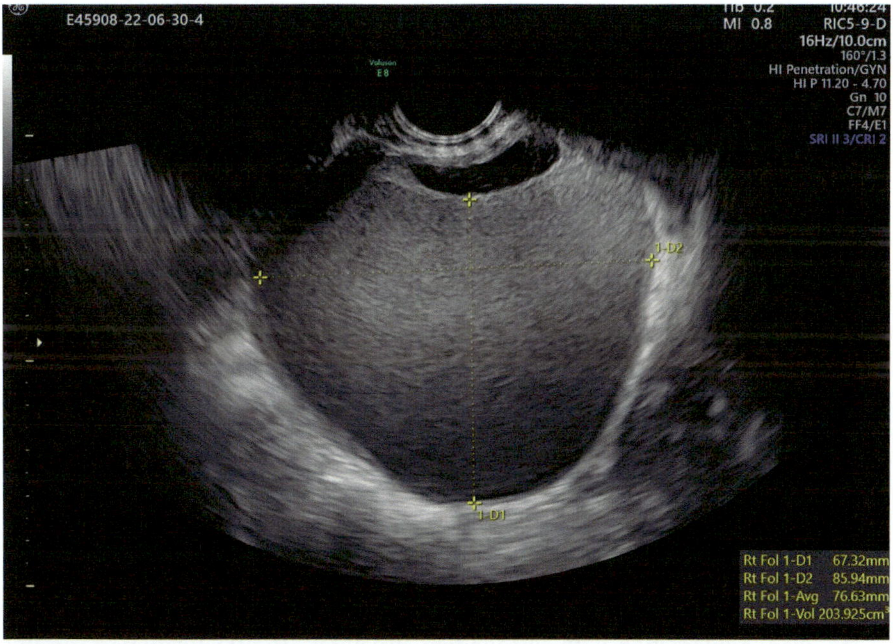

Fig. 5.3 Endometrioma cyst displaying typical "ground glass" echogenicity, featuring a cystic component with homogeneous low-level echogenicity

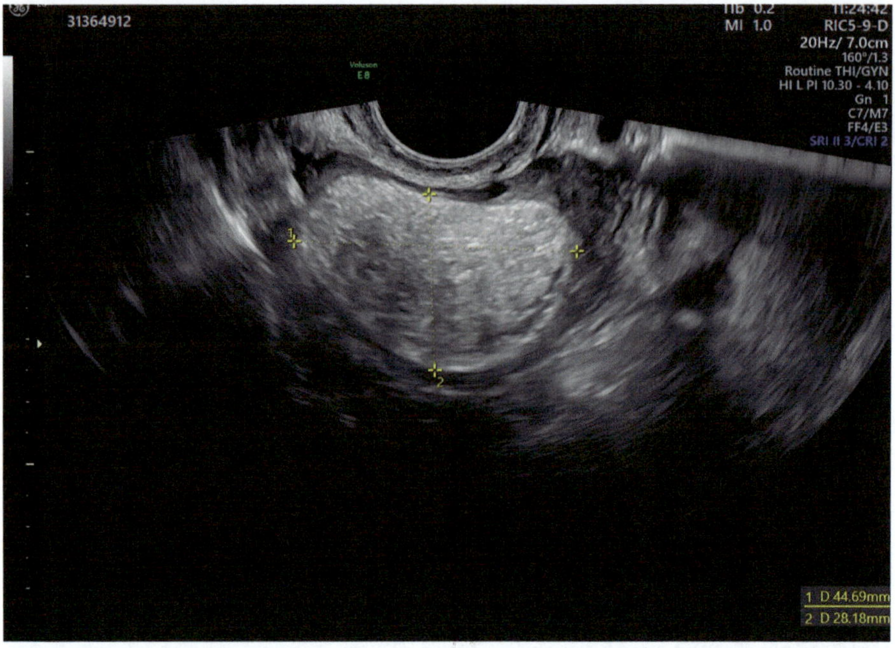

Fig. 5.4 Dermoid cyst showing the typical "snowball" appearance caused by the hyperechoic components within the cyst

presence of a dermoid cyst is not a barrier to assisted reproduction treatment success [12].

Hydrosalpinx, a condition involving the accumulation of fluid within the fallopian tube, can often be misdiagnosed as a paraovarian cyst during ultrasound examinations. This common diagnostic challenge arises due to overlapping imaging characteristics. However, hydrosalpinx typically presents a distinctive ultrasound appearance. In a sagittal view, it manifests as a unilocular, tubular (sausage-shaped) mass with thick, irregular walls, occasionally showing incomplete septa [9]. The content of a hydrosalpinx is anechoic, appearing dark on the ultrasound due to the clear fluid within. A unique feature seen in transverse sections is the 'beads-on-a-string' sign, which describes hyperechoic mural nodules measuring approximately 2–3 mm lining the inner wall of the tube (Fig. 5.5). The presence of a hydrosalpinx adversely affects IVF outcomes, reducing live birth rates by approximately 50% [13]. However, removing the hydrosalpinx can improve these outcomes. Therefore, it's important to be familiar with the ultrasound features of hydrosalpinx to ensure accurate diagnosis and appropriate treatment.

In the assessment of ovarian mobility, transvaginal ultrasound plays a pivotal role, particularly in predicting pelvic adhesions and detecting peritoneal endometriosis. The dynamic capabilities of this imaging technique allow for the evaluation of the ovary's interaction with surrounding structures. To effectively perform this assessment, first locate the ovary in both the midsagittal and transverse planes using

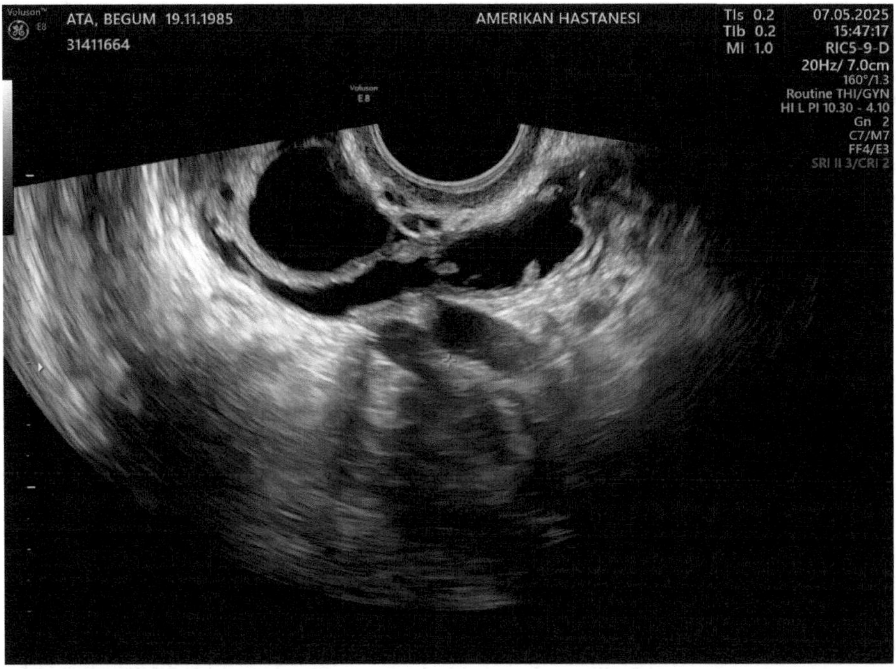

Fig. 5.5 Hydrosalpinx characterized by short round projections observed on the inner wall of the fluid-filled tubular structure

the ultrasound probe. Then, gently apply abdominal pressure in the ipsilateral fossa. A smoothly gliding ovary against the uterus and pelvic sidewall indicates a positive sliding sign, classifying the ovary as mobile [14]. In contrast, if the ovary does not move effortlessly against these structures, the sliding sign is negative, suggesting immobility. This lack of mobility can serve as a significant "red flag" for clinicians, highlighting women who may be at an increased risk for endometriosis [15]. By incorporating this examination into routine practice, practitioners can enhance their diagnostic capabilities and improve the early detection and management of endometriosis.

5.5 Ultrasound Assessment of the Uterus

In conducting a pelvic ultrasound examination, the initial step involves determining the orientation and movement characteristics of the uterus, specifically whether it is anteverted or retroverted, and assessing its mobility within the pelvic cavity. It is essential to understand that ultrasound is a dynamic imaging modality, capable of capturing real-time tissue movement and interaction. The baseline scan should include an assessment for the "sliding sign," a crucial dynamic indicator used to predict the presence of adhesions in the pelvic region [14].

The ultrasound transducer is initially introduced into the posterior vaginal fornix and gradually withdrawn to evaluate the movement of the rectum against both the posterior vaginal fornix and the posterior uterine wall in the mid-sagittal plane. Concurrently, external pressure is applied to the uterus via the examiner's left hand positioned on the patient's abdomen, which enhances the assessment of uterine and rectal mobility. A "negative sliding sign," characterized by the immobility of the rectum relative to the uterus and posterior vaginal fornix, suggests potential pelvic adhesions and may indicate the presence of endometriosis. Conversely, a "positive sliding sign," defined by noticeable rectal movement against the uterine wall, indicates the absence of significant adhesions [14].

5.5.1 Uterine Fibroids

Uterine fibroids are the most common benign gynecological tumors found in women of reproductive age. While most women with fibroids are asymptomatic, those who do experience symptoms typically report abnormal uterine bleeding and/or pelvic pain and pressure. Fibroids can also have reproductive implications, including infertility and adverse pregnancy outcomes [16].

The FIGO (International Federation of Gynecology and Obstetrics) classification system for uterine leiomyomas (fibroids) categorizes them based on their location within the uterus [17]. The relationship between fibroids and infertility remains a topic of debate. There is a general consensus on the impact of submucous fibroids (in the uterine cavity) and intramural fibroids that distort the uterine cavity on fertility. However, there is more controversy surrounding intramural fibroids, which are located within the uterine wall and do not distort the cavity [16]. Subserosal uterine fibroids (that are far from the cavity on the outside of the uterus) uterine fibroids are not felt to impact pregnancy rate.

On ultrasound, a uterine fibroid is classically characterized as a solid, round, well-defined, hypoechoic, heterogeneous lesion within the myometrium, often showing acoustic shadowing at the edge of the lesion, with or without internal fan-shaped shadowing [18] (Fig. 5.6). On color Doppler, the circumferential flow around the lesion is often visible [19]. All fibroids should be precisely measured, and their location within the myometrium should be identified and documented according to the FIGO classification system. Treatment strategies should be tailored to both patient and fibroid characteristics.

5.5.2 Adenomyosis

Adenomyosis is characterized by the proliferation of endometrial glands and stroma, which forms ill-defined lesions within the myometrium [20]. This benign condition is increasingly diagnosed in younger women who experience infertility. Adenomyosis can adversely affect in vitro fertilization outcomes, pregnancy rates, and live birth rates, while also increasing the risk of miscarriage [21]. Adenomyosis can also cause pelvic pain and painful periods. With advancements in non-invasive

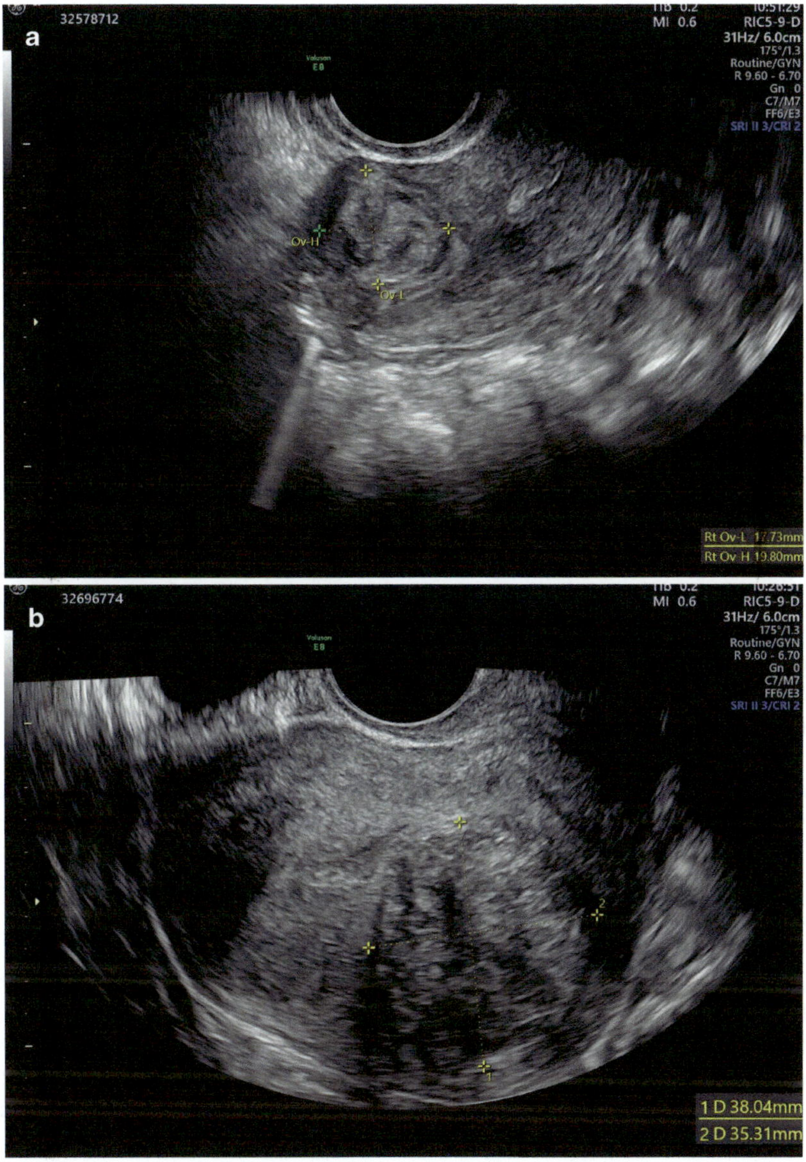

Fig. 5.6 2D TV US Imaging of Intramural Fibroids: (**a**) An intramural fibroid located at the fundus, which does not distort the uterine cavity. (**b**) An intramural fibroid situated in the posterior wall of the uterus, causing distortion of the uterine cavity

diagnostic techniques, such as MRI and transvaginal ultrasound (TVUS), adenomyosis has become a more recognizable condition in women of reproductive age.

According to the consensus on the revised definitions of the Morphological Uterus Sonographic Assessment (MUSA) features of adenomyosis, there are three direct and six indirect ultrasound features [19].

The direct ultrasound features include myometrial cysts, which are rounded or oval cystic spaces of any size within the myometrium; hyperechogenic islands, which are areas within the myometrium that are hyperechogenic and have no connection with the endometrium; and echogenic subendometrial lines and buds, which indicate invasion of endometrial tissue into the myometrium.

The indirect ultrasound features are a globular uterus, characterized by a uniformly enlarged, round uterus; asymmetrical myometrial thickening, which is uneven thickening of the myometrium; fan-shaped shadowing, which is shadowing that emanates from the myometrial lesions; translesional vascularity, characterized by the presence of blood vessels crossing the lesion, running perpendicular to the uterine cavity or serosa; irregular Junctional Zone (JZ), which involves disruption and irregularity in the normal appearance of the JZ; and an interrupted JZ, marked by the complete absence of a continuous JZ due to interference by lesions (Fig. 5.7). These features collectively help in the sonographic evaluation and diagnosis of adenomyosis. Diagnosis is typically made when at least one direct sign is present. However, when only indirect signs are present without any direct signs, a diagnosis cannot be conclusively made, leading to a classification of uncertainty. In such uncertain cases, further examination of the junctional zone using 3D transvaginal ultrasound (3D-TVUS) can be informative. If the junctional zone appears intact in these cases, adenomyosis can often be excluded, providing more clarity in diagnosis [19].

5.5.3 Endometrial Polyps/Intrauterine Adhesions

The assessment of the uterine cavity is another routine examination performed in patients with subfertility and infertility.

Endometrial polyps are benign outgrowths of the endometrial lining made up of glands, stroma, and blood vessels. They range in size and are often detected incidentally; however, they can sometimes present clinically with symptoms such as intermenstrual bleeding and metrorrhagia (heavy vaginal bleeding) or complicate fertility efforts [22]. The exact manner in which polyps affect fertility isn't entirely clear, but it is postulated that they may impede embryo implantation or create an unfavorable uterine environment [23]. The investigation generally begins with transvaginal ultrasound for initial visualization.

The 2D transvaginal ultrasound remains the first-line imaging modality, renowned for its capability to detect characteristic abnormalities in the endometrium, such as solitary homogeneous echogenic lesions that disrupt the normal mucosal contour, or an abnormally thickened endometrium that is atypical for the patient's age [24]. However, 3D ultrasound offers an enhanced perspective by

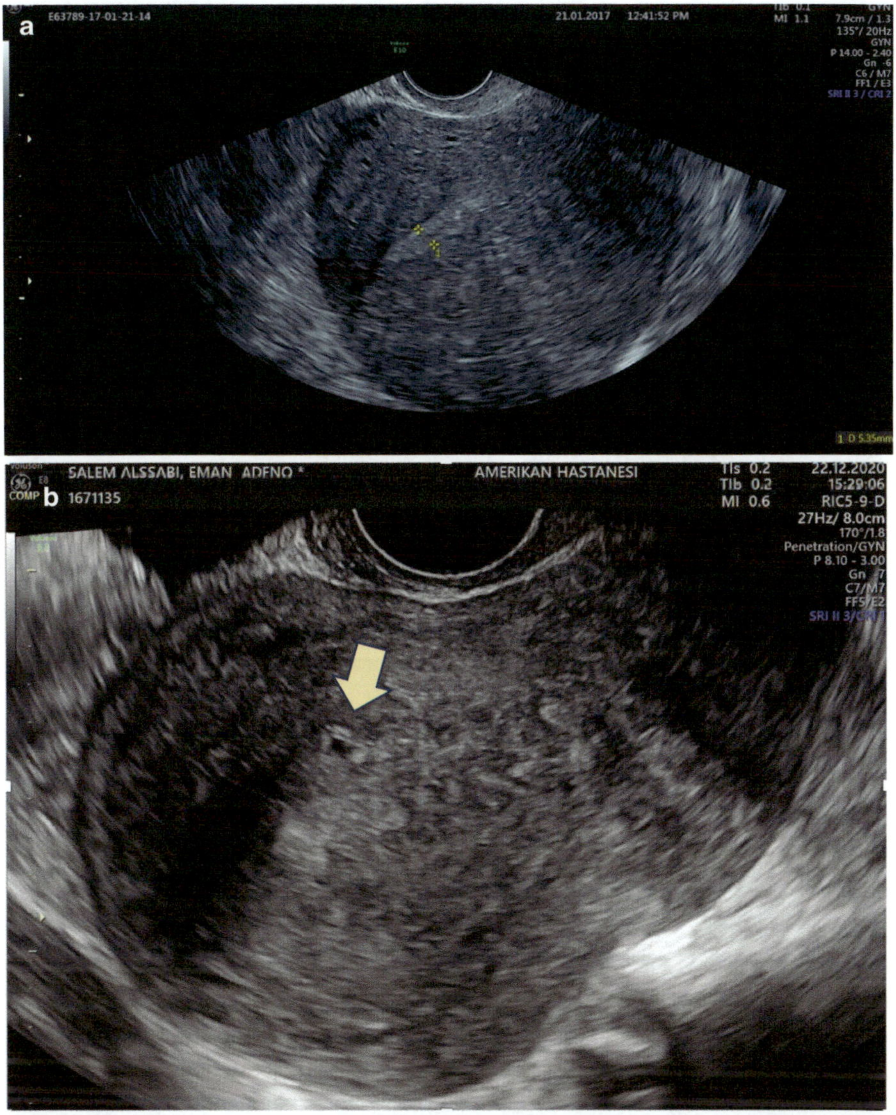

Fig. 5.7 Ultrasound features of Adenomyosis including a large globular uterus and myometrial cysts. (**a**) Myometrial asymmetry. (**b**) Myometrial cyst. (**c**) Echogenic subendometrial lines and buds. (**d**) Hyperechoic myometrial islands. (**e**) Fan shaped shadowing. (**f**) Translesional vascularity. (**g**) Interrupted junctional zone

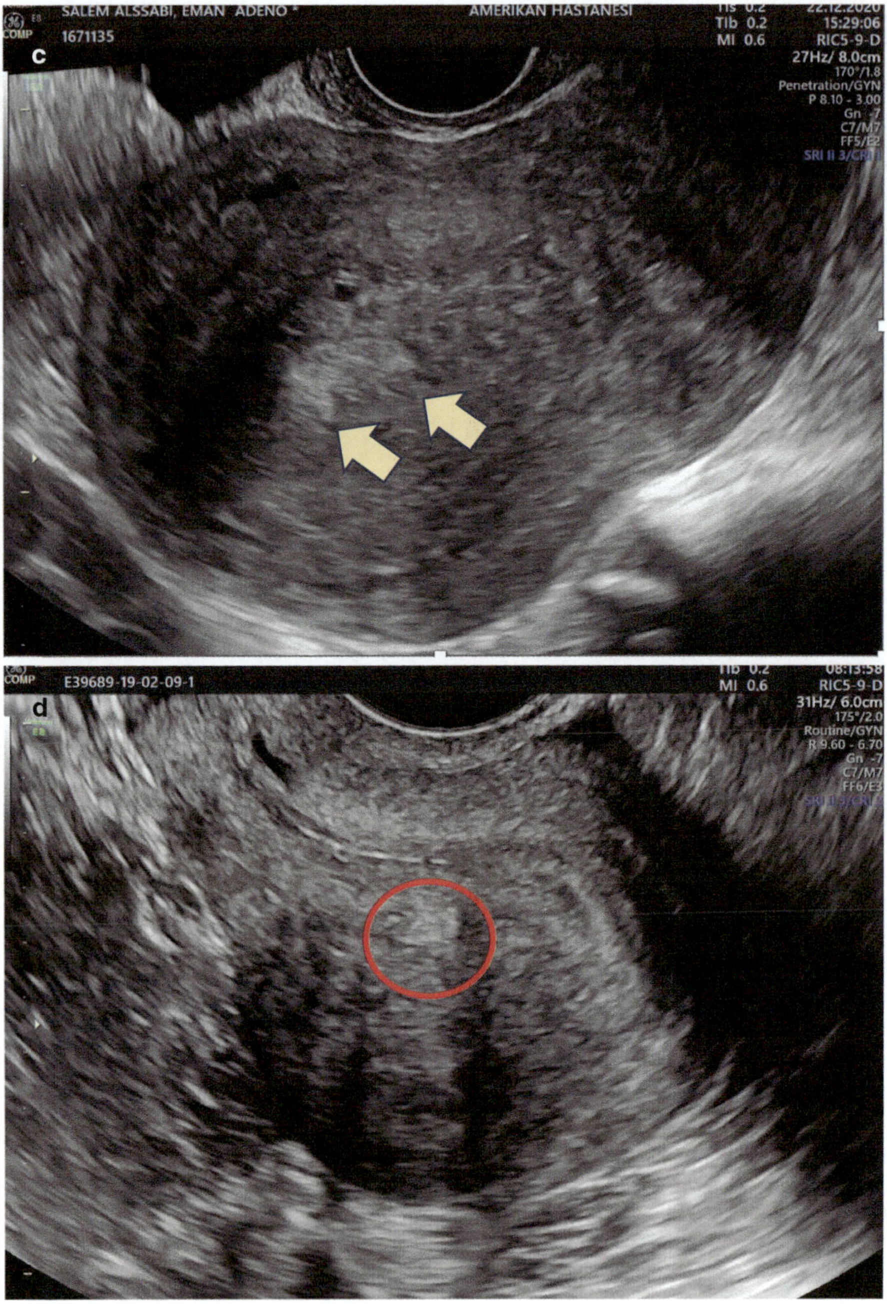

Fig. 5.7 (continued)

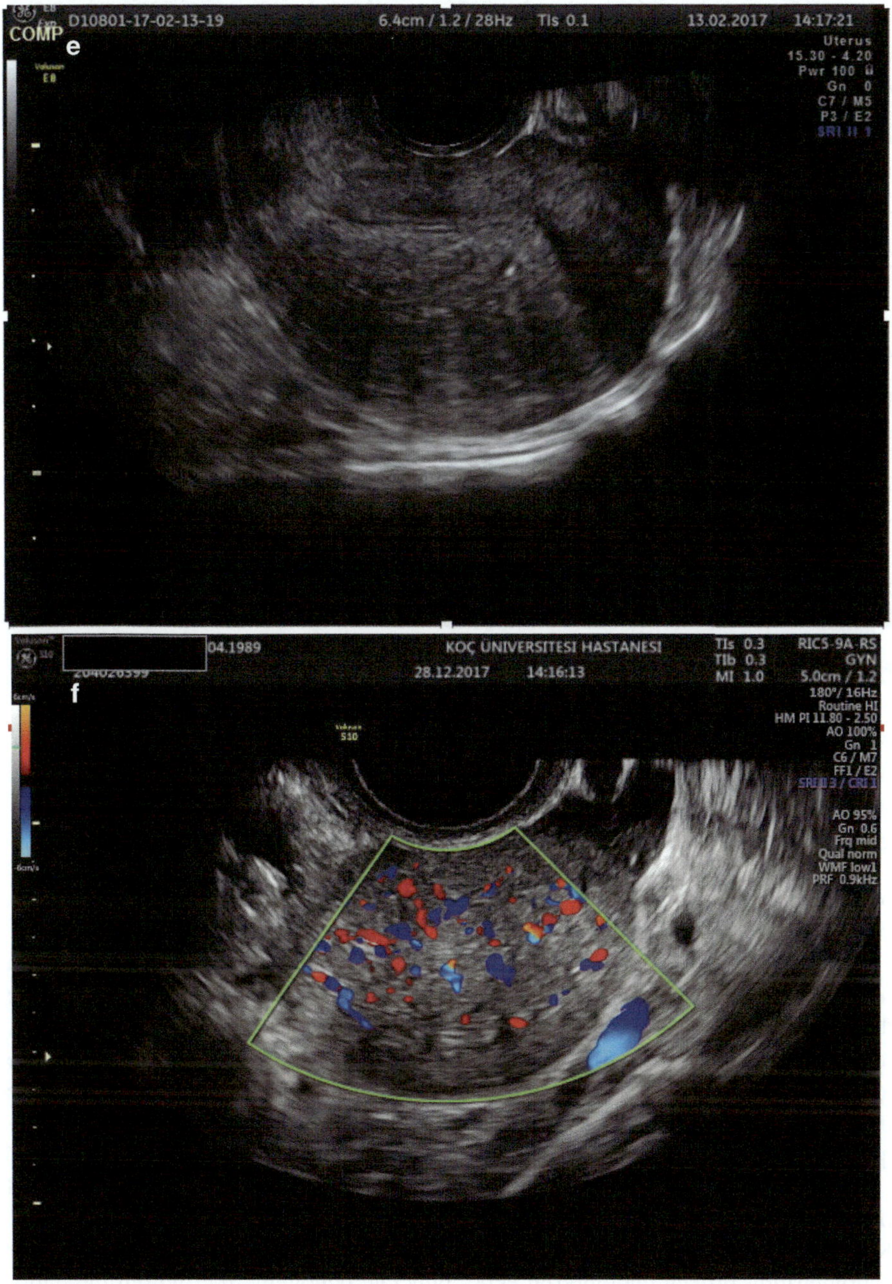

Fig. 5.7 (continued)

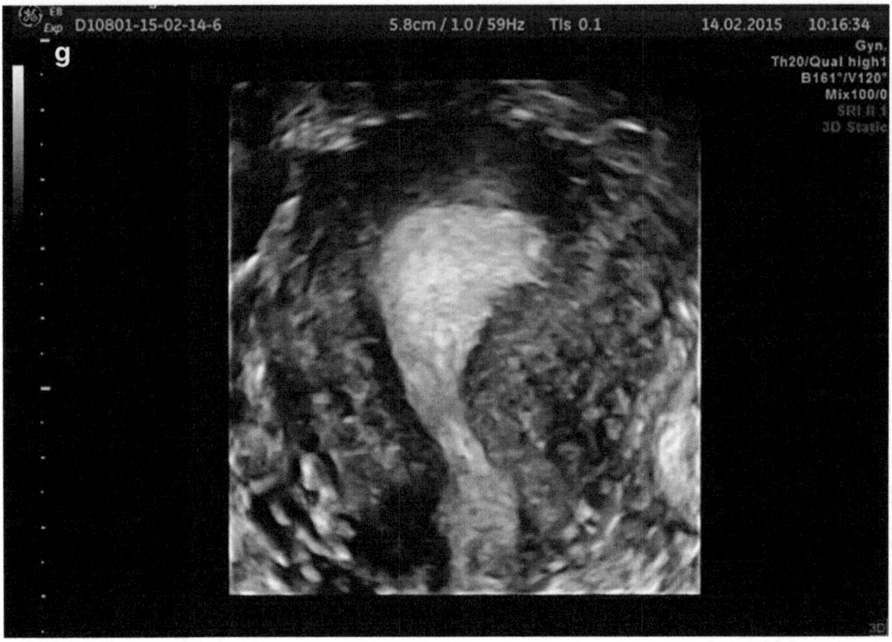

Fig. 5.7 (continued)

providing a comprehensive view of the polyp's size, shape, and exact location within the uterine cavity (Fig. 5.8). The coronal plane, in particular, is instrumental in not only bolstering diagnostic confidence but also facilitating patient understanding of their condition. These nuanced imaging insights are crucial for guiding clinical decision-making, particularly concerning the complexity of hysteroscopic polypectomy. By offering a clearer preoperative roadmap, ultrasound findings can significantly aid in surgical planning and assessment of procedure difficulty.

Intrauterine adhesions (IUAs) are notably more prevalent in women who have a history of multiple miscarriages [25]. The primary pathological event leading to the development of IUAs is damage to the endometrial stroma. When the stroma is lost, it is replaced by fibrous tissue, causing the adjacent endometrial surfaces to adhere to each other and form adhesions [26]. Menstrual disturbances are commonly the initial clinical signs of IUAs, but subfertility and recurrent miscarriage also frequently prompt women to seek medical assistance.

For diagnosing IUAs, two-dimensional (2D) ultrasound is a commonly used first-line imaging technique due to its ability to clearly visualize uterine structures. Key features suggestive of IUAs on 2D transvaginal ultrasound include an irregular endometrium, broken endometrial echo, punctate echogenic foci within the endometrium, an indistinct junction between the endometrium and myometrium, a thin endometrium that does not thicken with hormonal therapy, despite normal ovarian function and hormonal profiles, and rarely fluid in the cavity [27, 28].

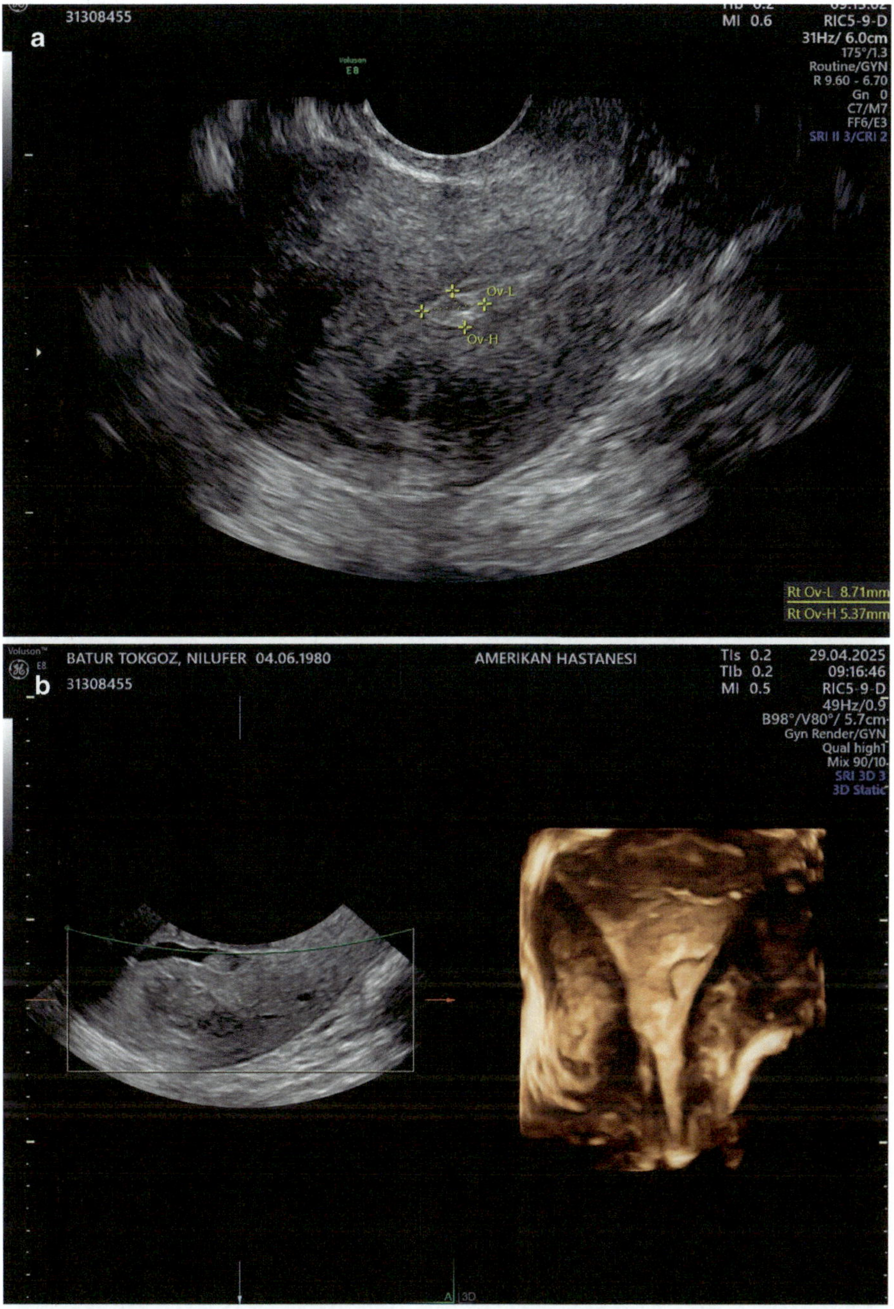

Fig. 5.8 (**a**) Focal thickening of endometrium indicative of endometrial polyp. (**b**) 3D ultrasound demonstrating a coronal view of the endometrial cavity, with the endometrial polyp located on the left lateral uterine wall

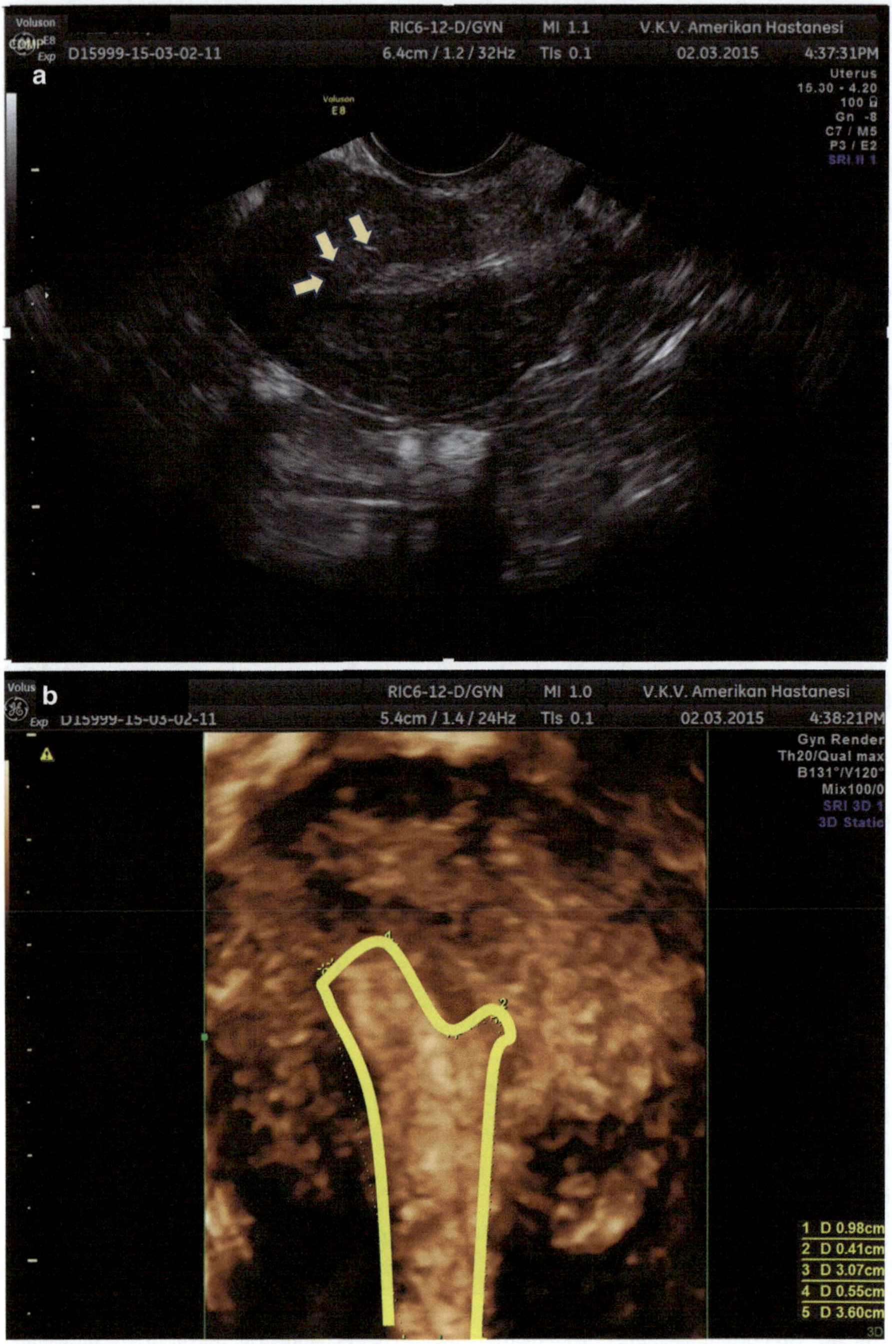

Fig. 5.9 (**a**) 2D transvaginal ultrasound revealing an irregular endometrium with a disrupted endometrial echo, suggestive of intrauterine adhesions. (**b**) 3D transvaginal ultrasound image of the same patient demonstrating a visible right cornu while the left cornu is not visualized. This finding is suggestive of intrauterine adhesions at the level of the left half of the fundus, including the cornual area

The 3D reconstruction of the uterine anatomy provides comprehensive panoramic views of the uterine cavity in the coronal plane, allowing for the visualization of focal obliterations (Fig. 5.9). It enables the identification of central bands of adhesions that cause partial or complete obliteration of the cavity, thereby effectively guiding hysteroscopic procedures.

5.6 Congenital Uterine Anomalies

Congenital uterine anomalies are more prevalent in infertile women (8%) and those with recurrent miscarriages (13.3%) compared to the general population (5.5%) [29]. The European Society of Human Reproduction and Embryology (ESHRE) and the American Society for Reproductive Medicine (ASRM) classify uterine anomalies based on the anatomical deviations that originate from the same embryological development [30, 31]. The uterine septum is the most common congenital uterine anomaly [32].

A systematic approach to 2D ultrasound involves capturing serial sagittal planes from beyond the outer margin of one side of the uterus to the other, including both the cervix and the uterine body, if feasible, as well as transverse planes from the cervix to beyond the uterine fundal level.

The visualization of a double endometrial complex on a transverse plane suggests a uterine septum [33]. To confirm the diagnosis, the external uterine contour should exhibit a convex, flat, or mildly concave configuration (ideally <1 cm), which can be challenging to assess with 2D ultrasound. An arcuate uterus is considered a variation of normal. A uterine septum is considered abnormal, which may increase the risks of pregnancy complications. Evaluating the internal and external fundal contours is crucial for diagnosing and correctly classifying a uterine anomaly as a septum, rather than a bicornuate uterus (two uteri). A uterus that appears to have two cavities could be either septate or bicornuate. This distinction is determined by evaluating the external contours of the uterine fundus (the top of the uterus), which is best visualized using a 3D ultrasound image. Additionally, measuring the fundal indentation is necessary to differentiate a septum from an arcuate uterus [34]. The coronal view, essential for diagnosing congenital uterine anomalies, is derived from a 3D dataset to assess both the shape of the uterine cavity and the fundal contours [35]. According to ESHRE guidelines, a septate uterus is indicated by an internal indentation at the fundal midline that exceeds 50% of the uterine wall thickness. In contrast, ASRM defines a septate uterus by an indentation depth of more than 1 cm and an indentation angle of less than 90°. To fully evaluate these diagnostic criteria, 3D ultrasound has become the modality of choice for diagnosing uterine anomalies, offering improved accuracy and detail in assessment (Fig. 5.10).

The coronal view, essential for diagnosing congenital uterine anomalies, is derived from a 3D dataset to assess both the shape of the uterine cavity and the fundal contours. According to ESHRE guidelines, a septate uterus is indicated by an internal indentation at the fundal midline that exceeds 50% of the uterine wall thickness [34]. On the other hand, ASRM defines a septate uterus by an indentation depth of more than 1 cm and an indentation angle of less than 90° [31]. To fully

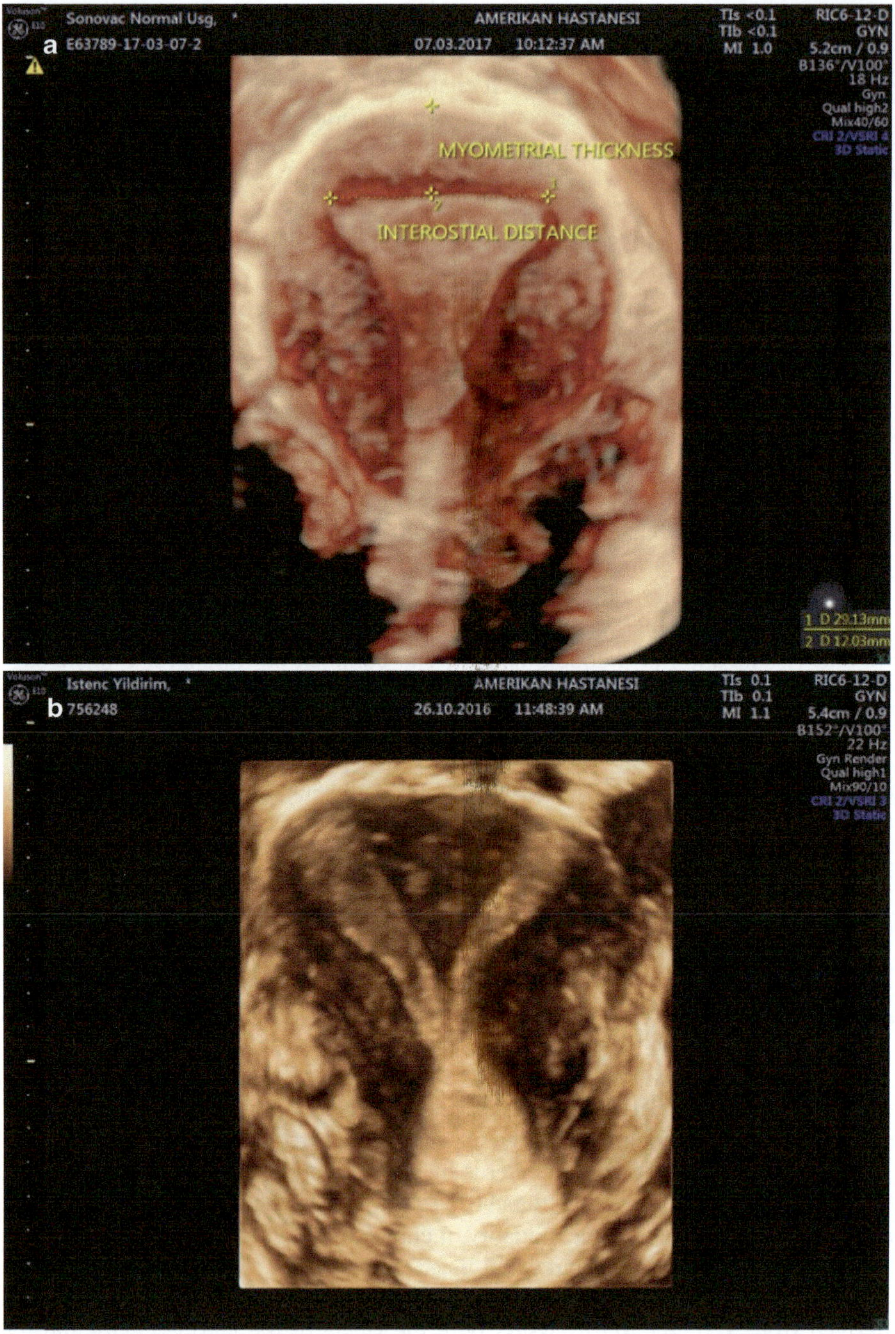

Fig. 5.10 (**a**) 3D US, coronal plane of normal uterus. (**b**) 3D US, coronal plane of uterus with septum

evaluate these diagnostic criteria, 3D ultrasound has become the modality of choice for diagnosing uterine anomalies, offering improved accuracy and detail in assessment.

5.7 Saline Sonogram

Saline infusion sonography is primarily used to detect structural abnormalities in the uterine cavity that could affect fertility or cause miscarriages. This includes uterine polyps, submucosal fibroids, and intrauterine adhesions. This procedure is also known as sonohysterography, hysterosonography, hydrosonography, or saline sonogram [36]. Saline Infusion Sonohysterography (SIS) is optimally timed to coincide with the early proliferative phase of a woman's menstrual cycle, typically right after menstruation but before ovulation [37]. Post-menstruation, the endometrial lining is thin, which allows for better visualization of the uterine cavity and any abnormalities, such as polyps or fibroids. A thin endometrial layer enhances contrast when the saline is infused, making it easier to identify lesions that might be isoechoic to the endometrial lining. Also conducting SIS before ovulation minimizes the risk of disrupting an early pregnancy, since it occurs prior to the implantation window. SIS is generally well-tolerated, though some patients may experience mild cramping or discomfort due to the insertion of fluid into the uterus. Providing patients with an understanding of what to expect can help alleviate anxiety and improve tolerance to the procedure. SIS is associated with a low complication rate. On rare occasions, patients might experience infection, such as endometritis, with an incidence of less than 1% [38]. To further minimize infection risk, sterile technique is used during the procedure. If the patient complains of pain, fever, or foul vaginal discharge starting one to 7 days after this procedure, they should be referred for evaluation for possible infection.

The procedure begins with a baseline transvaginal ultrasound to initially assess the uterus and ovaries.

A sterile speculum is inserted into the vagina, allowing visual access to the cervix
A thin catheter is gently inserted through the cervix into the uterine cavity
Sterile saline is then gradually infused into the uterine cavity through the catheter
As transvaginal ultrasound probe is inserted to capture images of the uterus, the saline expands the uterine cavity
The distension caused by the saline enhances visualization, allowing identification of abnormalities that may not be visible on a routine ultrasound.

In a normal SIS study, the endometrial lining appears symmetric and evenly surrounding the saline-filled uterine cavity (Fig. 5.11). Endometrial polyps appear as homogeneous polypoid lesions that are isoechoic to the endometrium (Fig. 5.12). Information about the size and location of the polyp can guide clinical intervention and assist the surgeon during hysteroscopic resection.

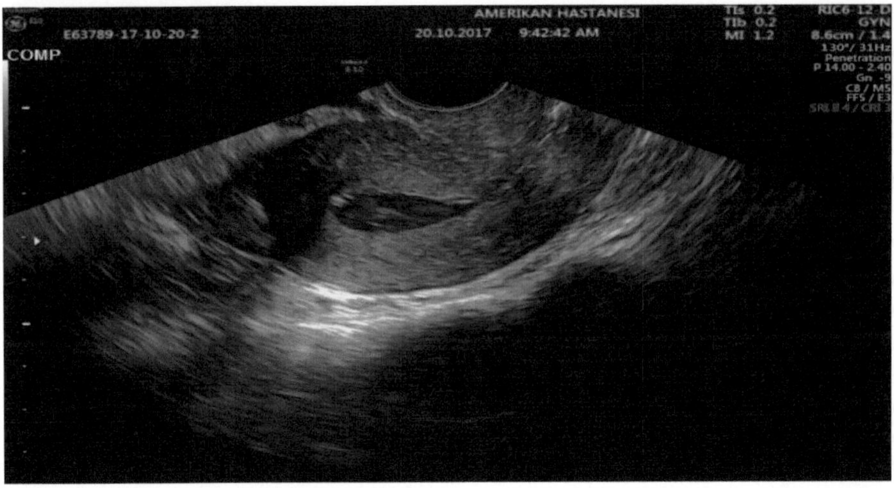

Fig. 5.11 Normal cavity noted by saline infusion sonography

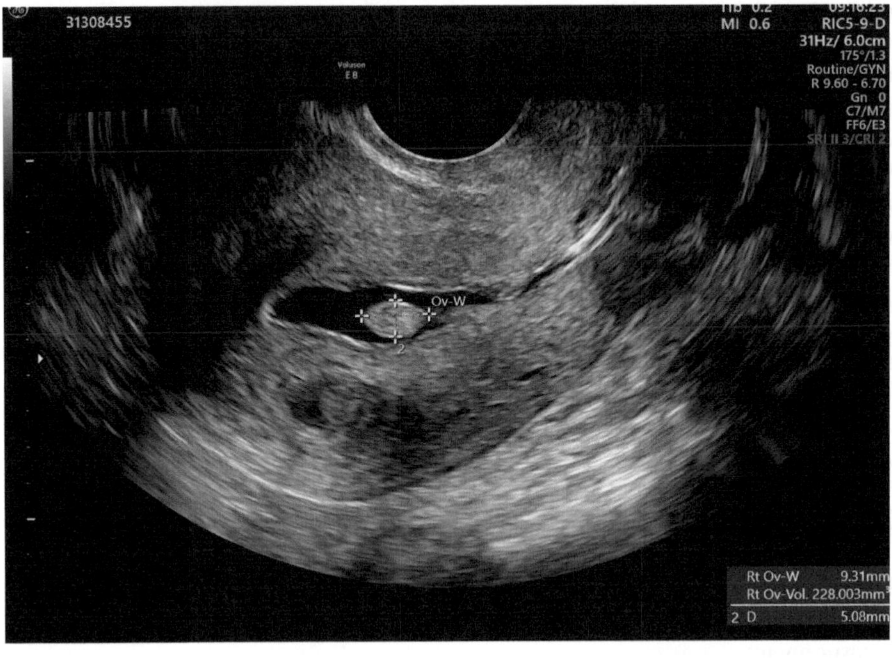

Fig. 5.12 Endometrial polyp originating from the posterior wall of the uterus, as identified by SIS

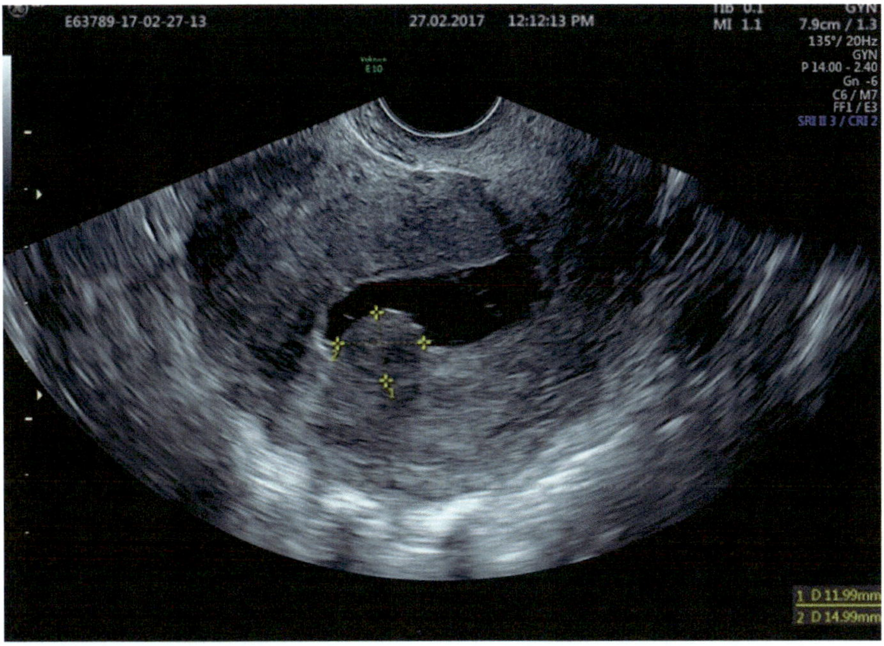

Fig. 5.13 Type 2 submucous fibroid located in the upper posterior part of uterine wall, as demostrated demonstrated by SIS

Submucous fibroids are benign uterine tumors composed of fibrous tissue and smooth muscle that protrude into the uterine cavity [37]. Fibroids appear as hypoechoic (darker or blacker image on ultrasound), round, and broad-based lesions on imaging, whereas endometrial polyps are seen as hyperechoic (lighter or a whiter image on ultrasound) masses compared to the myometrium [36] (Fig. 5.13). SIS is particularly useful for assessing the number, location, and extent of fibroids projecting into the cavity. Such information is crucial in determining the feasibility and potential difficulty of a hysteroscopic removal procedure, helping guide clinical decisions regarding the most appropriate treatment plan.

Intrauterine adhesions are frequently associated with infertility. Trauma to the endometrium from surgical procedures is a common cause of intrauterine adhesions (scar tissue known as Asherman's syndrome). Procedures such as dilation and curettage (D&C), myomectomy, removal of uterine septae, or any other intrauterine surgery can lead to the development of fibrous connective tissue bands within the uterine cavity [28]. Diagnosis starts with clinical suspicion and carried out with confirmatory SIS test. Echogenic bands are seen between the uterine walls [37]. The mainstay of treatment is hysteroscopic adhesiolysis, where the bands are carefully cut to restore the normal uterine architecture.

In summary, SIS is a valuable diagnostic tool due to its cost-effectiveness, ability to perform real-time evaluation, and efficacy in providing detailed information about uterine cavity with minimal discomfort or risk to the patient. It is frequently used as a first-line investigation before considering more invasive procedures.

5.8 Tubal Procedures

Tubal pathology (or blockage) is a major cause of female infertility, with a prevalence ranging from 11% to 30% [39]. This condition often arises from sexually transmitted infections, as well as previous surgeries or endometriosis. A clinical history may not always reveal tubal pathology since infections like chlamydia and gonorrhea can be asymptomatic. Consequently, evaluating the fallopian tubes is a standard component of the fertility work-up. Diagnostic laparoscopy with chromopertubation was once considered the gold standard for assessing tubal patency. However, it is no longer commonly performed due to its invasive nature and high cost. Hysterosalpingography (HSG) is still considered the first-choice test for assessing tubal patency during fertility work-ups [40, 41]. More recently, hystero-salpingo-foam sonography (HyFoSy) has been introduced as a more patient-friendly alternative [42].

5.8.1 Hysterosalpingography (HSG)

HSG involves a radiographic examination of the uterus and fallopian tubes. During the procedure, the patient lies on their back on the fluoroscopy table in the lithotomy position. After preparing the cervix, a tenaculum might be used to stabilize the cervix and position the uterus. The HSG catheter is then inserted through the endocervix. The balloon tip of the catheter may be inflated to help with uterine traction, prevent the contrast from leaking out, or to keep the catheter from being expelled accidentally. An iodinated contrast medium, either oil- or water-based, is introduced through the catheter into the uterine cavity. Radiographic images are periodically taken to observe the filling of the uterine cavity and fallopian tubes [43].

During a HSG, several key features of the fallopian tubes are evaluated, including their architecture, patency (whether they are open or blocked), the presence of any spillage of contrast material into the peritoneal cavity, and the distribution of this contrast intraperitoneally.

A normal hysterosalpingography (HSG) indicates that there is normal filling of the uterine cavity and fallopian tubes with the contrast medium, and that there is also free spillage of the contrast into the peritoneal cavity (Fig. 5.14).

The presence of a hydrosalpinx can adversely affect fertility outcomes, including the success rates of assisted reproductive technologies (ART) such as in vitro fertilization (IVF) [13]. A hydrosalpinx is a condition where the fallopian tube is blocked

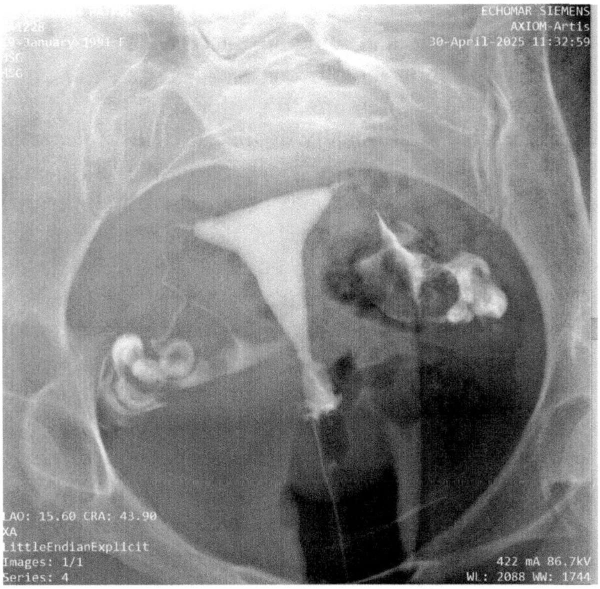

Fig. 5.14 HSG showing a normal uterine cavity with patent fallopian tubes

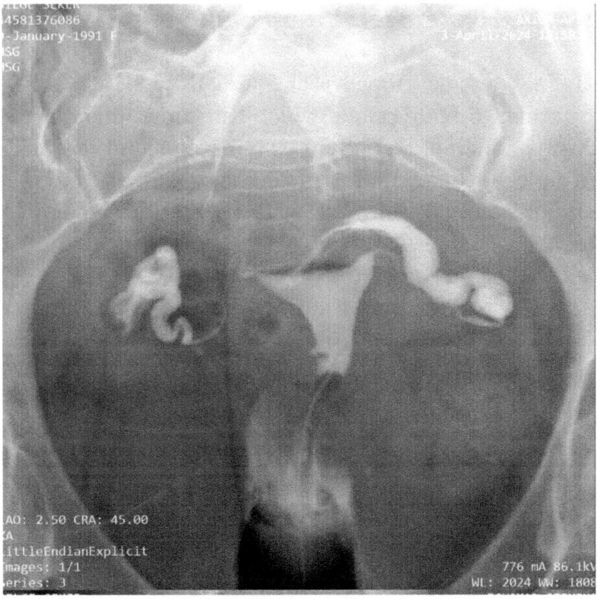

Fig. 5.15 Normal uterine cavity with a patent right fallopian tube and a distally blocked enlarged left fallopian tube, as detected by HSG

at the distal end, preventing the fluid normally produced in the tube from draining. On an HSG, a hydrosalpinx typically appears as a dilated tube that fills with contrast medium, but, crucially, there is an absence of free spillage of contrast into the peritoneal cavity, indicating that the tube is obstructed (Fig. 5.15).

In cases where there is a proximal tubal blockage, HSG can play a dual role as both a diagnostic and a therapeutic procedure. While the primary role of HSG is diagnostic, identifying blockages or abnormalities, it sometimes also has therapeutic benefits. The pressure from the contrast medium can occasionally reopen a blocked tube. Additionally, if the HSG identifies a proximal blockage, interventional radiology techniques can be employed, using selective catheterization to attempt to clear the blockage, providing further therapeutic benefit [44].

Hysterosalpingography (HSG) is generally considered safe in terms of radiation exposure when standard techniques are used. However, there is a small risk of adverse reactions to the iodinated contrast media used in the procedure. These reactions can range from mild symptoms, such as urticaria, to more severe reactions like bronchospasm and laryngeal edema [43].

For patients with a history of pelvic infection, it is common to prescribe an empirical antibiotic, such as doxycycline (100 mg orally twice daily for 5 days), as a precautionary measure to prevent infection. Despite these precautions, the incidence of HSG-related infections is reported to be around 3.1% [45]. They should be advised to contact their healthcare provider if they experience symptoms such as pelvic pain, unusual discharge, or fever after the HSG.

5.8.2 Hysterosalpingo-Foam Sonography (HyFoSY)

HyFoSy was developed as an alternative to HSG. It offers the advantage of avoiding exposure to both iodine, which can cause allergic reactions in some patients, and X-ray radiation. HyFoSy uses transvaginal ultrasound combined with the injection of an echogenic contrast medium (foam-gel) into the uterus and fallopian tubes. HyFoSy provides a more stable echogenic medium than other ultrasound-based tubal patency tests, such as Hysterosalpingo-contrast sonography (HyCoSy) which uses saline and air [46].

Similar to other procedures where solutions are injected into the uterine cavity, HyFoSy is ideally performed during the follicular phase of the menstrual cycle. This timing usually falls between day 6 and day 11, following the cessation of menstruation and before the onset of ovulation. Usually, the procedure is well tolerated and no painkillers are necessary.

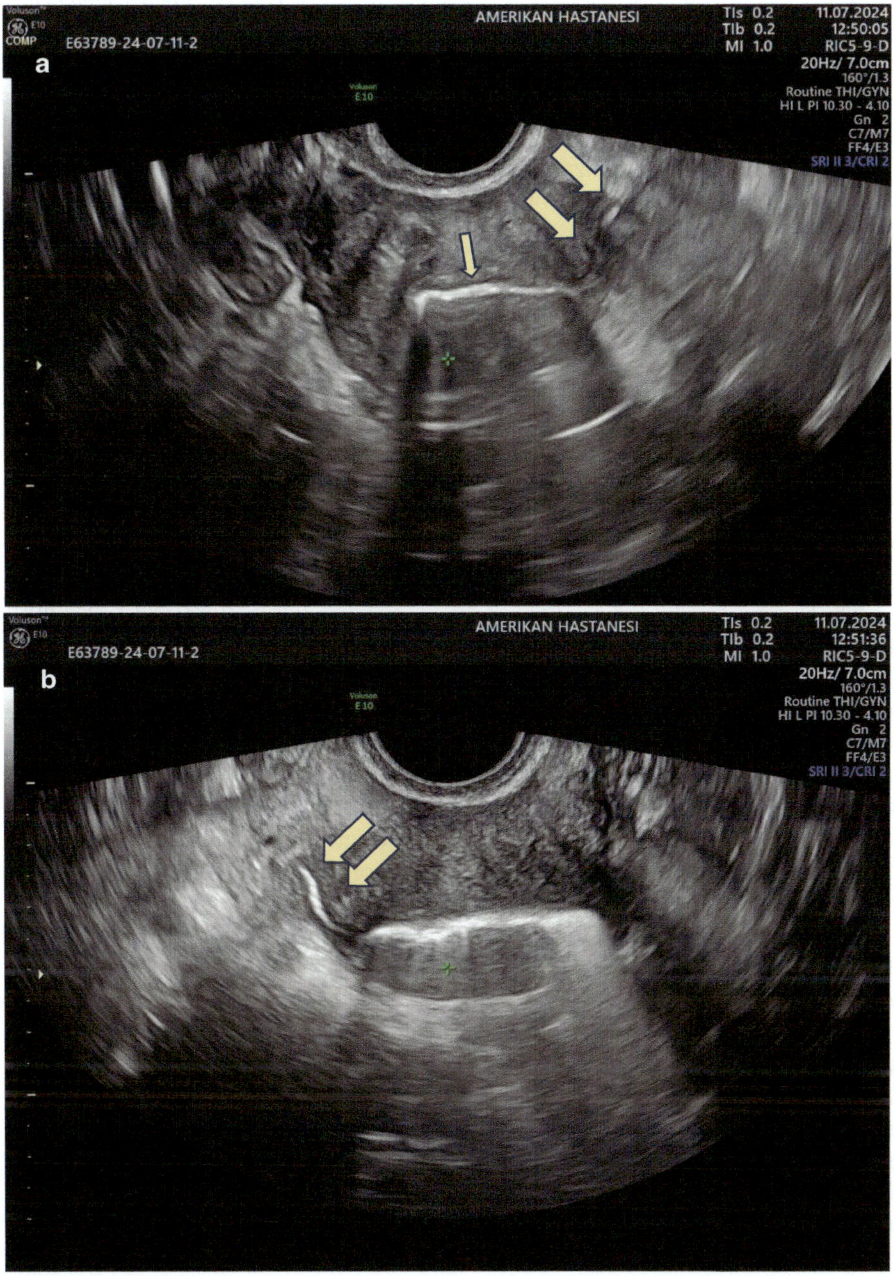

Fig. 5.16 2D HyFoSy. (**a**) Foam vissible in interstitial part and isthmus of the left tube. (**b**) Foam vissible in interstitial part isthmus and ampulla of the right tube

- A speculum is placed in the vagina and the cervix is cleaned.
- A fine sterile plastic catheter is then placed in the uterine cavity.
- Transvaginal scan is performed as the contrast (foam gel) is injected through the catheter.

The gel allows the visualization of the tube and the spillage around the ovaries. When the spilling is seen easily on both sides, the fallopian tubes are considered to be patent (Fig. 5.16).

HyFoSy is also considered to be less painful and less time-consuming than HSG and has been shown to be as effective as HSG [46–48].

5.9 Follicular Monitoring

The dose and type of gonadotropin for ovarian stimulation are selected based on the anticipated ovarian response, which is determined using baseline ultrasound findings. Several protocols are available to prevent a luteinizing hormone (LH) surge before the stimulated ovarian follicles mature. The most commonly used protocols are the GnRH agonist (long) protocol and the GnRH antagonist protocol.

The long protocol consists of two stages: pituitary suppression followed by ovarian stimulation. Pituitary suppression begins in the luteal phase of the cycle preceding the planned ovarian stimulation and continues for a minimum of 10 days before initiating stimulation medications. It is maintained throughout stimulation until the trigger shot is administered. While ultrasound confirmation is not required during the luteal phase, it is necessary to confirm downregulation with an ultrasound on day 2 or 3 of menses. During this evaluation, follicles are measured, and the presence of any larger than 10 mm could indicate asynchronous follicular response if treatment proceeds in that cycle. Serum estradiol levels below 30 pg/mL further verify downregulation before starting stimulation.

The GnRH antagonist protocol typically starts on day 2 or 3 of menstruation. For this protocol, it is crucial to confirm follicular synchronicity and that all follicles are smaller than 10 mm. Asynchronous follicular growth can increase the likelihood of cycle cancellation and result in a suboptimal response to ovarian stimulation as discussed earlier for GnRh agonist protocol.

Once the day 2–3 ultrasound confirms that conditions are optimal, exogenous gonadotropins are initiated to promote multi-follicular development. The primary goal is to obtain multiple mature, good-quality oocytes. Accurate monitoring of follicular size and number is crucial for a successful assisted reproductive treatment process [49]. During follicular tracking, the mean diameter of each follicle is measured, and their growth is closely followed (Fig. 5.17). The ultrasound image is frozen when the follicle diameter appears maximal, and the longest and widest follicle dimensions at 90-degree angles to each other are recorded. To ensure accuracy, the mean maximal follicle diameter is calculated by averaging measurements from at least two different dimensions.

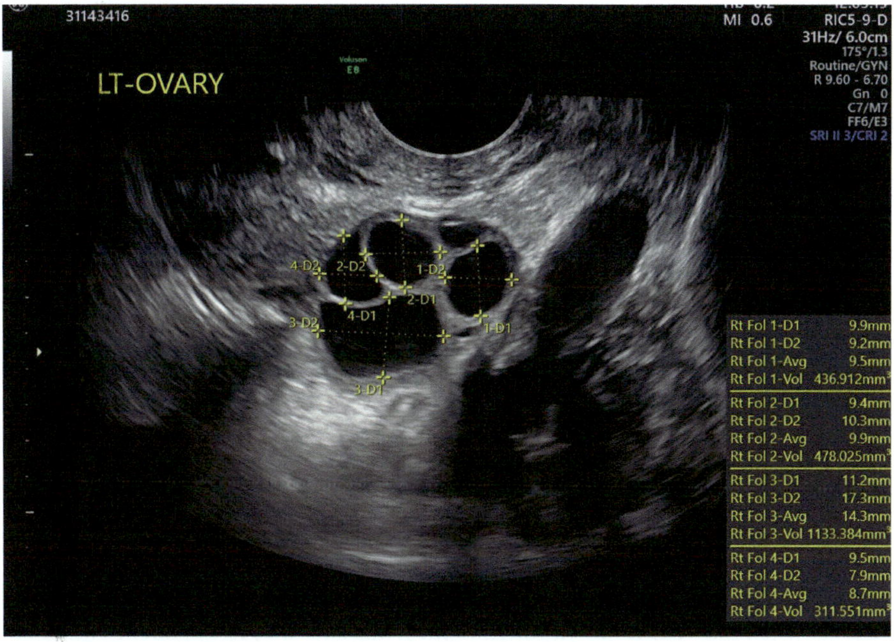

Fig. 5.17 Follicle measurements are taken along two perpendicular axes

The foundation of follicular tracking is to ensure that adequate stimulation is occurring and to identify patients at risk of ovarian hyperstimulation or insufficient follicle growth. Additionally, it is crucial to time final follicular maturation, which is essential for inducing the resumption of meiosis prior to oocyte retrieval.

Once a follicle grows beyond 10 mm, it is expected to grow at an average rate of approximately 1.69 ± 0.02 mm per day [50] or 1–2 mm per day. To enhance accuracy in tracking follicular development, serial ultrasonographic studies are conducted alongside regular serum measurements of estradiol, luteinizing hormone (LH), and progesterone levels. This dual approach continues until the follicles reach a size of 16–22 mm, at which point a trigger injection is administered to induce their final maturation [51]. Type of trigger is also chosen according to the number of follicles on the day of trigger. On the day of the trigger shot (usually human chorionic gonadotropin (hCG) or a gonadotropin releasing hormone (GnRH) agonist), if there are more than 17 follicles larger than 10 mm, the patient may be at increased risk for OHSS. Moreover, the estradiol (E2) level is also considered. High estradiol levels (>3500 pg/mL) combined with a large number of follicles increase the likelihood of developing OHSS [6].

The decision on which trigger medication to use, as well as its dosage, is critical in preventing OHSS and is based on comprehensive and final follicular measurement data.

5.10 Early Pregnancy Ultrasound

Post-embryo transfer, a patient can resume regular daily activities. Initial serum hCG is usually obtained 12 days after oocyte collection. In frozen embryo transfers, hCG is drawn 9 days after blastocyst transfer or 11 days after cleavage stage embryo. These timings align with an expected 4 weeks of gestational age in pregnancy.

Once a positive hCG result is obtained, a follow-up hCG test is performed 48-hours later to determine if the rise in hCG levels is consistent with a viable intrauterine pregnancy. The ratio of serum hCG at 48 hours compared to the initial level is predictive of pregnancy viability. A ratio greater than 1.66 (indicating an hCG rise of more than 66% at 48 hours) suggests a viable intrauterine pregnancy, whereas a ratio less than 0.87 (indicating an hCG decrease of more than 13%) suggests spontaneous pregnancy resolution [52].

If the rise in hCG is inappropriate, possible outcomes may include nonviable intrauterine pregnancy or an ectopic pregnancy.

Transvaginal ultrasound is the most useful imaging test for determining the location and viability of pregnancy. The hCG discriminatory zone is the serum hCG level above which a gestational sac should be visible when an intrauterine pregnancy is present. Studies show that a gestational sac was visualized in 80% of patients when the hCG level was at 1500 mIU/mL and in 99% of patients when the hCG level reached 3510 mIU/mL [53].

Anembryonic pregnancy, often referred to as a "blighted ovum," is a type of nonviable pregnancy characterized by the presence of a gestational sac that does not contain a yolk sac or embryo. This condition is diagnosed when no embryo is seen in a gestational sac with mean diameter ≥25 mm or ≥2 weeks after a scan showing gestational sac without yolk sac or embryo [54, 55].

Transvaginal ultrasound findings are crucial for accurately diagnosing an ectopic pregnancy and differentiating it from other possible conditions like a normal intrauterine pregnancy or ovarian cysts. The presence of a gestational sac containing a yolk sac or embryo located outside the uterus is the most specific ultrasonographic sign of an ectopic pregnancy [56]. Complex inhomogeneous extraovarian mass or an extraovarian mass containing an empty gestational sac are considered suggestive findings of an ectopic pregnancy [54, 57]. Fluid

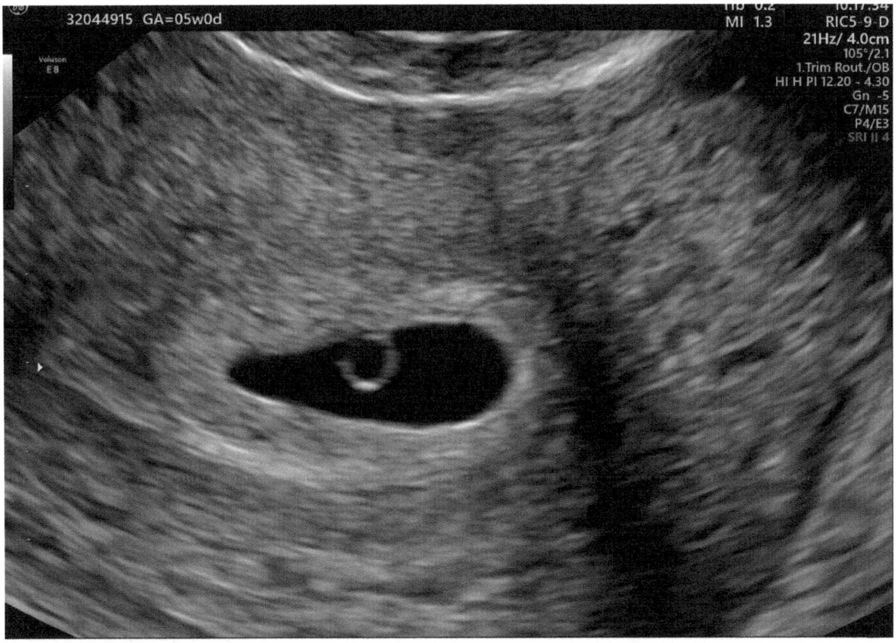

Fig. 5.18 A gestational sac with a yolk sac is visualized at 5 weeks of gestation

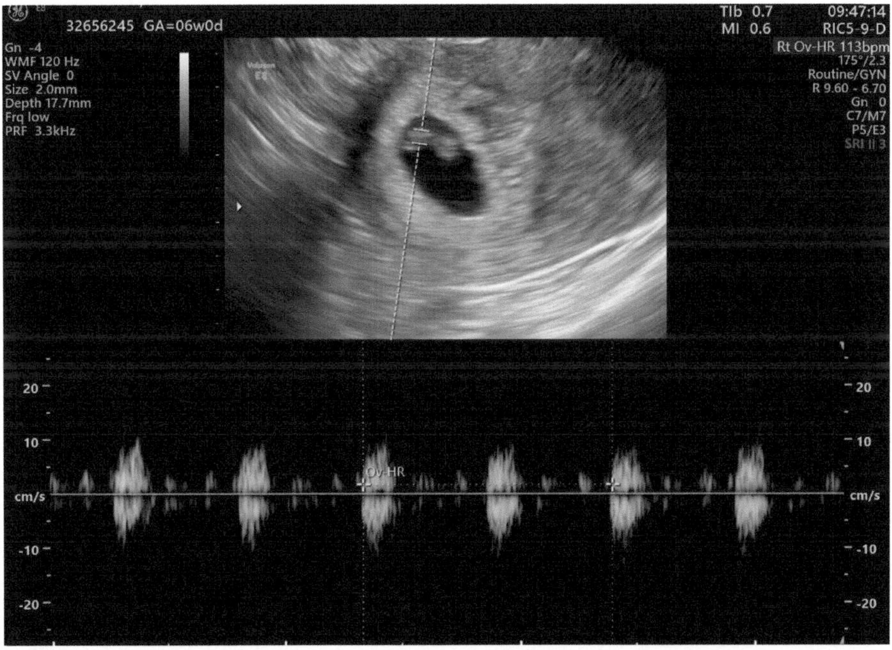

Fig. 5.19 Crown-rump length (CRL) measurement at 6 weeks of gestation, indicating the presence of a positive fetal heartbeat

with debris, consistent with blood, found in the pelvic cul-de-sac, is indicative of a ruptured ectopic pregnancy.

If the hCG test is positive and the rise in levels is appropriate, an ultrasound evaluation is typically scheduled approximately 4 weeks later, which corresponds to around 6 weeks of gestational age.

The gestational sac is the earliest sonographic indicator of an intrauterine pregnancy, typically detectable by 4.5 to 5 weeks of gestation [58]. Within the gestational sac, the yolk sac is the first anatomical structure to appear, providing confirmation of an intrauterine pregnancy. It is characterized by a spherical shape with a sonolucent center and an echogenic perimeter [59] (Fig. 5.18). The embryo is generally measurable at 6 to 7 weeks of gestation (Fig. 5.19).

Once a fetal heartbeat is detected, the patient is referred for early prenatal care and provided with information on healthy practices during early pregnancy.

5.11 Conclusion

In summary, the integration of ultrasound imaging into reproductive health has revolutionized the diagnosis and management of various gynecological conditions and infertility treatments. This non-invasive technique facilitates a thorough evaluation of reproductive anatomy and function, providing essential insights into ovarian reserve, uterine integrity, and fallopian tube patency. Throughout this chapter, we have highlighted the pivotal roles of baseline ultrasound, saline infusion sonography, and various tubal procedures in the comprehensive assessment of reproductive health.

The ability to monitor ovarian response during fertility treatments through ultrasonography not only optimizes patient outcomes but also enables timely interventions to mitigate risks associated with ovarian hyperstimulation syndrome (OHSS). Additionally, early pregnancy ultrasounds are crucial for confirming intrauterine pregnancies and identifying potential complications, such as ectopic pregnancies or anembryonic pregnancies, thereby guiding clinical decision-making.

References

1. Peck JD, et al. Lifestyle factors associated with histologically derived human ovarian non-growing follicle count in reproductive age women. Hum Reprod. 2016;31(1):150–7.
2. Hansen KR, et al. A new model of reproductive aging: the decline in ovarian non-growing follicle number from birth to menopause. Hum Reprod. 2008;23(3):699–708.
3. Practice Committee of the American Society for Reproductive Medicine. Electronic address, a.a.o. and M. Practice Committee of the American Society for Reproductive. Fertility evaluation of infertile women: a committee opinion. Fertil Steril. 2021;116(5):1255–65.
4. Coelho Neto MA, et al. Counting ovarian antral follicles by ultrasound: a practical guide. Ultrasound Obstet Gynecol. 2018;51(1):10–20.
5. Practice Committee of the American Society for Reproductive Medicine. Electronic address, a.a.o. and M. Practice Committee of the American Society for Reproductive. Testing and interpreting measures of ovarian reserve: a committee opinion. Fertil Steril. 2020;114(6):1151–7.

6. Practice Committee of the American Society for Reproductive Medicine. Electronic address, A.a.o. and M. Practice Committee of the American Society for Reproductive. Prevention and treatment of moderate and severe ovarian hyperstimulation syndrome: a guideline. Fertil Steril. 2016;106(7):1634–47.
7. Ferraretti AP, et al. ESHRE consensus on the definition of 'poor response' to ovarian stimulation for in vitro fertilization: the Bologna criteria. Hum Reprod. 2011;26(7):1616–24.
8. Jayaprakasan K, et al. Prediction of in vitro fertilization outcome at different antral follicle count thresholds in a prospective cohort of 1,012 women. Fertil Steril. 2012;98(3):657–63.
9. Andreotti RF, et al. O-RADS US risk stratification and management system: a consensus guideline from the ACR ovarian-adnexal reporting and data system committee. Radiology. 2020;294(1):168–85.
10. Exacoustos C, et al. Isolated ovarian endometrioma: a history between myth and reality. J Minim Invasive Gynecol. 2018;25(5):884–91.
11. Ghezzi F, et al. "Kissing ovaries": a sonographic sign of moderate to severe endometriosis. Fertil Steril. 2005;83(1):143–7.
12. Hernandez-Nieto C, et al. Conservative treatment versus surgical excision of ovarian dermoid cysts: impact on ovarian stimulation and IVF cycle success. Int J Gynaecol Obstet. 2020;148(3):392–8.
13. Zeyneloglu HB, Arici A, Olive DL. Adverse effects of hydrosalpinx on pregnancy rates after in vitro fertilization-embryo transfer. Fertil Steril. 1998;70(3):492–9.
14. Guerriero S, et al. Systematic approach to sonographic evaluation of the pelvis in women with suspected endometriosis, including terms, definitions and measurements: a consensus opinion from the international deep endometriosis analysis (IDEA) group. Ultrasound Obstet Gynecol. 2016;48(3):318–32.
15. Gerges B, et al. Sonographic evaluation of immobility of normal and endometriotic ovary in detection of deep endometriosis. Ultrasound Obstet Gynecol. 2017;49(6):793–8.
16. Erden M, et al. The effect of </=6 cm sized noncavity-distorting intramural fibroids on in vitro fertilization outcomes: a systematic review and meta-analysis. Fertil Steril. 2023;119(6):996–1007.
17. Munro MG, et al. The FIGO classification of causes of abnormal uterine bleeding in the reproductive years. Fertil Steril. 2011;95(7):2204–8, 2208 e1–3.
18. Palheta MS, Medeiros FDC, Severiano ARG. Reporting of uterine fibroids on ultrasound examinations: an illustrated report template focused on surgical planning. Radiol Bras. 2023;56(2):86–94.
19. Harmsen MJ, et al. Consensus on revised definitions of Morphological Uterus Sonographic Assessment (MUSA) features of adenomyosis: results of modified Delphi procedure. Ultrasound Obstet Gynecol. 2022;60(1):118–31.
20. Ferenczy A. Pathophysiology of adenomyosis. Hum Reprod Update. 1998;4(4):312–22.
21. Younes G, Tulandi T. Effects of adenomyosis on in vitro fertilization treatment outcomes: a meta-analysis. Fertil Steril. 2017;108(3):483–490 e3.
22. Nijkang NP, et al. Endometrial polyps: pathogenesis, sequelae and treatment. SAGE Open Med. 2019;7:2050312119848247.
23. Perez-Medina T, et al. Endometrial polyps and their implication in the pregnancy rates of patients undergoing intrauterine insemination: a prospective, randomized study. Hum Reprod. 2005;20(6):1632–5.
24. La Torre R, et al. Transvaginal sonographic evaluation of endometrial polyps: a comparison with two dimensional and three dimensional contrast sonography. Clin Exp Obstet Gynecol. 1999;26(3–4):171–3.
25. Hooker AB, et al. Systematic review and meta-analysis of intrauterine adhesions after miscarriage: prevalence, risk factors and long-term reproductive outcome. Hum Reprod Update. 2014;20(2):262–78.
26. Schenker JG. Etiology of and therapeutic approach to synechia uteri. Eur J Obstet Gynecol Reprod Biol. 1996;65(1):109–13.

27. Huang R, et al. Value of 2D ultrasonography in the diagnosis and evaluation of intrauterine adhesions - a prospective study. Reprod Biomed Online. 2024;49(2):103771.
28. Amin TN, Saridogan E, Jurkovic D. Ultrasound and intrauterine adhesions: a novel structured approach to diagnosis and management. Ultrasound Obstet Gynecol. 2015;46(2):131–9.
29. Chan YY, et al. The prevalence of congenital uterine anomalies in unselected and high-risk populations: a systematic review. Hum Reprod Update. 2011;17(6):761–71.
30. Grimbizis GF, et al. The ESHRE/ESGE consensus on the classification of female genital tract congenital anomalies. Hum Reprod. 2013;28(8):2032–44.
31. Practice Committee of the American Society for Reproductive Medicine. Electronic address, a.a.o. Evidence-based diagnosis and treatment for uterine septum: a guideline. Fertil Steril. 2024;122(2):251–65.
32. Valle RF, Ekpo GE. Hysteroscopic metroplasty for the septate uterus: review and meta-analysis. J Minim Invasive Gynecol. 2013;20(1):22–42.
33. Jayaprakasan K, Ojha K. Diagnosis of congenital uterine abnormalities: practical considerations. J Clin Med. 2022;11(5):1251.
34. Grimbizis GF, et al. The Thessaloniki ESHRE/ESGE consensus on diagnosis of female genital anomalies. Gynecol Surg. 2016;13:1–16.
35. Grigore M, et al. The added value of three-dimensional ultrasonography in uterine pathology. Exp Ther Med. 2021;22(5):1261.
36. Kumar K, et al. Utility of saline infusion sonohysterography in gynecology: a review article. Cureus. 2023;15(2):e35424.
37. Seshadri S, et al. The evolving role of saline infusion sonography (SIS) in infertility. Eur J Obstet Gynecol Reprod Biol. 2015;185:66–73.
38. Dessole S, et al. Side effects and complications of sonohysterosalpingography. Fertil Steril. 2003;80(3):620–4.
39. Nako Y, et al. A large study about reproductive factors that predict hysterosalpingography-identified tubal pathology: an insight into the necessity of preconception screening. J Clin Med. 2024;14(1):179.
40. Excellence, N.I.o.H.a. Fertility problems: assessment and treatment. 2017; Available from: www.nice.org.uk/guidance/cg156.
41. Infertility Workup for the Women's Health Specialist: ACOG Committee opinion, number 781 Obstet Gynecol. 2019;133(6):e377–84.
42. Maheux-Lacroix S, et al. Hysterosalpingosonography for diagnosing tubal occlusion in subfertile women: a systematic review with meta-analysis. Hum Reprod. 2014;29(5):953–63.
43. Saunders RD, Shwayder JM, Nakajima ST. Current methods of tubal patency assessment. Fertil Steril. 2011;95(7):2171–9.
44. Winfield AC, et al. Apparent cornual occlusion in hysterosalpingography: reversal by glucagon. AJR Am J Roentgenol. 1982;139(3):525–7.
45. Stumpf PG, March CM. Febrile morbidity following hysterosalpingography: identification of risk factors and recommendations for prophylaxis. Fertil Steril. 1980;33(5):487–92.
46. van Welie N, et al. Can hysterosalpingo-foam sonography replace hysterosalpingography as first-choice tubal patency test? A randomized non-inferiority trial. Hum Reprod. 2022;37(5):969–79.
47. Exacoustos C, et al. Can tubal flushing with Hysterosalpingo-Foam Sonography (HyFoSy) media increase women's chances of pregnancy? J Minim Invasive Gynecol. 2015;22(6S):S238.
48. Dreyer K, et al. Hysterosalpingo-foam sonography, a less painful procedure for tubal patency testing during fertility workup compared with (serial) hysterosalpingography: a randomized controlled trial. Fertil Steril. 2014;102(3):821–5.
49. Martins WP, et al. Ultrasound for monitoring controlled ovarian stimulation: a systematic review and meta-analysis of randomized controlled trials. Ultrasound Obstet Gynecol. 2014;43(1):25–33.
50. Baerwald AR, Walker RA, Pierson RA. Growth rates of ovarian follicles during natural menstrual cycles, oral contraception cycles, and ovarian stimulation cycles. Fertil Steril. 2009;91(2):440–9.

51. Wittmaack FM, et al. Effect of follicular size on oocyte retrieval, fertilization, cleavage, and embryo quality in in vitro fertilization cycles: a 6-year data collection. Fertil Steril. 1994;62(6):1205–10.
52. Condous G, et al. Failing pregnancies of unknown location: a prospective evaluation of the human chorionic gonadotrophin ratio. BJOG. 2006;113(5):521–7.
53. Connolly A, et al. Reevaluation of discriminatory and threshold levels for serum beta-hCG in early pregnancy. Obstet Gynecol. 2013;121(1):65–70.
54. Dogra V, Paspulati RM, Bhatt S. First trimester bleeding evaluation. Ultrasound Q. 2005;21(2):69–85; quiz 149–50, 153–4.
55. Doubilet PM, et al. Diagnostic criteria for nonviable pregnancy early in the first trimester. N Engl J Med. 2013;369(15):1443–51.
56. Webster K, et al. Ectopic pregnancy and miscarriage: diagnosis and initial management: summary of updated NICE guidance. BMJ. 2019;367:l6283.
57. Dialani V, Levine D. Ectopic pregnancy: a review. Ultrasound Q. 2004;20(3):105–17.
58. Bree RL, et al. Transvaginal sonography in the evaluation of normal early pregnancy: correlation with HCG level. AJR Am J Roentgenol. 1989;153(1):75–9.
59. Laing FC, Frates M. Ultrasound evaluation during the first trimester of pregnancy. In: Callen PW, editor. Ultrasonography in obstetrics and gynecology. Philadelphia: WB Saunders Co; 2000.

Controlled Ovarian Stimulation with or Without Intrauterine Insemination

6

Rose Mary Weidner

Acronyms

AMH	Anti-Mullerian Hormone
AFC	Antral Follicle Count
AI	Aromatase Inhibitor
ART	Assisted Reproductive Technology
ASRM	American Society for Reproductive Medicine
BhCG	Beta Human Chorionic Gonadotropin (pregnancy test result)
BMI	Body Mass Index
CC	Clomiphene Citrate
CFAS	Canadian Fertility and Andrology Society
COS	Controlled Ovarian Stimulation
CP	Clinical Pregnancy
CPR	Clinical Pregnancy Rate
ED	Emergency Department
EMT	Endometrial Thickness
ESHRE	European Society of Human Reproduction and Embryology
FDA	Food and Drug Administration
FSH	Follicle Stimulating Hormone
GnRH antagonist	Gonadotropin Releasing Hormone Antagonist
GND	Gonadotropins
HCG	Human Chorionic Gonadotropin

R. M. Weidner (✉)
McGill University Health Center Reproductive Center, Montreal, QC, Canada

McGill University Health Center, Montreal, QC, Canada
e-mail: rose-mary.weidner@muhc.mcgill.ca

M. Das, M. H. Dahan (eds.), *A Comprehensive Guide to Reproductive Health and Infertility Medicine for Nurses*, https://doi.org/10.1007/978-3-032-24372-0_6

HIV	Human Immunodeficiency Virus
HMG	Human Menopausal Gonadotropin
HSG	Hysterosalpingography
IM	Intramuscular
IUI	Intrauterine Insemination
IVF	In Vitro Fertilization
LBR	Live Birth Rate
LH	Luteinizing Hormone
LTZ	Letrozole (aromatase inhibitor)
MFI	Male Factor Infertility
MGP	Multiple Gestational Pregnancy
MPR	Multiple Pregnancy Rates
OHSS	Ovarian Hyper Stimulation Syndrome
OI	Ovulation Induction
OPK	Ovulation Predictor Kit
OS	Ovarian Stimulation
NORDS	Nordic Association of Andrology
PCO	Polycystic Ovaries
PR	Pregnancy Rate
rFSH	Recombinant Follicle-Stimulating Hormone
rhCG	Recombinant Human Chorionic Gonadotropin
SERM	Selective Estrogen Receptor Modulator
SET	Single Embryo Transfer
STI	Sexually Transmitted Infections
TI	Timed Intercourse
TMSC	Total Motile Sperm Count
TVUS	Transvaginal Ultra Sound
UEI	Unexplained Infertility
UI	Unexplained Infertility
U hCG	Urinary Human Chorionic Gonadotropin
U/S	Ultrasound
WHO	World Health Organization

6.1 Objectives

1. Review causes of infertility.
2. Explain the indications for use of intrauterine insemination (IUI).
3. Describe the optimal conditions for performing IUI treatments.
4. Identify the prerequisites for IUI.
5. Compare the varying treatment approaches that may be used: expectant management, timed intercourse (TI) with or without controlled ovarian stimulation (COS), IUI in a natural cycle, IUI with COS using oral or injectable medication.
6. Outline the phases of IUI treatment.

7. Follicle stimulation: Describe the protocols and different medication used in IUI with natural cycle or COS using clomiphene citrate (CC) and letrozole (LTZ), IUI using low dose or traditional gonadotropins recombinant follicle-stimulating hormone (rFSH) or human chorionic gonadotropin (HMG), IUI using a combination of oral and injectable hormones, or IUI using a gonadotropin-releasing hormone (GnRH) antagonist.
8. Explain ovulation monitoring of luteinizing hormone (LH testing) or through ultrasound (U/S) and the consequent timing for ovulation induction for IUI or timed intercourse.
9. Distinguish between the different types of methods used to prepare sperm for IUI.
10. Describe the IUI procedure.
11. Describe the indications for luteal support using progesterone.
12. Give the rationale for post-procedure teachings and interventions.
13. Explore the success rates of different treatments.
14. Describe the complications that may occur with IUI such as OHSS, multiple pregnancies, infection, spotting or cramping, ectopic pregnancy, or spontaneous abortion (SAB).
15. Elaborate on the role of the nurse in COS/IUI treatments.
16. Review the professional guidelines of ASRM CFAS, ESHRE, WHO.
17. Examine the newest trends in COS.

The acronyms used are listed at the end of the chapter.?or at the begining of the chapter as per editor preference.

6.2 Introduction

Infertility affects up to 15% of couples in childbearing age [1, 2]. The use of controlled ovarian stimulation (COS) is a cornerstone in fertility management. By pharmacologically stimulating the ovaries to produce multiple follicles, COS increases the chances of conception compared to natural cycles. While COS is often associated with in vitro fertilization (IVF), it is also commonly utilized alongside intrauterine insemination (IUI) or timed intercourse (TI).

Intrauterine insemination (IUI) or timed intercourse (TI) in a cycle with or without controlled ovarian stimulation (COS), using oral or injectable hormones, may be a good treatment option for couples or individuals trying to get pregnant. IUI treatments, compared to more advanced treatments like IVF, are less invasive and demanding physically, require less medication, and are more affordable. Couples or individuals availing of IUI may include those with unexplained infertility (UI), polyendocrine metabolic ovarian syndrome (PMOS), mild male factor infertility (MFI), or populations using donor sperm.

Intrauterine insemination (IUI) is an assisted reproductive technology (ART) that involves placing prepared sperm directly into the uterus at the time of ovulation to increase the chances of fertilization. This procedure increases the number of sperm that reach the egg by bypassing the cervix and making it easier for fertilization to occur. The aim of COS IUI should be to optimize success rates using low-cost means to accomplish a singleton pregnancy and to avoid the risk of a multiple gestational pregnancy (MGP).This chapter aims to guide fertility nurses on COS procedures using IUI from a clinical, educational, and emotional aspect.

6.2.1 Infertility Review

Infertility is defined as the inability to achieve a pregnancy after 12 months of unprotected and regular intercourse [1]. Infertility affects 1 in 6 to 7 couples worldwide [1, 2]. The infertility may be attributed to male, female, or unexplained causes [1].

In the *female* reproductive system, infertility may be caused by:

- *Blocked fallopian tubes* which may be a result of sexually transmitted infections (STIs) that were not treated, abdominal or pelvic surgery, complications from an abortion that was not safely done, or postpartum sepsis [1].
- *Disorders of the uterus* which may include endometriosis that can result in chronic inflammation, which in turn can cause scar tissue affecting the fallopian tubes, or the uterus may have congenital malformations such as a septate uterus or benign fibroids [1].
- *Ovarian disorders* such as polycystic ovaries (PCO) or other follicular disorders [1].
- *Endocrine disorders* that may manifest as an imbalance of reproductive hormones found in the hypothalamus and pituitary glands. Examples of these could be pituitary cancers or hypopituitarism [1].

In the *male* reproductive system, infertility may be caused by:

- *Mechanical obstruction* of the male reproductive tract that impedes the semen from being ejaculated. The blockage may occur in the ejaculatory duct or seminal vesicles and may be caused by injury or infection of the genital tract [1].
- *Hormonal disorders* that result in abnormal hormones found in the pituitary gland, hypothalamus, or testicles. Testosterone is one of the hormones that controls sperm production. Pituitary or testicular cancers are some examples of these disorders [1].
- *Failure of the testicles to produce sperm* due to varicoceles or from medical treatments such as chemotherapy that may impede the sperm-producing cells [1].
- *An abnormal sperm quality and function* that may cause an abnormal shape (morphology) or movement (motility) [1]. Anabolic steroids can cause abnormal sperm shape and sperm count [3].

6.2.2 Indications for Intrauterine Insemination (IUI)

IUI is used for a variety of infertility issues, including:

(a) *Mild Male Factor Infertility*
  - Mild male factor infertility (MFI) is defined as a low sperm count or poor motility, which can limit natural conception.
  - Rationale for IUI: Sperm processing before IUI selects the best sperm and will bypass cervical barriers with more chance of conception if two follicles are stimulated producing two oocytes compared to a spontaneous ovulation in which only one oocyte is released.

(b) *Unexplained Infertility*
  - Unexplained infertility (UI) is when all standard tests (tubal patency, ovulation, semen) are normal, but no pregnancy occurs. Approximately 15–30% of couples receive this diagnosis.
  - Rationale for IUI: IUI offers a controlled and enhanced chance of fertilization, particularly with multifolliculogenesis.

(c) *Ovulatory Dysfunction*
  - Ovulatory dysfunction occurs when a woman has irregular menstrual cycles or anovulation which is the absence of ovulation (e.g., PMOS).
  - Rationale for IUI: IUI is combined with ovulation induction to time insemination precisely.

(d) *Donor Insemination*
  - Donor insemination (DI) is used for single women, for same-sex couples, or for those with severe male infertility.
  - Rationale for IUI: Sperm from an approved donor bank is used. Rigorous standards are used to screen the donor and test the sperm in accordance with regulatory standards and the sperm donor is usually fertile.

(e) *Immunological Infertility*
  - Immunological infertility occurs when there is a presence of anti-sperm antibodies in the male or female.
  - Rationale for IUI: IUI may help reduce exposure to antibodies by using washed sperm.

(f) *Cervical Factor Infertility*
  - Cervical factor infertility may occur in the presence of a thick or hostile cervical mucus that might inhibit sperm passage.
  - Rationale for IUI: IUI places sperm directly into the uterus, bypassing this obstacle [4].

(g) *Sexual Dysfunction*
  - Sexual dysfunction such as erectile dysfunction or ejaculatory disorders may lead to lack of sexual intercourse.
  - Rationale for IUI: IUI allows potential conception by using collected sperm without intercourse.

(h) *Serodiscordant Couples*
  - Serodiscordant couples are defined as having one partner who is affected by a viral infection such as HIV, hepatitis C [5], or hepatitis B and the other partner is not affected.
  - Rationale for IUI: Sperm washing separates sperm from the seminal fluid and is then used for intrauterine insemination hoping to decrease chances of transmission to the female or avoiding unprotected intercourse for the male when he is negative for the infection. Washed sperm for IUI is more commonly used to prevent Hepatitis and HIV infection in Europe than it is in North America when IVF and ICSI are often preferred.

6.2.3 Optimal Conditions for IUI Treatment

Certain conditions are felt to provide the best possibility of achieving a pregnancy. These conditions are:

- The number of spermatozoa with progressive motility present in the ejaculate total motile sperm count (TMSC) should be above 9–15 million post-wash [5].
- The female should have patency of both fallopian tubes but can get pregnant with unilateral tubal patency if there are no signs of pelvic adhesions [5].
- Female age should be <40 as females over 40 years of age have decreased pregnancy rates. However, the rates may be higher if using donor sperm [5].
- No diagnosis of endometriosis, although minimal or mild endometriosis may also be an indicator for IUI [4].
- Short duration of infertility [6] (less than 3 years).
- BMI < 30 kg/m^2 or < 18.5 kg/m^2 [7].
- AFC > 5 [8].

6.2.4 Prerequisites for IUI

Before IUI, a thorough evaluation will ensure that the couple is suitable for this treatment. The following assessments may be done:

(a) *Tubal Patency*
  - Tubal patency looks to establish that at least one fallopian tube should be open to proceed with IUI.
  - Tests used to assess tubal patency: *hysterosalpingography (HSG)*, *sonohysterosalpingography (HYCOSY)*, *diagnostic laparoscopy*.

(b) *Ovarian Reserve Assessment*
  - Examining the ovarian reserve will determine if the woman has a good number of eggs left.

- This can be done by using the following: Blood tests to document FSH and AMH levels and an Ultrasound (U/S) to measure the *Antral Follicle Count* (AFC), these tests are usually done between day 2–5 of the menstrual cycle.
- In one study, AMH monitoring was found to be superior to FSH monitoring in predicting high and good responders to COS. FSH was found to be a better indicator for predicting egg quality [9]. In another study, it was found that women <35 year of age with a low AMH conceived as often as the same aged females with a normal AMH. This study also agreed that AMH influenced the ovarian response and not the pregnancy success rates. The response was no different in women with low AMH versus normal AMH when using oral COS, but when using injectable gonadotropins, the women with low AMH levels needed higher doses [10].

(c) *Semen Analysis*
- The results of a semen analysis should meet certain minimum criteria (e.g., total motile sperm count >5 million).
- Semen samples with poor parameters may be unsuitable unless processed optimally.
- In a published guideline, they were unable to define a clear guideline as to the lower cutoff levels of pre- and post-washed sperm in which IUI should be held [11].

6.2.5 Treatment Approaches

Once the individual or couples have conducted the required testing, different treatment options may be chosen based on the likely hood of success as assessed by the physician or due to patient preferences.

(a) *Expectant management in unexplained infertility (UI):* defined as not intervening but rather waiting.
- The cumulative pregnancy rate over 2 years may be as high as 72% in young women <35. It decreases in women >35 (45%) and is 30% in couples with >5 years of UI [12].
- In couples with a good prognosis (age and duration of infertility), expectant management can be effective [13].
- Expectant management could be effective in women <35 years of age with a shorter infertility duration.
- Therefore, expectant management would not be beneficial for women >35 or with infertility >5 years. Most centers would initiate care after 3 years of infertility.

(b) *Controlled ovarian stimulation (COS) or natural cycle with or without ovulation induction (OI)*
- In COS, the female is given medication that stimulates follicle growth using oral clomiphene citrate (CC) or letrozole (LTZ), or injectable recombinant

follicle-stimulating hormone (rFSH) or human menopausal gonadotropin (HMG) agents. The hope is that more than one follicle may grow.

- In a natural cycle, no medication is used to stimulate the follicle growth and only one dominant follicle matures.
- Monitoring includes ultrasound and hormone levels such as luteinizing hormone (LH) and progesterone (P4) to estimate ovulation. Estradiol (E2) levels may be monitored to correlate with follicle growth.
- Ovulation may occur naturally, but to predict this, one can measure serum LH and P4 levels or by using ovulation predictor kits (OPK) or blood tests. In most cases, ovulation predictor kits measure urine LH levels only, and a level above 20 IU/L is considered positive. Some women with PMOS can have such a level without ovulating in the presence of a lack of folliculogenesis. If too much fluid is consumed, levels may test as negative despite ovulation having occurred using urinary tests.
- Once ovulation is imminent, ovulation induction may be done by administering a "trigger shot" of human chorionic gonadotropin (HCG) medication.

(c) *Intrauterine Insemination (IUI) or Timed Intercourse (TI)*

- In preparation for IUI, sperm is "washed" and inserted into the uterus close to ovulation. Washing removes dead sperm, inflammatory cells, and prostaglandins which would cause strong uterine contractions expelling the sperm if placed directly in the uterus without preparation.
- During TI, intercourse is timed to correspond to expected ovulation.
- Timing: either IUI or TI is planned for 0–40 hours after hCG trigger or 24 hours post-LH surge [11, 14, 15].
- *Luteal support* with progesterone is often prescribed, especially in cycles in which injectable gonadotropins (GND) are administered.

6.2.6 Phases of IUI Treatment

Phases of IUI treatment are listed below but will be explained in more detail later.

(a) *Follicular stimulation*

- Follicular growth of oocytes occurs naturally or via controlled ovarian stimulation (COS).

(b) *Ovulation induction*

- Ovulation induction may need to be performed by injecting human chorionic gonadotropin (hCG) medication or ovulation may occur naturally. The female patient may be monitored by vaginal ultrasounds(U/S) to determine the size of the follicle(s), or ovulation can be measured by measuring LH and P4 levels [16].

(c) *Sperm preparation*
- Sperm preparation is performed by using one of the following techniques: swim-up technique, density gradient centrifugation or simple wash.

(d) *Insemination*
- IUI is performed by placing a catheter into the uterus via the cervix. The catheter is attached to a syringe and a small amount, 0.3 mL to 0.5 mL, of spermatozoid is inserted into the uterus.

(e) *Post-procedure care*
- Once the procedure is completed, the woman can remain on bedrest immediately after the procedure for up to 10–15 minutes or may go on with her regular activities.
- *Luteal support* which involves a progesterone supplement (vaginally or intramuscular) can be administered post-ovulation/IUI the following day or 7–8 days post-ovulation/IUI.
- A beta human chorionic gonadotropin (BhCG) test either done by a urine or blood sample is done 14–16 days post-IUI or post-TI. The timing of the sample may vary from clinic to clinic. A woman will be considered 4 weeks pregnant at this time.
- A viability ultrasound (U/S) is usually scheduled between week 6 and 7 of gestation, follow-up U/S may be conducted as per clinic policy, and a referral to an obstetrician is given for follow-up.
- If complications occur, further blood tests, U/S, or interventions may be required. This will be discussed in the section dealing with complications.
- If the pregnancy test is negative, the patient may repeat cycles of IUI as ordered.
- Patients are asked to follow up with their doctor if the amount of IUIs ordered has been unsuccessful or if there were complications.
- The physicain may order additional IUI cycles or may decide to order further investigations. The physiican and patient or couple may decide to progress to In Vitro Fertilization (IVF).

6.2.7 Follicle-Stimulating Protocols

Physiology of Ovulation and the Rationale for COS

The natural menstrual cycle is governed by complex hormonal feedback mechanisms involving the hypothalamus, pituitary gland, and ovaries. Typically, one dominant follicle develops under the influence of follicle-stimulating hormone (FSH) and luteinizing hormone (LH), culminating in ovulation around mid-cycle (day 14 in a 28-day cycle). In a regular menstrual cycle, an LH surge usual occurs 11–16 days prior to menstruation [5].

COS artificially modulates this hormonal interplay to promote the development of multiple follicles, increasing the probability of fertilization and conception. By carefully administering exogenous agents, COS overcomes suboptimal endogenous hormonal responses, treats anovulatory disorders, and enhances the efficiency of conception attempts, particularly in unexplained infertility, mild male factor infertility, and ovulatory dysfunctions [14].

Ovarian stimulation may occur naturally without any follicle-stimulating medication or with COS, which may include oral or injectable hormones that can be taken to increase the number of oocytes (eggs) available.

(a) *Natural Cycle IUI*
- In natural cycle IUI, no medication is administered. It is only used for women with regular ovulation.
- *Advantages*: Low-cost, low multiple pregnancy rates.
- *Disadvantages*: Low success rates unless no contact with sperm.

(b) *Clomiphene Citrate (CC)*

Clomiphene citrate (CC), a selective estrogen receptor modulator (SERM), inhibits estrogen receptors in the hypothalamus, resulting in increased secretion of gonadotropin-releasing hormone (GnRH) and subsequent FSH and LH release with follicular development [17–19].

This is a first-line oral agent.
- *Dose:* 50–150 mg daily for 5 days, starting on cycle day 2–5 [15, 18, 20].
- *Advantages*: Low cost, ease of use.
- *Disadvantages*: Potential anti-estrogenic effects on endometrium and cervical mucus, lower pregnancy rates compared to newer agents.
- *Nursing consideration:* monitor for mood swings, visual disturbances, and thin endometrial lining which may decrease implantation [18, 20]. Common side effects may include hot flashes, abdominal distention, breast tenderness, nausea, and headache [21]. Should not be taken for more than 12 months in a lifetime since it can then raise the risks of ovarian cancers.

(iii) *Letrozole*

Another oral option is letrozole (LTZ) which is an aromatase inhibitor (AI) that reduces estrogen production, therefore stimulating FSH release [20].
- This treatment option is favored in women with polyendocrine metabolic ovarian syndrome (PMOS) or CC-resistant cases.
- However, it is important to note that LTZ is not approved by the Food and Drug Administration (FDA) in the USA for ovulation induction.
- This is the medication of choice for PMOS in Australia and in most countries including the USA.
- *Dose:* 2.5–7.5 mg daily for 5 days starting from day 2–5 [15, 20]. Most women do not receive more than 5 mg daily.

- *Benefits:* LTZ tends to produce more monofollicular cycles and thus is found to have a lower multiple pregnancy rates compared to clomiphene citrate [22].
- *Other Advantages:* LTZ has been found to exhibit better endometrial thickness and improved cervical mucus than seen with clomiphene citrate [23].
- *Evidence*: Multiple randomized trials and meta-analyses have demonstrated higher live birth rates with letrozole compared to CC, particularly among anovulatory women [22, 23].
- *Nursing consideration:* LTZ is preferred in patients with PMOS due to the low risk of multiple gestational pregnancy and better endometrial response and higher live birth rates than CC [22, 23]. Side effects are usually mid to moderate and may consist of hot flashes, increased sweating, fatigue, joint pain, headache, swelling, back pain, and nausea [21].

(d) *Gonadotropins (FSH, HMG)*

Injectable gonadotropins (GND) include recombinant follicle-stimulating hormone (rFsh) or urinary-derived human menopausal gonadotropins (hMG). These GNDs directly stimulate the follicular growth in the ovaries [24].

Injectable gonadotropins directly stimulate the ovaries and are associated with a higher number of developing follicles.

- *Starting Dose:* initial low doses of 37.3 and 75 IU subcutaneously daily are started between days 2 and 4 of the cycle. The injections may be titrated based on ovarian response and body weight and increased at 5–7 day intervals [5].
- A low dose is preferred over conventional (>150 IU) dose GND due to the increased risk of multiple gestational pregnancy (MGP) with the later [11, 14].
- *Protocols:* Medication can be increased or decreased based on the patient's reponse. A low-dose protocol is preferred over traditional doses [13].
- Most evidence supports the use of progesterone to support the luteal phase after GND IUI or intercourse cycles. This is usually started 1–3 days post-insemination and should be continued until 7 to 12 weeks of pregnancy. It can be delivered as vaginal, oral, or injectable medications depending on what is available in your local area.
- *Advantages*: GND injections yield a higher ovulation rate and maybe higher pregnancy rates [25].
- *Disadvantages*: GND injections show an increased risk of multiple gestation and ovarian hyperstimulation syndrome (OHSS), are costly, and need intensive monitoring to avoid the above risks [11, 14].
- *Nursing consideration:* GND protocols require careful monitoring to avoid ovarian hyperstimulation syndrome (OHSS) and comprehensive injection training and support. *Educate patients* on medication schedules and possible

side effects of medication or OHSS symptoms. *Teach medication side effects*: hot flashes, mood swings, abdominal bloating, injection site reactions [26]. *Teach about OHSS symptoms:* nausea, vomiting, rapid weight gain, more severe ascities, thrombosis, renal failure [26]. *Teach and review injection techniques:* nurses or pharmacists may teach and review the injection techniques.

(e) *Combined protocols*
- Combines oral medication such as CC or LTZ with injectable gonadotropins (low dose).
- This aims to optimize follicular growth while minimizing the risks and costs associated with high-dose gonadotropins.
- *Advantages*: Multiple studies have shown increased pregnancy rates with combined LTZ and low dose GND [20, 27].
- *Disadvantages*: one of the disadvantages may be the cost of the GND injections as well as the complexity of injections versus oral medication.
- *Nursing considerations*: the nursing considerations would be the same for the oral and GND protocols above.

(f) *GnRH Antagonist use*

A Growth hormone relasing (GnRH) antagonist is a synethetic decapeptide. The antagonist causes a negative feedback effect of estrogen, which blocks the pituitary release of GnRH. This delays the early surge of LH which prevents premature ovulation and extends FSH-dependent follicular growth. It has been found to have a negative response on the oocytes [20].
- A GnRH antagonist may be added in the final days of stimulation once a lead follicle attains 12–14 mm to prevent premature ovulation, although this is not commonly done.
- This ensures that insemination can be properly timed and avoids cycle cancelation due to early ovulation.

Monitoring During the Treatment Cycle

- *Ultrasound*: Transvaginal ultrasounds (TVUS) are done for follicular tracking to track dominant follicle growth. A vaginal ultrasound is performed on day two or three of the menstrual cycle to rule out factors such as a functional cyst (benign cyst) [5] that may contraindicate starting the cycle and again between day 9 and 10 (of a 28 day cycle) or two days before an expected natural luteinizing hormone (LH) surge which usually occurs 16 days before the expected start of menstruation [5]. Further transvaginal ultrasounds (TVUS) may be required until the size of the lead follicle(s) measures 17-18 mm, which may indicate impending ovulation. A cycle may be cancelled if there are too many large follicles (i.e., 3 or more follicle >16 mm) [28, 29].
- The TVUS also measures the endometrial thickness (EMT) which ideally should be >7 mm to 8 mm, although some studies have shown that patients can still get pregnant with a thin endometrial lining. The studies state that it is the pattern of the endometrium that is most important for implantation rates [30, 31].

- TVUS is performed with an empty bladder. The average size of the follicles is measured as well as the endometrial thickness (EMT). The EMT is measured in the sagittal plane at the thickest portion near the fundus [30].
- *Hormone levels*: Follicle-stimulating hormone (FSH) and anti-Mullerian hormone (AMH) levels are usually assessed prior (usually every 12 months or as indicated) to commencing fertility treatment in order to guide the treatment and chosen medication and dose. During COS or natural cycle, the following may be tested: estradiol (E2) level—produced by the follicle(s), it is important for endometrial preparation, and it corresponds to follicle growth and size; luteinizing hormone (LH) level—triggers ovulation; and progesterone (P4) level—increases in the luteal phase.

6.2.8 Ovulation Induction and Timing of Insemination/ Timed Intercourse

Timing is critical:

- *Ovulation can be estimated via two ways:* via *TVUS* by measuring the size of the follicle(s) can be measured by a serum level or as a positive LH result in a urine test.
- *TVUS* estimates ovulation to be imminent when a lead follicle measures between 17 and 20 mm diameter.
- LH testing can be tested via a blood sample; the result is considered positive if there is a 180% rise from the baseline level, usually over 18 IU/L [5].
- *LH measurements*: In the early follicular phase, LH often hovers between 1.9 and 12.5 IU/L. As ovulation approaches, it can catapult to anywhere in the vicinity of 8.7 to 76.3 IU/L. In the luteal phase, it usually declines to around 0.5–16.9 IU/L.
- *LH testing kit*: an LH testing kit is a monitoring kit than can be procured from a pharmacy that allows the patient to begin monitoring for an LH surge starting 4–6 days before expected ovulation. The LH surge usually occurs 24–36 hours before ovulation. The kits come with test strips that one must urinate on and will show up as a positive result or a darker line on the strip. To avoid missing the LH surge, it is recommended to use the ovulation predictor kit (OPK) 2–4 days before expected LH surge. It is recommended to test twice a day (in the morning and evening, roughly 12 hours apart).
- Ovulation can be natural or induced (with an HCG injection) and ovulation usually occurs 24–36 hours afterward.
- *Optimal trigger*: the optimal time to trigger is when the ultrasound measurement of a dominant follicles is between 17 and 20 mm diameter.
- *Urinary Human Chorionic Gonadotropin (uhCG) injection* (using hCG 5000–10,000 IU or recombinant hCG (rhCG) such as Ovidrel 250 micrograms) is administered subcutaneously or intramuscularly. The injection will induce ovulation which will occur about 24–36 hours later.

- IUI is done 24–36 hours after hCG administration or following a detected LH surge. IUI can be done between 0 and 40 hours [11, 14].
- *Single vs. Double IUI*: Some advocate for two IUIs in a cycle, but evidence is mixed. ASRM and ESHRE recommend a single IUI [11, 14], as the evidence is insufficient to show that a double IUI increases pregnancy rates [11].
- It is important to teach that the egg lives for only 24 hours after ovulation; however, the sperm can live up to 5 days in the female reproductive tract.

6.2.9 Semen Preparation Techniques

The goal of sperm preparation is to isolate the *most motile and morphologically normal sperm.*

(a) *Swim-Up Technique*
  - In this technique, the sperm swim into a medium, separating from debris and immotile sperm.
  - This works best with a patient with good initial sperm motility.

(b) *Density Gradient Centrifugation*
  - In this process, the semen is layered over density media and centrifuged.
  - This is good for poor-quality samples.

(c) *Simple Wash*
  - This is a basic method; the wash removes seminal plasma.

All methods aim to minimize reactive oxygen species (ROS) and improve sperm concentration [32, 33].

The ideal period of abstinence prior to supplying the semen sample for IUI or for TI varies. The WHO guidelines advocate for abstinence from 2 to 7 days, and the Nordic Association of Andrology (NORDA) and the European Society of Human Reproduction and Embryology (ESHRE) recommend 2–4 days of abstinence. Some guidelines favor shorter periods of abstinence ≤ 1 day. It was found that shorter periods of abstinence resulted in a decrease in sperm volume and sperm concentration but an increase in progressive motility and velocity. It was found that an increase in pregnancy rates occurred with those with abstinence of <3 days, with the highest pregnancy rates being with abstinence of <2 days [33].

6.2.10 The IUI Procedure

- The procedure is performed in a clinic, usually without anesthesia. It is usually a painless, albeit uncomfortable procedure and analgesics are not required.
- A speculum is inserted into the vagina in order to visualize the cervix.
- A fine catheter is inserted through the cervix to deposit sperm into the uterine cavity.

- The fine plastic catheter is attached to a small syringe containing 0.3 mL to 0.5 mL of the "prepared sperm." The sperm is pushed into the catheter which then deposits the sperm into the uterus, therefore inseminating the patient.
- On rare occasion, the spermatozoid may be put inside the proximal vagina.
- The woman may rest for a few minutes afterward, or between 10 and 15 minutes, although this practice has not been proven to increase success in IUI [11, 34].
- A patient may have mild cramping and spotting following the procedure.
- IUI is believed to increase the density of the gametes (sperm or eggs) at the site of fertilization even if there are abnormalities with the sperm or cervical mucus [4].

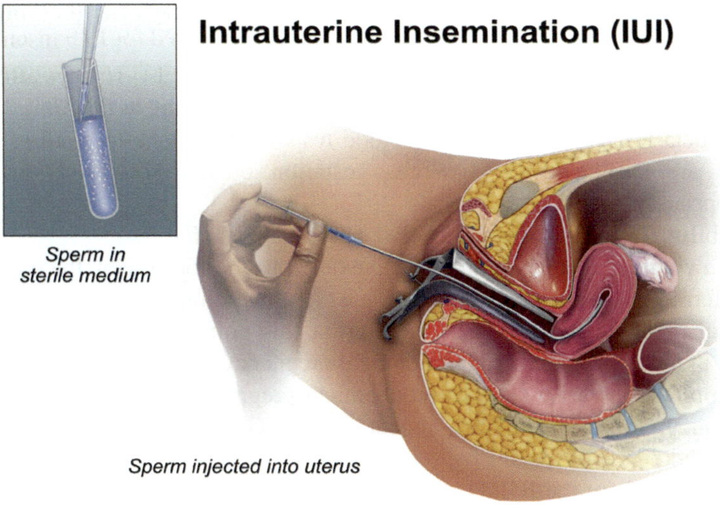

"IUI"by BruceBlaus; licensed under CC BY-SA 4.0 [35]

6.2.11 Luteal Support

- Once a patient has ovulated (the release of the egg(s)), the corpus luteum forms from the empty egg follicle(s) and begins producing progesterone. The corpus luteum is a temporary gland that helps support the beginning of a pregnancy if conception occurs during that cycle. Progesterone works by thickening the uterine lining and creating a good environment for a fertilized egg to implant.
- In a large study systemic review, a meta-analysis found that gonadotropin IUI cycles may benefit from supplemental progesterone. This is thought to be due to the decrease of the exogenous corpus luteum function of GND IUI cycles. This does not seem to affect CC IUI, therfore, it is believed that progesterone is not indicated in CC IUI cycles [36].

- Some clinics may choose to offer luteal support for the IUI cycles, especially GND cycles. Progesterone may be given orally, vaginally, or intramuscularly (IM) starting on the day following IUI or TI or it may be commenced mid-luteal, day 7 post-IUI.

6.2.12 Post-procedure Care

- The patient may choose to stay lying down for10–15 minutes post-procedure, but the literature does not show proof that this will increase pregnancy [11, 34].
- In a study examining seminal regurgitation and pregnancy rates, it was found that seminal regurgitation during IUI did not relate to pregnancy rates [37].
- Regular activity is not prohibited post-IUI. The clinic may offer their own opinions on this.
- A urine or beta hCG (pregnancy) blood test may be done 14–16 days after IUI or TI. The pregnancy is considered to be at 4 weeks gestation at this time.
- If the beta test is positive, serum blood tests may be done to confirm that the levels are sufficient for 4 weeks gestation or that the levels are rising appropriately.
- A viability TVUS may be done between weeks 6 and 7.
- Once a viable pregnancy with a positive heartbeat has been seen, the patient may be referred to their obstetrician for care. At this point, it may be considered a clinical pregnancy (CP). The follow-up at this point may vary from clinic to clinic in terms of follow-up for a clinical pregnancy.
- If complications arise such as biochemical pregnancy, miscarriage, or ectopic pregnancy; follow up TVUS, repeat beta hCG, or other follow up may be warranted.
- In the case where the IUI/TI was unsuccessful, another cycle of treatment may be repeated if ordered.
- Follow-up with the physician may be needed and further treatment cycles of IUI planned, more investigation ordered, or the patient my move on to in vitro fertilization (IVF).

6.2.13 Success Rates

- The success rates of IUI may be between 10 and 20% per cycle, depending on various factors.
- Most pregnancies occur within the first *3–6 cycles*.
- The cumulative success increases with repeated attempts but plateaus over time.

Factors affecting success:

- *Female age* (best under 35).
- *Infertility duration* (shorter duration = better outcomes), usually less than 5 years.

- *Ovulation induction method* (hCG trigger or LH monitoring).
- *Endometrial thickness* (8–12 mm considered optimal).
- *Post-wash motile sperm count* ≥ 5 million.

6.2.14 Complications

Although rare, the following complications may occur:

(a) *Ovarian Hyperstimulation Syndrome (OHSS)*
   - More common with gonadotropins.
   - Ranges from mild to life-threatening.
   - This occurs when there are many follicles and a high level of E2. This syndrome causes third spacing which can cause ascites and hemoconcentration with an increased risk of thrombolytic incidents.
   - If the patient has an excessive number of follicles, the clinician may decide to cancel the cycle. If this occurs, it is important to frame the cancellation as a preventive measure and not a failure.
   - *Nurses' role*: Teach the patient the following symptoms: may have bloating in abdominal region, may have swelling of the hands and feet, shortness of breath, nausea and vomiting, concentrated urine (from dehydration brought on by fluid shift).
   - *Teach:* about monitoring for symptoms and when to call the clinic or go to the emergency departments (ED). Follow the clinic guidelines.

(b) *Multiple Pregnancy*
   - Especially with multiple follicles. Higher-order multiple pregnancy (3 or more) places the mother and fetuses at greater risk.
   - Associated risks: preterm birth, low birth weight, pregnancy complications.
   - The doctor and patient may choose to cancel the cycle. If the cycle is cancelled, advise to use protection or abstinence until the next menses occurs. gestation may be recommendeted to the patient/couple to avoid the risks of multiple fetuses.
   - *Nurses' role*: teach about the importance of adhering to instructions and explain the reality of risks of multiple pregnancies. Listen to patient(s) and allow to express themselves.

(c) *Infection*
   - Endometritis or other infections can occur although rare. This can be prevented by sterile technique and testing for sexually transmitted infections (STIs) prior to treatment.
   - *Nurses' role*: teaching for signs and symptoms of infection. Assure that STI testing results are documented, and that if positive, the patients have been treated (female and male).

(d) *Spotting or Cramping*
- Spotting or cramping is minor and self-limiting. May have slight cramping post-procedure. May have spotting approximately 5 days post-IUI or TI at time of implantation.
- *Nurses' role:* it is important to teach if cramping gets worse and becomes painful or if spotting becomes very heavy with bright red bleeding to go to emergency department (ED) or follow the clinic's protocol for possible pregnancy loss.

(e) *Pregnancy loss*
- Biochemical pregnancy occurs when an initial pregnancy test may be positive, but the levels may diminish with time or show no viable yolk sac at viability U/S.
- Spontaneous abortion (SAB) of miscarriage. Usually, the beta hCG levels are followed to assure they are diminishing in the absence of a suspected ectopic pregnancy. At times, medication (such as Cytotec) may be ordered if incomplete SAB or if products of conception (POC) are retained in utero, and a dilation and curettage (D &C) may be needed.
- *Nurses' role:* It is important to advise to go to ER or follow the clinic's protocol if cramping and bleeding get worse (a lot of pain and heavy bleeding). Patients are advised to go to ED in case of extreme pain and heavy bleeding (filling a pad every hour for more than 2 hours).
- Offer support and empathy to the patient(s).

(f) *Ectopic pregnancy*
- Pregnancy not in utero, may be in fallopian tubes, or other. in the case of an ectopic pregnancy with no fetus in utero, medication or surgery may be indicated. if there is a viable fetus AND an ectopic pregnacy, the ectopic pregnacy may be removed surgically, to allow the viable fetus to surive.
- *Nurses' role:* It is important to teach the signs of ectopic pregnancy and ruptured ectopic pregnancy such as increasing pain, severe bleeding, abdominal distention, passing out. Patient should be taught to go to ED in case of any of these symptoms.

(g) *Emotional and Psychological Impact*
- Anxiety, depression, and emotional exhaustion are common. The psychological strain of the treatments may impair adherence and outcomes [38].
- *Nurses' role:* Provide a safe environment that allows the patient(s) to verbalize what they are experiencing. Offer empathy and referrals to counselling if necessary [38].

6.2.15 Role of the Fertility Nurse

Fertility nurses play an indispensable role throughout the COS process.

Patient Educator
The nurse educates by:

- Demonstrating medication administration [39]. It is important to base teaching on the patients' health literacy levels and emotional readiness.
- Clarifying monitoring schedules and procedures [39].
- Setting realistic expectations for treatment outcomes [39].

Risk Manager
The nurse manages by:

- Vigilant surveillance for complications [39].
- Preventive strategies to minimize risks [39].

Emotional Support Provider
The nurse provides support by:

- Using active listening techniques
- Recognizing and validating strategies and emotional responses such as frustration and grief [38]
- Offering coping and mental health referrals and resources [38].

Ethical Advocate
The nurse advocates by:

- Ensuring informed consent [40].
- Protecting patient confidentiality [40].
- Balancing treatment goals with patient autonomy and well-being. It is important to respect patient choices regarding continuation or cancellation.

Care Coordinator
The nurse coordinates by:

- Facilitating communication among the interdisciplinary team [39]
- Streamlining logistics involving labs, pharmacies, and scheduling

Patient Education Points
Medication Management
The nurse will:
- Provide clear demonstration of medication administration and provide written instructions [39].
- Emphasize the importance of timing accuracy for optimal outcomes [39].
- Assure understanding of medication calendars and provide reminders.

Side Effect Awareness
The nurse will take the time with the patient to:
- Differentiate between the expected versus concerning symptoms [41].

Monitoring Compliance

The nurse will emphasize the:

- Importance of punctual attendance for ultrasounds and blood draws [39].

Lifestyle Guidance

The nurse will provide:

- Recommendations for hydration, moderate exercise, and stress management [39].
- Advice against vigorous activities to prevent ovarian torsion [39].
- Guidelines for limiting caffeine and alcohol intake.

Ethical Considerations

Risk of Multiples

The nurse will have:

- Informed discussions about the risks of high-order multiples and cancellation policies [40].

Access and Equity

The nurse will:

- Recognize and address financial barriers to fertility treatments [40].
- Advocate for insurance coverage and patient assistance programs.

Emotional Burdens

The nurse will:

- Integrate psychosocial support and mental health resources into care planning [38].
- Ensure equitable emotional support access regardless of socioeconomic status.

6.2.16 Guidelines or Recommendations

Canadian Fertility and Andrology Society (CFAS)

Only the recommendations, rather than what is not recommended, are highlighted.

CFAS recommends:

(a) In couples with a good prognosis (and duration of infertility), expectant management can be effective [13].
(b) IUI with oral agents is an appropriate treatment in couples with unexplained infertility (UI) and is more effective than expectant management [13].
(c) LTZ or CC can be used as an oral agent for IUI [13].
(d) GND can be offered to couples with UI [13].
(e) Patients need to be aware that GND/IUI is associated with increased pregnancy rates (PR) and multiple pregnancy rates (MPR) [13].
(f) IVF can be used as an elective first-line treatment in UI, in order to assure single embryo transfer (SET), and decreased MPR [13].
(g) IVF should be offered to couples with UI if 3 cycles of OS/IUI have failed [13].

American Society of Reproductive Medicine (ASRM)
Only the most relevant recommendations and what is not recommended are highlighted.

Recommendations:

(a) It is recommended to use CC with IUI in UI [14].
(b) It is recommended to use LTZ with IUI as an alternative to CC/IUI (LTZ not approved by FDA) [14].
(c) It is not recommended to use CC or LTZ plus conventional GND/IUI as it may increase the PR as well as the MPR [14].
(d) It is not recommended to use low-dose GND with IUI as it is no more effective than COS with CC and LTZ/IUI and it is more complex and more expensive [14].
(e) It is not recommended to use conventional GND with IUI, as it increases not only PR but also MPR [14].
(f) It is recommended to do a single IUI between 0 and 36 hours post-hCG in IUI [14].
(g) It is recommended that couples do 3–4 cycles of COS with oral medication with IUI and move to IVF rather than COS with GND and IUI [14].

European Society of Human Reproduction and Embryology (ESHRE)
Only the most relevant recommendations are highlighted.

Recommendations:

(a) Twelve months of regular unprotected intercourse is recommended before testing [42].
(b) The discussion to start active treatment over expectant management is based upon the prognosis of the couple in UI [42].
(c) IUI with COS is recommended as the first line of treatment for UI [42].
(d) Care is needed to avoid OHSS and MPR if low-dose GND/IUI is used [42].
(e) IVF is not recommended over IUI [42].
(f) The decision to use IVF is individualized to patient characteristics such as age/duration of infertility, previous treatments, and previous pregnancies [42].

World Health Organization (WHO)—Global Recommendations
Recommendations:

(a) Couples with UI and a good prognosis of becoming pregnant in the next 12 months (>30%) should be recommended for expectant management for 6 months before IUI [11].
(b) Couples with poor sperm quality only not recommended for or against IUI [11].
(c) Couples with UI, IUI in natural cycle should not be offered [11].
(d) Couples with UI and male with with TMSC above 10 million and pregnancy is <30%recommendation for COS/IUI [11].
(e) It is not possible to define clear lower cutoff levels for pre–/post-wash sperm below which IUI should not be attempted [11].

(f) If using hCG trigger shot, a singe IUI is recommended 24–40 hours later [11].
(g) IUI in a natural cycle should be performed one day after and the LH surge [11].
(h) During an IUI cycle, singlee insemination is recommended over a double insemination as no evidence has shown increase in PR [11].
(i) Women having IUI should be offered 10–15 minutes of bedrest after the procedure [11].
(j) Three cycles of IUI should be indicated for UI [11].
(k) There is insufficient evidence to recommend the number of cycles of IUI to undergo.
(l) There is little evidence regarding the choice of semen preparation (swim-up, gradient wash, or centrifugation) [11].
(m) To avoid multiple gestational pregnancies (MGP), two or more fetuses in COS/IUI, IUI should be withheld if 2 dominant follicle >15 mm or 5 folliclesof 10 mm or more at the time of hCG injection or LH surge [11].
(n) If GND is used in IUI, 75 IU or less should be used to avoid an increased risk of MGP, even though it may increase the PR [11].
(o) CC and LTZ are acceptable alternatives with IUI as they decrease the MGP rate as well as the cost of treatment, although they have lower PR [11].
(p) Adding GnRH to GND in COS/IUI is not recommended as it increases PR as well as MGP rates and is costly [11].
(q) An alternative to cycle cancellation can be follicle aspiration to decrease MGP rates [11].
(r) Evidence does not support informing individuals undergoing COS/IUI of the possibility of pre-term and low birth weight babies in singleton and twin pregnancies versus those without fertility treatments [11].

6.2.17 Emerging Trends in COS

The following trends are emerging in COS, and it is important to keep abreast of the newest developments to keep current.

Mild Stimulation Strategies
This trend could:

- Reduce gonadotropin doses to lower OHSS risk and enhance patient comfort [43].
- Offer cost-effective and patient-friendly approaches to treatment.

Personalized Medicine
These trends may already be in place but could be common moving forward.

- Using AMH levels and antral follicle counts to guide dosing [44].
- Introducing pharmacogenomic studies that aim to tailor stimulation protocols further [44].
- Using Artificial intelligence tools to predict optimal protocols.

New Adjuvant Therapies
Some physicians may already be suggesting these supplements to patients.

- Coenzyme Q10 supplementation for oocyte quality improvement [43].
- DHEA administration for poor responders [43].
- Use of melatonin and growth hormone in adjuvant settings.

6.3 Conclusion

COS with IUI is an affordable first-line first-line treatment for certain patients once they have been appropriately worked up and followed by a physician experienced with IUI procedures and protocols, success rates and risks [1, 11, 13, 14]. COS IUI is ideal for couples experiencing infertility caused by mild male factor, anovulation, unexplained infertility, inability to have intercourse (due to physical or psychological factors), and being single, same-sex couples, and a serodiscordant couple, for example, one partner having HIV [5].

IUI is noninvasive and cost-effective and is often used before resorting to complex methods like IVF. COS using oral medication such as clomiphene citrate (CC) and LTZ is recommended by many medical organizations as the first line of treatment, when expectant management has failed [11, 13, 14, 42]. Gonadotropins such as rFSH and hMG can be used in low doses or conventional doses, which have been found to increase risks of multiple gestational pregnancy (MGP) [45, 46].

Evidence to suppport the best approach has yet to be conclusive for ovulation in the best approach for ovulation maturation and induction (LH surge versus hCG administration) [5]. Luteal support in gonadotropin cycles is felt to improve live birth rate but has not been proven in cycles using oral medication [5].

Reproductive medicine seeks to offer effective, low-cost treatment and live births with the least amount of risk. Studies seek to find the best methods and guideline to indicate future success while minimizing risks.

Bibliography

1. World Health Organization. Infertility. May 22, 2024.https://www.who.int/news-room/fact-sheets/detail/infertility.
2. Templeton A. Infertility-epidemiology, aetiology and effective management. Health Bull (Edinb). 1995;53:294–8.
3. Gore AC, Chappell VA, Fenton SE, et al. EDC-2: the Endocrine Society's second scientific statement on endocrine-disrupting chemicals. Endocr Rev. 2015;36(6):E1–E150. https://doi.org/10.1210/er.2015-1010.
4. Van Voorhis BJ, Barnett M, Sparks AE, Syrop CH, Rosenthal G, Dawson J. Effect of the total motile sperm count on the efficacy and cost-effectiveness of intrauterine insemination and in vitro fertilization. Fertil Steril. 2001;75:661–8. https://doi.org/10.1016/s0015-0282(00)01783-0. PMID: 11287015.

5. Soares SR, Santos-Ribeiro S. Ovarian stimulation and intrauterine insemination. In: Dahan MH, editor. Handbook of current and novel protocols for the treatment of infertility. 1st ed. San Diego: Elsevier Science & Technology; 2023. p. 93–103.
6. Hansen KR, Eisenberg E, Baker V, Hill MJ, Chen S, Talken S, et al. Midluteal progesterone: a marker of treatment outcomes in couples with unexplained infertility. NICHD Reproductive Medicine Network, editor. J Clin Endocrinol Metab. 2018;103(7):2743–51.
7. Zheng J, Cai J, Liu L, Guo Y, Sun J, Ren J. Low BMI is associated with poor IUI outcomes: a retrospective study in 13,745 cycles. J Assist Reprod Genet. 2022;39(12):2819–25. https://doi.org/10.1007/s10815-022-02658-y. Epub 2022 Nov 21. PMID: 36411395; PMCID: PMC9790829.
8. Chang MY, Chiang CH, Chiu TH, Hsieh TT, Soong YK. The antral follicle count predicts the outcome of pregnancy in a controlled ovarian hyperstimulation/intrauterine insemination program. J Assist Reprod Genet. 1998;15(1):12–7. https://doi.org/10.1023/a:1022518103368. PMID: 9493060; PMCID: PMC3468200.
9. Butler WJ, Pico A, Hawkins KC, Younis AI. Discordance between day-3 follicle stimulating hormone & anti-mullerian hormone is predictive of clinical pregnancy during fertility treatment. Gynecol Endocrinol. 2021;37(9):798–801.
10. Tiegs AW, Sun L, Scott RT, Goodman LR. Comparison of pregnancy outcomes following intrauterine insemination in young women with decreased versus normal ovarian reserve. Fertil Steril. 2020;113(4):788–796.e4.
11. Cohlen B, Bijkerk A, Van Der Poel S, Ombelet W. IUI: review and systematic assessment of the evidence that supports global recommendations. Hum Reprod Update. 2018;24(3):300–19. https://doi.org/10.1093/humupd/dmx041.
12. Hull MG, Glazener C M, Kelly N J, Conway D I, Foster P A, al Hinton RA e. Population study of causes, treatment, and outcome of infertility. Br Med J (Clin Res Ed). 1985;291:1693. https://doi.org/10.1136/bmj.291.6510.1693.
13. Buckett W, Sierra S. The management of unexplained infertility: an evidence-based guideline from the Canadian Fertility and Andrology Society. Reprod Biomed Online. 2019;39(4):633–40. https://doi.org/10.1016/j.rbmo.2019.05.023.
14. Penzias A, Bendikson K, Falcone T, Hansen K, Hill M, Jindal S, Mersereau J, et al. Evidence-based treatments for couples with unexplained infertility: a guideline. Fertil Steril. 2020;113(2):305–22. https://doi.org/10.1016/j.fertnstert.2019.10.014.
15. Danhof NA, Wang R, van Wely M, van der Veen F, Mol BWJ, Mochtar MH. IUI for unexplained infertility—a network meta-analysis. Hum Reprod Update. 2020;26(1):1–15. https://doi.org/10.1093/humupd/dmz035.
16. Alanya Tosun S, Ergun B, Gokmen Karasu AF, Ozkaya E, Gurbuz T. The utility of detecting ovulation to predict success in ovulation induction and intrauterine insemination cycles - a prospective observational study. Ginekol Pol. 2021;92(12):860–4.
17. Goldstein SR, Siddhanti S, Ciaccia AV, Plouffe L Jr. A pharmacological review of selective oestrogen receptor modulators. Hum Reprod Update. 2000;6:212–24.
18. Ritter J, Flower R, Henderson G, Loke YK, MacEwan D, Rang H. Rang & Dale's pharmacology. 9th ed. Philadelphia: Elsevier; 2019.
19. The Practice Committee of the American Society for Reproductive Medicine. Use of clomiphene citrate in infertile women: a committee opinion. Fertil Steril. 2013;100(2):341–8. https://doi.org/10.1016/j.fertnstert.2013.05.033.
20. Taiyeb AM, Haji AI, Ibraheem ZO, Alsakkal GS. Pregnancy outcomes following different protocols of controlled ovarian hyperstimulation in couples undergoing intrauterine insemination. Clin Exp Pharmacol Physiol. 2021;48(8):1070–9.
21. Goenka ML, Goenka D, Chakraborty S. Iomiphene/letrozole stimulation in intrauterine insemination. 2012. https://doi.org/10.5005/jp/books/11638_15.
22. Huang S, Du X, Wang R, Li R, Wang H, Luo L, et al. Ovulation induction and intrauterine insemination in infertile women with polycystic ovary syndrome: a comparison of drugs. Eur J Obstet Gynecol Reprod Biol. 2018;231:117–21.

23. Akbari S, Ayazi Roozbahani M, Ayazi Roozbahani F. Comparing of letrozole versus clomiphene citrate combined with gonadotropins in intrauterine insemination cycles. Iran J Reprod Med. 2012;10(1):29–32. PMID: 25242971; PMCID: PMC4163260.
24. Fauser BC, Devroey P. Reproductive biology and ovarian stimulation. Trends Endocrinol Metab. 2003;14(5):236–42.
25. Quintero RB, Urban R, Lathi RB, Westphal LM, Dahan MH. A comparison of letrozole to gonadotropins for ovulation induction, in subjects who failed to conceive with clomiphene citrate. Fertil Steril. 2007;88(4):879–85.
26. https://www.reproductivefacts.org/news-and-publications/fact-sheets-and-infographics/side-effects-of-injectable-fertility-drugs-gonadotropins/.
27. Dias CMF, Vitorino GBT, Furlan SMP, Reis RMD, de Sa Rosa Silva ACJ, Mendes MC, et al. Intrauterine insemination: prognostic factors. JBRA Assist Reprod. 2024;28(2):254–62.
28. Tang Y, He QD, Zhang TT, Wang JJ, Huang SC, Ye Y. Controlled ovarian stimulation should not be preferred for male infertility treated with intrauterine insemination: a retrospective study. Reprod Biol Endocrinol. 2021;19(1):45.
29. Thomas S, Sebastian T, Karthikeyan M, Mangalaraj AM, Aleyamma TK, Kamath MS. Effectiveness of spontaneous ovulation as monitored by urinary luteinising hormone versus induced ovulation by administration of human chorionic gonadotrophin in couples undergoing gonadotrophin-stimulated intrauterine insemination: a randomised controlled trial. BJOG. 2019;126(Suppl 4):58–65.
30. Liu KE, Hartman M, Hartman A. Management of thin endometrium in assisted reproduction: a clinical practice guideline from the Canadian Fertility and Andrology Society. Reprod Biomed Online. 2019;39(1):49–62.
31. Quaas AM, Gavrizi SZ, Peck JD, Diamond MP, Legro RS, Robinson RD, et al. Endometrial thickness after ovarian stimulation with gonadotropin, clomiphene, or letrozole for unexplained infertility, and association with treatment outcomes. Eunice Kennedy Shriver National Institute of Child Health and Human Development Reproductive Medicine Network, editor. Fertil Steril. 2021;115(1):213–20.
32. Boomsma CM, Cohlen BJ, Farquhar C. Semen preparation techniques for intrauterine insemination. Cochrane Database Syst Rev. 2019;10(10):CD004507. https://doi.org/10.1002/14651858.CD004507.pub4. PMID: 31612995; PMCID: PMC6792139.
33. Ayad BM, Van der Horst G, Du Plessis S. Revisiting the relationship between the ejaculatory abstinence period and semen characteristics. Int J fertil Steril [Internet]. 2018 Jan [cited 2025 Mar 21];11(4). Available from: https://doi.org/10.22074/ijfs.2018.5192.
34. Cordary A, Braconier A, Guillet-May F, Morel O, Agopiantz M, Callec R. Immobilization versus immediate mobilization after intrauterine insemination; a systemic review and meta-analysis. J Gynecol Obstet Human Reprod. 2017;46:747–51.
35. "IUI" by BruceBlaus is licensed under CC BY-SA 4.0. To view a copy of this license, visit https://creativecommons.org/licenses/by-sa/4.0/?ref=openverse.
36. Hill MJ, Whitcomb BW, Lewis TD, Wu M, Terry N, et al. Progesterone luteal support after ovulation induction and intrauterine insemination: a systematic review and meta-analysis. Fertil Steril. 2013;100:1373–80. https://doi.org/10.1016/j.fertnstert.2013.06.034.
37. Craig LB, Arya S, Burks HR, Warta K, Jarshaw C, Hansen KR, Peck JD. Relationship between semen regurgitation and pregnancy rates with intrauterine insemination. Fertil Steril. 2021;116(6):1526–31. Available in PMC 2022 Dec 01. https://doi.org/10.1016/j.fertnstert.2021.07.1183.
38. Maheshwari A, Hamilton M, Bhattacharya S. Effect of female age on the diagnostic categories of infertility. Hum Reprod. 2008;23(3):538–42.
39. Practice Committee of the American Society for Reproductive Medicine. Use of exogenous gonadotropins for ovulation induction in anovulatory women: a committee opinion. Fertil Steril. 2020;113(1):66–72.
40. Nastri CO, Teixeira DM, Moroni RM, Leitão VMS, Martins WP. Ovarian hyperstimulation syndrome: pathophysiology, staging, prediction and prevention. Ultrasound Obstet Gynecol. 2015;45(4):377–93.

41. Papanikolaou EG, Verpoest W, Fatemi H, Staessen C, Bourgain C, Smitz J, et al. A novel method of triggering oocyte maturation after co-treatment with a gonadotropin-releasing hormone (GnRH) antagonist in high responders. Fertil Steril. 2005;83(6):1613–6.
42. The Guideline Group on Unexplained Infertility, Romualdi D, Ata B, Bhattacharya S, Bosch E, Costello M, et al. Evidence-based guideline: unexplained infertility. Human Reproduction. 2023;38(10):1881–90.
43. Macklon NS, Stouffer RL, Giudice LC, Fauser BC. The science behind 25 years of ovarian stimulation for in vitro fertilization. Endocr Rev. 2006;27(2):170–207.
44. Grynberg M, Labrosse J. Ovarian reserve testing: necessary but confusing. BJOG. 2019;126(3):253–6.
45. Diamond MP, Legro RS, Coutifaris C, Alvero R, Robinson RD, Casson P, Christman GM, Ager J, Huang H, Hansen KR, Baker V. Letrozole, gonadotropin, or clomiphene for unexplained infertility. N Engl J Med. 2015;373(13):1230–40.
46. Zolton JR, Lindner PG, Terry N, DeCherney AH, Hill MJ. Gonadotropins versus oral ovarian stimulation agents for unexplained infertility: a systematic review and meta-analysis. Fertil Steril. 2020;113(2):417–25.

Pharmacotherapy: Adjuvant Pharmacotherapy in Fertility Care for Men and Women

7

Ashley Ulker and LaTasha B. Craig

7.1 Introduction

The live birth rate for in vitro fertilization (IVF) in the United States in 2022 for women aged 35–37 was 31%, meaning that 69% of patients did not achieve a live birth [96] in this age group. This statistic highlights the potential emotional and financial challenges associated with IVF. As a result, both healthcare providers and patients are motivated to explore strategies to optimize each and every IVF cycle. However, many of the adjunct treatments, or "add-ons," lack strong evidence to support their utility and may increase the overall cost of treatment. Achieving the balance between patient autonomy while providing evidence-based care can be challenging, as failure to discuss these options with patients could also be seen as paternalistic and may deny them the access to potentially beneficial therapies [109]. In this chapter, we will review the evidence behind some of the most common IVF adjuvant therapies, both over the counter and prescribed, that aim to improve outcomes for female and male patients undergoing IVF. Table 7.1 summarizes these recommendations.

A. Ulker
The Section of Reproductive Endocrinology & Infertility, Department of Obstetrics & Gynecology, University of Oklahoma Health Sciences Center, Oklahoma City, OK, USA
e-mail: Ashley-UlkerSarokhan@ouhsc.edu

L. B. Craig (✉)
The Section of Reproductive Endocrinology & Infertility, Department of Obstetrics & Gynecology, University of Oklahoma Health Sciences Center, Oklahoma City, OK, USA

The University of Oklahoma College of Medicine, Oklahoma City, OK, USA
e-mail: LaTasha-Craig@ou.edu

M. Das, M. H. Dahan (eds.), *A Comprehensive Guide to Reproductive Health and Infertility Medicine for Nurses*, https://doi.org/10.1007/978-3-032-24372-0_7

Table 7.1 Summary of adjuvant pharmacotherapy in IVF for women

	Dosage	Timing	Proposed mechanism	Recommendation
Growth hormone	4–24 IU	Initiate cycle day 21 prior to stimulation—stimulation day 8	Increase IGF-1 (folliculogenesis, embryogenesis)	May consider in poor responders
DHEA	25 mg TID, 75 mg/qday	Pretreatment 2–3 months	Increase IGF-1 (folliculogenesis)	May consider in poor responders
Coenzyme Q 10	200–600 mg qday	Pretreatment 2–3 months	Antioxidant	May consider in poor responders
Testosterone	2.5–12.5 mg/qday	Pretreatment 2–4 weeks	Increase follicular responsiveness	May consider in poor responders
Aspirin	75–100 mg/qday	Beginning with stimulation versus prior to embryo transfer	COX inhibitor, increase blood flow, decrease clot	Do not recommend; benefit not demonstrated
Corticosteroids	Methylprednisolone 4–16 mg/day Prednisolone 5–60 mg/day Dexamethasone 0.5–1 mg/day	Initiate at the start of COH to 4 days prior to transfer	Suppress androgen levels, increase IGF-1	Do not recommend; benefit is not demonstrated
Vitamin D	600 IU/day if not deficient; higher doses may vary, but not to exceed 4000 IU/day	Daily for at least 30 days	Follicle recruitment, folliculogenesis, embryogenesis, implantation	May consider for other health indications
Myo-inositol	1–4 mg/day 40:1 myo-inositol to D-chiro-inositol	Pretreatment 2–3 months or daily	Insulin sensitization, antioxidant	May consider in women with PMOS for other comorbidities

7.2 Growth Hormone: Females

Growth hormone (GH) is involved in reproductive physiology, and it is capable of influencing processes such as steroidogenesis, folliculogenesis, and embryogenesis. This is done mainly through its ability to increase circulating insulin-like growth factor-1 (IGF-1) levels, which helps augment the gonadotropin effect on granulosa and theca cells [36, 121]. It has been used off-label as adjuvant therapy for IVF or controlled ovarian stimulation (COH) for patients classified as "poor responders" or those who are anticipated to have low oocyte yield.

There are several observational studies that suggest that GH may improve outcomes in poor responders undergoing IVF [44, 55, 56, 76]. However, the randomized controlled trials (RCTs) and meta-analyses on the subject have yielded inconsistent results [23, 24, 50, 53, 114, 123].

A 2021 Cochrane review evaluated the use of GH as an adjunctive treatment in IVF and included 16 RCTs (n = 1352 women) [97]. Two RCTs evaluated GH in routine use, and 14 studied GH in poor responders. This review found limited evidence supporting the benefit of GH in improving IVF success, largely due to the heterogeneity in analyses, poor reporting of study methods, imprecise data, and variability. A 2023 systematic review and meta-analysis assessed 10 RCTs performed in China (n = 852 infertile women with DOR) and found that GH was associated with increased clinical pregnancy rates (CPR; RR 1.63, 95% CI 1.31–2.03, $p < 0.001$) and a greater number of oocytes retrieved (mean difference = 0.91, 95% CI 0.47–1.35, $p > 0.0001$) [60, 61]. Finally, a 2023 meta-analysis included 16 RCTs (2323 women with POR defined by Bologna criteria) undergoing different adjuvant treatment strategies prior to IVF [dehydroepiandrosterone (DHEA), CoQ10, GH, transcutaneous electrical acupoint stimulation (TEAS)] [123]. Eight RCTs were evaluated, and GH was second only to DHEA in terms of improving the number of oocytes retrieved and the high-quality embryo rate, but there was no significant benefit in improving the CPR and live birth rate (LBR). However, because the doses and regimens of GH in the trials were variable, the effects on pregnancy outcomes are uncertain.

The inherent heterogeneity between studies is a common limitation when attempts are made to combine available RCTs and interpret the data. There are differences in the definition of a poor responder, variation in the dose and timing of GH administration, stimulation protocols, and outcome measures. For providers, it is important to note that there is no standard recommended dose or timing of GH administration. These studies discussed starting injectable GH anywhere from cycle day 21 prior to ovarian stimulation to starting on stimulation day 8 of IVF. Dosages varied depending on frequency of administration and were between 4 and 25 IU daily. Growth hormone may also add significant cost to an already costly treatment, especially in those patients without insurance coverage. Lastly, it is important to discuss with patients the off-label use of this medication during IVF cycles. GH may be considered in poor responders undergoing IVF; however, there is no definitive evidence of improved outcomes currently available.

7.3 DHEA: Females

Dehydroepiandrosterone (DHEA) is an endogenous androgen primarily produced by the zona glomerulosa of the adrenal cortex, as well as by the ovarian theca cells and through peripheral conversion [99]. Early studies indicated that DHEA acts as a prohormone in the ovarian steroidogenesis pathway and may also increase IGF-1, thereby having similar potential properties to growth hormone with regard to improving follicular development [21, 71]. DHEA supplementation for the purpose of "anti-aging properties" has been explored since the early 2000s [16].

Wiser et al. performed one of the first RCTs on DHEA supplementation with IVF in 2010 and found a significantly higher LBR in the DHEA-supplemented group. However, their primary outcome measure was not LBR, and only 7 total pregnancies were reported. Subsequent RCTs have demonstrated mixed results, with some showing no difference in ovarian response markers or total oocytes retrieved with DHEA supplementation [3, 113, 115, 116], while others have demonstrated improvements in both categories [51, 118]. One of the larger studies included 140 women undergoing IVF with intracytoplasmic sperm injection (ICSI) with poor ovarian response (POR) according to the Bologna criteria and reported higher CPR, ongoing pregnancy rate, number of retrieved oocytes, and fertilization rate in those supplemented with DHEA [51]. Another study that compared pregnancy outcomes in patients between the ages of 36 and 40 years old ($n = 109$) found that DHEA supplementation increased LBR significantly [101, 102].

Several meta-analyses done on this topic provide varied results. Some suggest that DHEA has a positive effect on women with diminished ovarian reserve (DOR) undergoing IVF [58, 90, 112, 119]. Xu et al. [112] included those with DOR, poor responders, and normal responders and demonstrated a significant increase in CPR (RR = 1.25; 95% CI 1.01–1.61; $P = 0.04$) and LBR (RR1.76; 95% CI 1.17–2.63; $P = 0.006$) [112]. A 2016 meta-analysis included 16 studies and 2323 POR patients by Bologna criteria to evaluate adjuvant treatments, and the authors concluded that DHEA had the greatest advantage in improving implantation rate, high-quality embryo rate, and the number of retrieved oocytes when compared to the other adjuvant treatments [112]. Other meta-analyses, however, have concluded that DHEA use is not associated with higher CPR [14, 70, 81, 84].

Further studies powered to detect a difference in LBR are still needed in order to determine the benefit of DHEA supplementation. The dose utilized is either 25 mg by mouth three times per day versus 75 mg by mouth once a day for up to 3 months prior to IVF. Although it is important to counsel patients on potential side effects, which include hair loss, hirsutism, and changes in voice, these effects are negligible at these suggested doses. There may be a potential benefit to DHEA supplementation, but definitive clinical benefit has yet to be demonstrated, as current evidence is inconsistent [52].

7.4 Testosterone: Females

Androgen receptor gene expression has been demonstrated to be present in primary follicles and increasing gradually in preantral follicles. Testosterone is an androgen that may therefore augment follicular responsiveness to FSH by upregulating FSH receptors on granulosa cells. Given this proposed mechanism of action, testosterone has been proposed as an adjuvant therapy prior to IVF in patients who are anticipated to be poor responders [62, 116].

Some smaller RCTs have demonstrated improvements in CPR and LBR with testosterone prior to stimulation in poor responders, but they vary with regard to timing, route, and dosage and were not powered to detect a difference in LBR

[15, 28, 48, 49, 64]. A 2015 Cochrane review concluded that pre- or co-treatment with testosterone was associated with higher LBR but found no difference in outcomes after removing studies at risk of performance bias [69]. A 2019 meta-analysis included 7 studies, 5 of which looked at LBR and 2 of which did not, and found a higher LBR (RR 2.29, 95% CI 1.31–4.01, $P = 0.004$), CPR (RR 2.32, 95% CI 1.47–3.64, $P = 0.0003$), total number of oocytes retrieved (mean difference = 1.28, 95% CI 0.83–1.73, $P < 0.00001$), mature oocytes (mean difference = 0.96, 95% CI 0.28–1.65, $P = 0.006$), and total number of embryos (mean difference 1.17, 95% CI 0.67–1.67, $P < 0.00001$) in the group receiving testosterone [75]. However, there are several limitations, which include difference in the outcomes calculated, small number of studies, heterogeneity, and different definitions of DOR between studies.

The T-TRANSPORT trial is the first multicenter multinational double-blind placebo-controlled RCT aiming to detect differences in CPR between testosterone transdermal gel or placebo for the treatment of poor responders in 290 poor responders meeting Bologna criteria. Only preliminary data is available as a published abstract, and results indicate that CPR and ovarian stimulation outcomes (number of oocytes retrieved, embryos, and mature oocytes) did not differ between groups, and there were several adverse events that led to treatment discontinuation [68].

The doses vary between studies and include transdermal testosterone gel (10–25 mg/day) and transdermal patches 2.5–5.5 mg/day. Timing is also variable from several days to several weeks prior to ovarian stimulation. There are potential side effects that should be communicated to patients, which include symptomatic hyperandrogenemia and diminished oocyte response. These symptoms can include acne, hair loss, and oily skin. The strongest evidence available indicates no difference in CPR, though remaining data is pending, and further studies are needed in which the primary outcome measure is LBR in order to draw conclusive results.

7.5 Aspirin: Females

Acetylsalicylic acid, commonly known as aspirin, works by inhibiting cyclooxygenase in platelets, thereby reducing prostaglandin synthesis. In low doses it also promotes vasodilation (enlargement of the blood vessels) by blocking the production of thromboxane A2. Due to its resulting effect on blood flow, it has been studied as an adjunct in IVF, with the potential to enhance ovarian blood flow and uterine vascularity and receptivity. It has particularly been studied in couples with recurrent pregnancy loss (two or more miscarriages) or implantation failure, under the same hypothesis that improved blood flow and reduced thrombosis could enhance pregnancy outcomes [47].

One of the largest RCTs includes 1380 IVF cycles and compared LBR in an unselected IVF population undergoing fresh embryo transfer [108]. They found that the group receiving 75 mg of aspirin daily (from transfer until pregnancy test) had higher LBR [108]. Conversely, a 2009 RCT compared groups taking 100 mg daily aspirin versus placebo prior to stimulation and found no difference in CPR or LBR between groups [54]. Two other RCTS of 193 and 487 participants found no significant difference in CPR [26] or LBR [33] between aspirin and placebo. Similarly, a Cochrane review of 13 studies (n = 2653) confirmed the aforementioned findings and did not find an improvement in outcomes for unselected infertile population undergoing IVF [94]. The EAGeR trial, a large double-blinded RCT, evaluated the benefits of aspirin supplementation in women who previously had 1–2 pregnancy losses and found no difference in LBR (58% vs 53%, $P = 0.984$) or pregnancy loss (13% vs 12%, $p = 0.7812$) between groups [89]. Due to the lack of compelling evidence, adjuvant aspirin is not recommended to improve IVF outcomes (ASRM Committee opinion).

7.6 Corticosteroids: Females

Corticosteroids are steroid hormones produced by the adrenal cortex and include both glucocorticoids and mineralocorticoids. Glucocorticoids, such as prednisolone and dexamethasone, have been studied as fertility treatments since the 1980s, specifically for someone with PMOS undergoing controlled ovarian hyperstimulation. These hormones may improve ovarian response by reducing elevated androgen levels, which can negatively affect folliculogenesis. They may also promote the production of growth factors such as IGF-1 and have effects similar to GH [41].

Regarding ovarian stimulation, a 2001 RCT with 290 women undergoing IVF demonstrated that 1 mg of dexamethasone reduced the IVF cancellation rate due to poor ovarian response but did not improve implantation or ongoing pregnancy rate [45]. A 2017 Cochrane review of only 2 studies (n = 310) [31, 45], found insufficient evidence that glucocorticoids improve CPR or LBR during ovarian stimulation for subfertile couples undergoing IVF [41]. This study included both patients with PMOS and those who were normal responders, not those who were specifically at risk of poor response.

Regarding implantation, a RCT from 2003 involving 360 cycles compared daily prednisolone (10 mg for 4 weeks starting on stimulation day 1) to no treatment and found no significant difference in number of mature oocytes retrieved, pregnancy rates, or implantation rates [105]. A subsequent Cochrane review of 14 studies (n = 1879) found no evidence that glucocorticoids improved pregnancy rates. Additionally, a meta-analysis of the 3 studies that included LBR found no difference between groups [13]. Finally, a 2023 meta-analysis of 9 studies (n = 1391) found no significant improvement in the LBR, miscarriage rate, ectopic pregnancy rate, or implantation rate between glucocorticoid supplementation during IVF versus control group.

There was variability regarding dosing and timing of glucocorticoid treatment in different studies. Another limitation of the available evidence is that many studies were not powered to detect a difference in LBR due to a small sample size. The typical dose ranged from methylprednisolone 4–16 mg/day, prednisolone 5–60 mg/day, to dexamethasone 0.5–1 mg/day. Possible side effects of systemic steroid use include hypertension, hypokalemia, and osteoporosis, though these are typically dose- and duration-dependent. Given the current evidence, glucocorticoids are not recommended for routine use for the purpose of improving ovarian stimulation or implantation (ASRM Committee Opinion). Side effects of glucocorticoid use in the short term include weight gain, water retention, and initiation or aggravation of diabetes. Patients complaining of excessive thirst and urination should be referred for a follow up with the physician, possibly representing uncontrolled blood sugar levels.

7.7 Inositol: Females

Inositol is a polyalcohol that is found in 9 different stereoisomer forms. Two of these, myo-inositol and D-chiro-inositol, have been shown to improve insulin sensitivity by mediating post-receptor effects of insulin. Increased insulin resistance is commonly observed in women with PMOS, so inositol has been postulated to benefit this population. Inositol also has antioxidant properties that may reduce oxidative damage to cells. It is commonly found in beans, fruits, and nuts, but can also be produced endogenously and can be purchased as an over-the-counter supplement [72].

An early study investigating inositol and PMOS found improvement in insulin sensitivity and ovulation when 1200 mg of D-chiro-inositol was taken for 6–8 weeks [72]. Several subsequent studies have also demonstrated potential benefits of myo-inositol for those with PMOS [19, 22, 32, 78]. Unfer et al. established that the number of mature oocytes was higher with myo-inositol when compared with D-chiro-inositol, in PMOS patients undergoing IVF [106]. It was then discovered that women normally had a myoinositol: D-chiroinositol ratio of 40:1, and supplementation with that ratio was superior to D-chiro-inositol alone [18, 74].

A 2017 meta-analysis including 7 RCTS ($n = 935$) found that pretreatment with myo-inositol increases CPR, decreases miscarriage, and increases the proportion of good-quality embryos in women with PMOS undergoing IVF [120]. A 2018 Cochrane review included 13 RCTs with 1472 patients with PMOS compared pretreatment with inositol to placebo, no treatment, another antioxidant, a fertility agent, or another type of inositol [92]. The authors found significant increase in CPR in those receiving myoinositol versus D-chiroinositol, though the analysis included only the previously mentioned study by Unfer et al., so there was insufficient evidence to determine if myo-inositol supplementation was beneficial in women undergoing IVF with PMOS.

Myo-inositol has typically been given in 1–4 g/day doses; however, there is no established preferred dose. Clinical trials done for different diagnoses have documented doses ranging from 4 to 30 g/day with only the risk of mild GI symptoms at doses >12 g/day [18]. Existing data does not show definite benefit in terms of clinical pregnancy or live birth in women undergoing IVF, but there is some evidence to suggest that myo-inositol may improve other outcomes in women with PMOS, like diabetes and cardiovascular disease, due to its insulin sensitizing properties. Inositols are relatively inexpensive and accessible, but patients should be counseled on the appropriate formulation to purchase (40:1 myoinositol to chiro-inositol), as an increased D-chiro inositol may actually be detrimental [18]. Metformin is another insulin-sensitizing medication used in women with PMOS. Since the mechanism of action has overlap with inositol, combining both has not been shown to offer further benefit, and one or the other is usually chosen. The benefit of inositol is that it usually has less gastrointestinal complaints than does metformin. Although intestinal upset with inositol can also occur and often resolves with time.

7.8 Vitamin D: Females

Vitamin D is a steroid hormone best known for promoting bone mineralization and maintaining calcium and phosphorus homeostasis, but its role in reproduction has also been demonstrated [66, 117]. There are several proposed ways in which it may affect reproductive physiology, including follicle recruitment through AMH regulation, folliculogenesis, and embryogenesis [66, 117]. Vitamin D may also increase ovarian steroid hormone production, and deficient levels may impair implantation and placentation [8, 57, 79]. Despite its known association with fertility, the evidence supporting its benefit in ART is mixed [77, 85].

In 2010, a correlation was demonstrated between follicular fluid and serum 25OH-D levels in women undergoing IVF, specifically that patients achieving clinical pregnancy had a significantly higher follicular fluid 25O HD level [77]. A 2012 retrospective cohort study of 188 infertile women undergoing IVF found that vitamin D deficiency was associated with lower pregnancy rates, but overall ovarian stimulation parameters were unchanged [85] which prompted the idea that vitamin D status may be more involved in implantation. However, a prospective cohort study of 280 frozen embryo transfers found comparable CPR between vitamin D replete, insufficient, and deficient women [107].

A 2022 meta-analysis including 10 studies (4 RCTs $n = 666$ and 6 observational $n = 6997$) found that women diagnosed with vitamin D deficiency had increased risk of miscarriage compared with women who were vitamin D replete (OR 1.94, 95% CI 1.25–3.02). However, there were several limitations with this study, including low overall study quality as well as study heterogeneity [100]. A subsequent 2023 meta-analysis, which included 12 studies, found that vitamin D supplementation improved the clinical pregnancy rate of infertile women but did not alter the implantation or biochemical pregnancy rate. The dosing used in the studies ranged significantly from 560 daily to 600,000 IU once, in both oral and IM forms and daily and weekly and monthly dosing. The extreme dosing was only used in one study that may have skewed results. These authors support the use of vitamin D supplementation (1000–10,000 IU) daily for >30 days [65].

Unfortunately, there is no clear evidence that vitamin D supplementation will improve IVF outcomes. Vitamin D supplementation continues to be recommended for those who are deficient, as it does serve many other functions in reproductive-aged women, but the evidence regarding pregnancy outcomes is inconsistent. Vitamin D is usually taken as 1000 to 2000 units daily or 10,000 units weekly; overweight patients may require higher doses to have normal blood levels. Excessive intake of vitamin D can be a teratogen resulting in fetal abnormalities. As such, if intake is very high, this risk should be discussed with the patient.

7.9 Vitamin D: Males

Vitamin D receptors and enzymes for vitamin D metabolism have been found in testes, the male reproductive tract, and sperm. This finding lends biologic plausibility to the potential role of vitamin D deficiency in male factor infertility [7, 12]. Observational data is mixed, demonstrating positive correlations in some studies [1, 5, 6, 34, 37, 38, 40, 83, 104, 113, 122] but not all studies [73, 82, 86, 101, 102]. Only a few studies have included data on pregnancy outcomes, and those have conflicting results [73, 101, 102].

A cross-sectional study of 1248 infertile men found that both vitamin D deficiency and low ionized calcium are significantly associated with poorer semen quality and altered sex steroid levels in infertile men [38]. A single-center triple-blinded RCT randomized 330 men with male factor infertility and vitamin D insufficiency to either high-dose vitamin D supplementation or placebo, and no difference in semen parameters or LBR was found between groups. A subgroup analysis of oligospermic men in this study, however, did demonstrate an increased LBR in the treatment group (35.6% vs. 18.3% pg% CI 1.6–32.9%) [39].

A 2022 systematic review included 53 studies, 32 of which focused on the effect of vitamin D on sperm parameters. A positive correlation between vitamin D serum levels and total or progressive sperm motility was found, and this relationship persisted in the general population as well as infertile men. None of these studies examined effects on LBR. The included studies were also of poorer quality, smaller, and had high levels of heterogeneity in study design, making it difficult to make comparisons, and for this reason no statistical analysis of these results was performed [2].

While there is some evidence to suggest an association with fertility and adequate vitamin D levels, there is inadequate evidence to support the supplementation of vitamin D for improvement of pregnancy outcomes or semen analysis parameters (see Table 7.2). Larger prospective studies are needed to be able to draw meaningful conclusions from the data.

Table 7.2 Summary of adjuvant pharmacotherapy in IVF for men

	Dosage	Timing	Proposed mechanism	Recommendation
Antioxidants	Variable formulations	Pretreatment × 3 months	Decrease ROS, DNA fragmentation	Benefit is not demonstrated
Coenzyme Q 10	200–600 mg qday	Pretreatment × 3 months	Antioxidant	Benefit is not demonstrated
Vitamin D	600 IU/day if not deficient; higher doses may vary, but not to exceed 4000 IU/day	Daily for at least 30 days	Improve semen quality	May consider for other health indications

7.10 COQ10: Females

Coenzyme Q10, or CoQ10, is a naturally occurring antioxidant that decreases with age. It is hypothesized to lead to decreased free radical damage in developing oocytes, which may in turn lead to better-quality oocytes and decreased risk of aneuploidy [42, 67]. This relationship between antioxidant levels and poor oocyte quality is well studied, which is why CoQ10 has been proposed as an adjuvant to improve outcomes in poor responders [9, 10]. It is also a mitochondrial nutrient. Mitochondria are the power plants of eggs, and mitochondria levels and function are decreased in older women (defined as 35 years of age or older). As such, CoQ10 has been used to improve mitochondrial function.

There are few good-quality studies on this subject. Bentov et al. conducted a double blind-placebo controlled RCT aimed to compare aneuploidy rates in patients getting CoQ10 versus placebo and found no significant difference in aneuploidy or CPR between the groups. The study was terminated before reaching the target number of participants, however, and thus was underpowered [11]. A second RCT in 2014 included 101 women with clomiphene-resistant PMOS and compared pregnancy outcomes in those getting CoQ10 with clomiphene versus clomiphene alone and found significant improvement in ovulation and CPR in the study group [27]. A 2020 Cochrane review, which included the aforementioned studies, found no improvement in LBR with antioxidants compared with placebo but did show improvement in CPR with COQ10 supplementation. These authors found that there was only low- to very low-quality evidence to suggest that antioxidant use may provide benefit for subfertile women [93].

A 2018 RCT (n = 169) compared the number of high-quality embryos from IVF between those who received CoQ10 versus placebo amongst young patients with DOR and found that the CoQ10 group had a greater number of high-quality embryos for transfer ($p = 0.03$), yet no difference in LBR [111]. A 2020 meta-analysis including 5 RCTs ($n = 449$) found that CoQ10 resulted in an increased CPR, and that this effect remained significant when women with poor ovarian response and PMOS were analyzed separately. There was no significant difference between groups regarding LBR [30].

COQ10 is a relatively low-cost, low risk intervention with a plausible utility. However, more robust research is needed in order to make overarching recommendations. Safety data shows that the studied doses are safe (200–600 mg/day) which is reassuring [35]. It may have the potential to improve outcomes for poor responders, but additional research is needed before its routine recommendation to meaningfully improve outcomes. Occasionally patients will complain of difficulty sleeping on CoQ10, and moving the medication to the morning can help with this issue.

7.11 COQ10: Males

Evidence suggests that oxidative stress may play a role in the etiology of male infertility as well. The imbalance between reactive oxygen species and protective antioxidants could lead to abnormal sperm parameters and high levels of sperm DNA fragmentation. Therefore, using antioxidants to combat excessive oxidative stress in the treatment of infertility is a common recommendation [59].

An RCT from 2009 included 212 infertile men with idiopathic oligoasthenoteratospermia that were randomly assigned to CoQ10 versus placebo during a 26-week period followed by a 30-week treatment-free phase. They found significant improvement in sperm concentration and motility in the CoQ10 group and a positive correlation between treatment duration with CoQ10 and sperm count as well as sperm motility and morphology. They also found an improvement in reproductive hormone levels, including testosterone, suggesting CoQ10 may be a beneficial adjunct in the treatment of male infertility [87].

A systematic review and meta-analysis from 2021 included 20 studies looking at 3 different antioxidants (selenium, carnitine, and CoQ10). They found improvement in semen parameters, including motility and sperm concentration; however this improvement was not seen in pregnancy rates. The poor quality of the studies is a major limitation [91]. A 2022 meta-analysis included 23 RCTs and 10 different antioxidants (n = 1917). Only 12 of these studies reported the pregnancy rate and found no statistical difference between treatment and placebo with regard to this [59].

While this evidence surrounding male infertility and CoQ10 is encouraging, further studies are needed in order to draw a meaningful conclusion with regard to the effect on pregnancy and LBR (Table 7.2).

7.12 Antioxidants: Males

There are many antioxidants being marketed to treat male infertility, and there is biological plausibility to support their supplementation. Oxidative stress can cause structural modifications to the sperm plasma membrane, which may interfere with sperm motility, the acrosome reactions, and sperm-oocyte fusion [4, 98]. It may also cause DNA breaks, damaging the nuclear and mitochondrial genome and "DNA fragmentation." Studies have shown that subfertile men have higher levels of reactive oxygen species and lower antioxidant levels in their semen compared with fertile men [17, 43, 124]. Antioxidants may then theoretically decrease oxidative stress and potentially improve sperm motility and reduce DNA fragmentation.

A 2019 Cochrane meta-analysis found a higher LBR with antioxidants when compared to placebo (OR 3.61; 95% CI 1.27–10.29) but no statistically significant difference in the CPR [95]. However, when studies at high risk of bias were removed from the analysis, there was no evidence of increased LBR [95]. The authors conclude that there is low-quality evidence from 7 small RCTs suggesting antioxidant supplementation in subfertile males may improve LBR; however, the current evidence is inconclusive.

The MOXI (Males, Antioxidants, and Infertility) trial was an NICHD-funded multicenter RCT trial to assess whether antioxidants would improve male infertility without the use of ART. 171 patients were randomized to either placebo or an antioxidant formula (vitamin C, vitamin E, selenium, carnitine, folic acid, lycopene, or vitamin D) for at least 3 months and up to 6 months. In the internal pilot study, the use of antioxidant combination did not result in a significant improvement in semen parameters after 3 months of therapy, compared to placebo. Furthermore, men with asthenospermia or high DNA fragmentation did not exhibit improvement in motility or decrease in DNA fragmentation. Though not powered to examine differences in pregnancy rates, those who received an antioxidant were not more likely to conceive during natural conception or insemination cycles. Overall, antioxidant treatment was not found to improve semen parameters or DNA integrity in infertile males, so the trial was discontinued [98].

Despite the volume of supplements available for purchase, there is compelling evidence to actually dissuade patients from pursuing them (Table 7.2). Despite being widely available and inexpensive, most antioxidants are uncontrolled by regulation and evidence for their effectiveness is not certain. The evidence surrounding antioxidants is inconclusive at best. Healthcare professionals should try to prevent patients from further financial burden of empiric therapy with over-the-counter antioxidant nutraceuticals.

7.13 Conclusion

There appears to be a common theme reflected in the review of adjuvant therapies for IVF: larger RCTs are necessary before most of these treatments can be routinely recommended for the purpose of improving reproductive outcomes. The population of patients pursuing IVF is often a vulnerable group, willing to try any "add-on" that offers a chance at improved outcomes. For this reason, it's important to become familiar with the literature available in order to best counsel patients and provide realistic expectations. It is essential to avoid overselling a certain treatment based on anecdotal evidence, as this may lead to even more emotional and financial expense. It is possible that some of these adjuvants may become part of routine care, especially for specific patient populations, but until robust evidence is available, the use of such clinical adjuncts in routine practice should be approached with caution.

References

1. Abbasihormozi SH, Kouhkan A, et al. Association of vitamin D status with semen quality and reproductive hormones in Iranian subfertile men. Andrology. 2017;5:113–8.
2. Adamczewska D, Słowikowska-Hilczer J, Walczak-Jędrzejowska R. The association between vitamin D and the components of male fertility: a systematic review. Biomedicine. 2022;11(1):90. https://doi.org/10.3390/biomedicines11010090. PMID: 36672602; PMCID: PMC9912266.
3. Agarwal R, et al. Evaluation of dehydroepiandrosterone supplementation on diminished ovarian reserve: a randomized, double-blinded, placebo-controlled study. J Obstet Gynaecol India. 2017;67(2):137–42.
4. Aitken RJ. Generation of reactive oxygen species, lipid peroxidation, and human sperm function. Biol Reprod. 1989;41:183–97.
5. Akhavizadegan H, Karbakhsh M. Comparison of serum vitamin D between fertile and infertile men in a vitamin D deficient endemic area: a case-control study. Urologia. 2017;84:218–20.
6. Arab A, Hadi A, Moosavian SP, Askari G, Nasirian M. The association between serum vitamin D, fertility and semen quality: a systematic review and meta-analysis. Int J Surg. 2019;71:101–9. https://doi.org/10.1016/j.ijsu.2019.09.025.
7. Banks N, Sun F, Krawetz SA, Coward RM, Masson P, Smith JF, Trussell JC, Santoro N, Zhang H, Steiner AZ. Male vitamin D status and male factor infertility. Fertil Steril. 2021;116(4):973–9. https://doi.org/10.1016/j.fertnstert.2021.06.035. Epub 2021 Jul 18. PMID: 34289935; PMCID: PMC8561776.
8. Barrera D, et al. Calcitriol affects hCG gene transcription in cultured human syncytiotrophoblasts. Reprod Biol Endocrinol. 2008;6:3.
9. Ben-Meir A, et al. Coenzyme Q-dependent mitochondrial respiratory chain activity in granulosa cells is reduced with aging. Fertil Steril. 2015a;104(3):724–7.
10. Ben-Meir A, et al. Coenzyme Q10 restores oocyte mitochondrial function and fertility during reproductive aging. Aging Cell. 2015b;14(5):887–95.
11. Bentov Y, Hannam T, Jurisicova A, Esfandiari N, Casper RF. Coenzyme Q10 supplementation and oocyte aneuploidy in women undergoing IVF-ICSI treatment. Clin Med Insights Reprod Health. 2014;8:31–6. Published 2014 Jun 8. https://doi.org/10.4137/CMRH.S14681.
12. Blomberg Jensen M. Vitamin D and male reproduction. Nat Rev Endocrinol. 2014;10(3):175–86. https://doi.org/10.1038/nrendo.2013.262. Epub 2014 Jan 14. PMID: 24419359.
13. Boomsma CM, Keay SD, Macklon NS. Peri-implantation glucocorticoid administration for assisted reproductive technology cycles. Cochrane Database Syst Rev. 2012;6:CD005996.
14. Bosdou JK, Venetis CA, Kolibianakis EM, Toulis KA, Goulis DG, Zepiridis L, et al. The use of androgens or androgen-modulating agents in poor responders undergoing in vitro fertilization: a systematic review and meta-analysis. Hum Reprod Update. 2012;18(2):127–45. https://doi.org/10.1093/humupd/dmr051.
15. Bosdou JK, Venetis CA, Dafopoulos K, Zepiridis L, Chatzimeletiou K, Anifandis G, Mitsoli A, Makedos A, Messinis IE, Tarlatzis BC, Kolibianakis EM. Transdermal testosterone pretreatment in poor responders undergoing ICSI: a randomized clinical trial. Hum Reprod. 2016;31(5):977-85. https://doi.org/10.1093/humrep/dew028. Epub 2016 Mar 7. PMID: 26956551
16. Burger HG. Androgen production in women. Fertil Steril. 2002;77(Suppl. 4):S3–5.
17. Bykova M, Athayde K, Sharma R, Jha R, Sabanegh E, Agarwal A. P-597. Defining the reference value of seminal reactive oxygen species in a population of infertile men and normal healthy volunteers. Fertil Steril. 2007;88(Suppl 1):S305.
18. Carlomagno G, Unfer V, Roseff S. The D-chiro-inositol paradox in the ovary. Fertil Steril. 2011;95(8):2515–6.

19. Chiu TT, Tam PP. A correlation of the outcome of clinical in vitro fertilization with the inositol content and embryotrophic properties of human serum. J Assist Reprod Genet. 1992;9(6):524–30.
20. Casson PR. Dehydroepiandrosterone supplementation augments ovarian stimulation in poor responders: a case series. Hum Reprod. 2000;15(10):2129-2132. https://doi.org/10.1093/humrep/15.10.2129
21. Casson PR, Lindsay MS, Pisarska MD, Carson SA, Buster JE. Dehydroepiandrosterone supplementation augments ovarian stimulation in poor responders: a case series. Hum Reprod. 2000;15(10):2129-32. https://doi.org/10.1093/humrep/15.10.2129. PMID: 11006185.
22. Chiu TT, et al. Follicular fluid and serum concentrations of myo-inositol in patients undergoing IVF: relationship with oocyte quality. Hum Reprod. 2002;17(6):1591–6.
23. Cozzolino M, et al. Growth hormone cotreatment for poor responders undergoing in vitro fertilization cycles: a systematic review and meta-analysis. Fertil Steril. 2020a;114(1):97–109.
24. Cozzolino M, et al. How vitamin D level influences in vitro fertilization outcomes: results of a systematic review and meta-analysis. Fertil Steril. 2020b;114(5):1014–25.
25. de Fried EP, Bossi NM, Notrica JA, Levin MV. Vitamin-d treatment does not improve pregnancy rates in patients undergoing art: a prospective, randomized, double-blind placebo-controlled trial. Fertil Steril. 2013;100(3):S493–4. 48.
26. Dirckx K, Cabri P, Merien A, Galajdova L, Gerris J, Dhont M, De Sutter P. Does low-dose aspirin improve pregnancy rate in IVF/ICSI? A randomized double-blind placebo controlled trial. Hum Reprod. 2009;24(4):856-60. https://doi.org/10.1093/humrep/den476. Epub 2009 Jan 8. PMID: 19131401.
27. El Refaeey A, Selem A, Badawy A. Combined coenzyme Q10 and clomiphene citrate for ovulation induction in clomiphene-citrate-resistant polycystic ovary syndrome. Reprod Biomed Online. 2014;29(1):119–24.
28. Fabregues F, et al. Transdermal testosterone may improve ovarian response to gonadotrophins in low-responder IVF patients: a randomized, clinical trial. Hum Reprod. 2009;24(2):349–59.
29. Ferraretti AP, et al. ESHRE consensus on the definition of 'poor response' to ovarian stimulation for in vitro fertilization: the Bologna criteria. Hum Reprod. 2011;26(7):1616–24.
30. Florou P, Anagnostis P, Theocharis P, Chourdakis M, Goulis DG. Does coenzyme Q(10) supplementation improve fertility outcomes in women undergoing assisted reproductive technology procedures? A systematic review and meta-analysis of randomized-controlled trials. J Assist Reprod Genet. 2020;37(10):2377–87. https://doi.org/10.1007/s10815-020-01906-3.
31. Fridström M, Carlström K, Sjöblom P, Hillensjö T. Effect of prednisolone on serum and follicular fluid androgen concentrations in women with polycystic ovary syndrome undergoing in-vitro fertilization. Hum Reprod. 1999;14(6):1440–4. https://doi.org/10.1093/humrep/14.6.1440.
32. Gerli S, et al. Randomized, double blind placebo-controlled trial: effects of myo-inositol on ovarian function and metabolic factors in women with PCOS. Eur Rev Med Pharmacol Sci. 2007;11(5):347–54.
33. Haapsamo M, et al. Low-dose aspirin therapy and hypertensive pregnancy complications in unselected IVF and ICSI patients: a randomized, placebo-controlled, double-blind study. Hum Reprod. 2010;25(12):2972–7.
34. Hammoud AO, Meikle AW, et al. Association of 25-hydroxy-vitamin D levels with semen and hormonal parameters. Asian J Androl. 2012;14:855–9.
35. Hidaka T, et al. Safety assessment of coenzyme Q10 (CoQ10). Biofactors. 2008;32(1-4):199–208.
36. Hull KL, Harvey S. Growth hormone: roles in female reproduction. J Endocrinol. 2001;168(1):1–2.
37. Jensen MB, Bjerrum PJ, et al. Vitamin D is positively associated with sperm motility and increased intracellular calcium in human spermatozoa. Hum Reprod. 2011;26:1307–17.
38. Jensen MB, Lawaetz JG, et al. Vitamin D deficiency and low ionized calcium are linked with semen quality and sex steroid levels in infertile men. Hum Reprod. 2016;31:1875–85.
39. Jensen MB, Lawaetz JG, et al. Effects of vitamin D supplementation on semen quality, reproductive hormones, and live birth rate: a randomized clinical trial. J Clin Endocrinol Metab. 2018;103:870–81.

40. Jueraitetibaike K, Ding Z, et al. The effect of vitamin D on sperm motility and the underlying mechanism. Asian J Androl. 2019;21:400–7.
41. Kalampokas T, Pandian Z, Keay SD, Bhattacharya S. Glucocorticoid supplementation during ovarian stimulation for IVF or ICSI. Cochrane Database Syst Rev. 2017;3(3):CD004752. https://doi.org/10.1002/14651858.CD004752.pub2. PMID: 28349525; PMCID: PMC6464567.
42. Kalen A, Appelkvist EL, Dallner G. Age-related changes in the lipid compositions of rat and human tissues. Lipids. 1989;24(7):579–84.
43. Kamath MS, Mascarenhas M, Franik S, Liu E, Sunkara SK. Clinical adjuncts in in vitro fertilization: a growing list. Fertil Steril. 2019;112(6):978–86. https://doi.org/10.1016/j.fertnstert.2019.09.019.
44. Keane KN, et al. Single center retrospective analysis of growth hormone supplementation in IVF patients classified as poor-prognosis. BMJ Open. 2017;7(10):e018107.
45. Keay SD, et al. Low-dose dexamethasone augments the ovarian response to exogenous gonadotrophins leading to a reduction in cycle cancellation rate in a standard IVF programme. Hum Reprod. 2001;16(9):1861–5.
46. Kessopoulou E, Powers HJ, Sharma KK, Pearson MJ, Russell JM, Cooke ID, et al. A double-blind randomized placebo cross-over controlled trial using the antioxidant vitamin E to treat reactive oxygen species associated male infertility. Fertil Steril. 1995;64:825–31.
47. Khairy M, et al. Aspirin in women undergoing in vitro fertilization treatment: a systematic review and metaanalysis. Fertil Steril. 2007;88(4):822–31.
48. Kim CH, Howles CM, Lee HA. The effect of transdermal testosterone gel pretreatment on controlled ovarian stimulation and IVF outcome in low responders. Fertil Steril. 2011;95(2):679–83.
49. Kim CH, et al. Ovarian features after 2 weeks, 3 weeks and 4 weeks transdermal testosterone gel treatment and their associated effect on IVF outcomes in poor responders. Dev Reprod. 2014;18(3):145–52.
50. Kolibianakis EM, Venetis CA, Diedrich K, Tarlatzis BC, Griesinger G. Addition of growth hormone to gonadotrophins in ovarian stimulation of poor responders treated by in-vitro fertilization: a systematic review and meta-analysis. Hum Reprod Update. 2009;15(6):613–22. https://doi.org/10.1093/humupd/dmp026.
51. Kotb MM, Hassan AM, AwadAllah AM. Does dehydroepiandrosterone improve pregnancy rate in women undergoing IVF/ICSI with expected poor ovarian response according to the Bologna criteria? A randomized controlled trial. Eur J Obstet Gynecol Reprod Biol. 2016;200:11–5.
52. Kroboth PD, et al. DHEA and DHEA-S: a review. J Clin Pharmacol. 1999;39(4):327–48.
53. Kyrou D, Kolibianakis EM, Venetis CA, Papanikolaou EG, Bontis J, Tarlatzis BC. How to improve the probability of pregnancy in poor responders undergoing in vitro fertilization: a systematic review and meta-analysis. Fertil Steril. 2009;91(3):749–66. https://doi.org/10.1016/j.fertnstert.2007.12.077.
54. Lambers MJ, et al. Low-dose aspirin in non-tubal IVF patients with previous failed conception: a prospective randomized double-blind placebo-controlled trial. Fertil Steril. 2009;92(3):923–9.
55. Lan KC, et al. Growth hormone supplementation may improve the pregnancy rate and endometrial receptivity among women aged more than 40 years undergoing in vitro fertilization. Biom J. 2019;42(6):411–6.
56. Lee YX, Shen MS, Tzeng CR. Low dose growth hormone adjuvant treatment with ultra-long ovarian stimulation protocol in poor responders showed non-inferior pregnancy outcome compared with normal responders. Front Endocrinol. 2019;10:892.
57. Lerchbaum E, Rabe T. Vitamin D and female fertility. Curr Opin Obstet Gynecol. 2014;26(3):145–50.
58. Li J, Yuan H, Chen Y, Wu H, Wu H, Li L. A meta-analysis of dehydroepiandrosterone supplementation among women with diminished ovarian reserve undergoing in vitro fertilization or intracytoplasmic sperm injection. Int J Gynaecol Obstet. 2015;131(3):240–5.
59. Li KP, Yang XS, Wu T. The effect of antioxidants on sperm quality parameters and pregnancy rates for idiopathic male infertility: a network meta-analysis of randomized controlled trials.

Front Endocrinol (Lausanne). 2022;13:810242. https://doi.org/10.3389/fendo.2022.810242. PMID: 35265037; PMCID: PMC8898892.

60. Lin G, Zhong X, Li S, Xu L. Clinical evidence of growth hormone for infertile women with diminished ovarian reserve undergoing IVF: a systematic review and meta-analysis. Front Endocrinol (Lausanne). 2023a;14:1215755. https://doi.org/10.3389/fendo.2023.1215755. PMID: 38027219; PMCID: PMC10663944.
61. Lin L, Li T, Chen L, Sha C, Gao W, Wei H, Zhu X. Glucocorticoid supplementation during ovulation induction for assisted reproductive technology: a systematic review and meta-analysis. J Matern Fetal Neonatal Med. 2023b;36(2):2227310. https://doi.org/10.1080/14767058.2023.2227310. PMID: 37385781.
62. Lossl K, et al. Biological and clinical rationale for androgen priming in ovarian stimulation. Front Endocrinol. 2020;11:627.
63. Marian G, Showell R, Mackenzie-Proctor V, Jordan R, Hodgson C, Farquhar C. Inositol for subfertile women with polycystic ovary syndrome. Cochrane Database Syst Rev. 2018;(12):CD012378. https://doi.org/10.1002/14651858. CD012378.pub2
64. Massin N, et al. Effects of transdermal testosterone application on the ovarian response to FSH in poor responders undergoing assisted reproduction technique–a prospective, randomized, double-blind study. Hum Reprod. 2006;21(5):1204–11.
65. Meng X, Zhang J, Wan Q, Huang J, Han T, Qu T, Yu LL. Influence of vitamin D supplementation on reproductive outcomes of infertile patients: a systematic review and meta-analysis. Reprod Biol Endocrinol. 2023;21(1):17. https://doi.org/10.1186/s12958-023-01068-8. PMID: 36737817; PMCID: PMC9896710.
66. Merhi ZO, et al. Circulating vitamin D correlates with serum antimullerian hormone levels in late-reproductiveaged women: women's interagency HIV study. Fertil Steril. 2012;98(1):228–34.
67. Miles MV, et al. Age-related changes in plasma coenzyme Q10 concentrations and redox state in apparently healthy children and adults. Clin Chim Acta. 2004;347(1-2):139–44.
68. Montoya-Botero P, Rodriguez-Purata J, Polyzos NP. Androgen supplementation in assisted reproduction: where are we in 2019? Curr Opin Obstet Gynecol. 2019;31(3):188–94.
69. Nagels HE, Rishworth JR, Siristatidis CS, Kroon B. Androgens (dehydroepiandrosterone or testosterone) for women undergoing assisted reproduction. *Cochrane Database of Systematic Reviews*. 2015;11:CD009749. https://doi.org/10.1002/14651858.CD009749.pub2. Accessed 15 July 2026
70. Narkwichean A, Maalouf W, Campbell BK, Jayaprakasan K. Efficacy of dehydroepiandrosterone to improve ovarian response in women with diminished ovarian reserve: a meta-analysis. Reprod Biol Endocrinol. 2013;11:44. https://doi.org/10.1186/1477-7827-11-44.
71. Narkwichean A, Jayaprakasan K, Maalouf WE, Hernandez-Medrano JH, Pincott-Allen C, Campbell BK. Effects of dehydroepiandrosterone on in vivo ovine follicular development. Hum Reprod. 2014;29(1):146-54. https://doi.org/10.1093/humrep/det408. Epub 2013 Nov 20. PMID: 24256992
72. Nestler JE, et al. Ovulatory and metabolic effects of D-chiro-inositol in the polycystic ovary syndrome. N Engl J Med. 1999;340(17):1314–20.
73. Neville G, Martyn F, Kilbane M, O'Riordan M, Wingfield M, McKenna M, McAuliffe FM. Vitamin D status and fertility outcomes during winter among couples undergoing in vitro fertilization/intracytoplasmic sperm injection. Int J Gynaecol Obstet. 2016;135(2):172–6. https://doi.org/10.1016/j.ijgo.2016.04.018. Epub 2016 Jul 30. PMID: 27530219.
74. Nordio M, Basciani S, Camajani E. The 40:1 myo-inositol/D-chiro-inositol plasma ratio is able to restore ovulation in PCOS patients: comparison with other ratios. Eur Rev Med Pharmacol Sci. 2019;23(12)
75. Noventa M, et al. Testosterone therapy for women with poor ovarian response undergoing IVF: a meta-analysis of randomized controlled trials. J Assist Reprod Genet. 2019;36(4):673–83.
76. Ob'edkova K, et al. Growth hormone co-treatment in IVF/ICSI cycles in poor responders. Gynecol Endocrinol. 2017;33(Suppl. 1):15–7.
77. Ozkan S, et al. Replete vitamin D stores predict reproductive success following in vitro fertilization. Fertil Steril. 2010;94(4):1314–9.

78. Papaleo E, et al. Myo-inositol in patients with polycystic ovary syndrome: a novel method for ovulation induction. Gynecol Endocrinol. 2007;23(12):700–3.
79. Parikh G, et al. Vitamin D regulates steroidogenesis and insulin-like growth factor binding protein-1 (IGFBP-1) production in human ovarian cells. Horm Metab Res. 2010;42(10):754–7.
80. Practice Committee of the American Society for Reproductive Medicine. Electronic address, A.a.o. and M. Practice committee of the American society for reproductive. The role of immunotherapy in in vitro fertilization: a guideline. Fertil Steril. 2018;110(3):387–400.
81. Qin JC, Fan L, Qin AP. The effect of dehydroepiandrosterone (DHEA) supplementation on women with diminished ovarian reserve (DOR) in IVF cycle: evidence from a meta-analysis. J Gynecol Obstet Hum Reprod. 2017;46(1):1–7. https://doi.org/10.1016/j.jgyn.2016.01.002.
82. Ramlau-Hansen CH, Moeller UK, et al. Are serum levels of vitamin D associated with semen quality? Results from a cross-sectional study in young healthy men. Fertil Steril. 2011;95:1000–4.
83. Rehman R, Lalani S, et al. Association between vitamin D, reproductive hormones and sperm parameters in infertile male subjects. Front Endocrinol. 2018;9:607.
84. Richardson A, Jayaprakasan K. The use of androgen priming in women with reduced ovarian reserve undergoing assisted reproductive technology. Semin Reprod Med. 2021;39(5–06):207–19. https://doi.org/10.1055/s-0041-1735646.
85. Rudick B, et al. Characterizing the influence of vitamin D levels on IVF outcomes. Hum Reprod. 2012;27(11):3321–7.
86. Rudnicka A, Adoamnei E, et al. Vitamin D status is not associated with reproductive parameters in young Spanish men. Andrology. 2020;8:323–31.
87. Safarinejad MR. Efficacy of coenzyme Q10 on semen parameters, sperm function and reproductive hormones in infertile men. J Urol. 2009;182(1):237–48. https://doi.org/10.1016/j.juro.2009.02.121. Epub 2009 May 17. PMID: 19447425.
88. Schachter M, Raziel A, Strassburger D, Rotem C, Ron-El R, Friedler S. Prospective, randomized trial of metformin and vitamins for the reduction of plasma homocysteine in insulin-resistant polycystic ovary syndrome. Fertil Steril. 2007;88(1):227–30. https://doi.org/10.1016/j.fertnstert.2006.11.071.
89. Schisterman EF, et al. Preconception low-dose aspirin and pregnancy outcomes: results from the EAGeR randomised trial. Lancet. 2014;384(9937):29–36.
90. Schwarze JE, Canales J, Crosby J, Ortega-Hrepich C, Villa S, Pommer R. DHEA use to improve likelihood of IVF/ICSI success in patients with diminished ovarian reserve: a systematic review and meta-analysis. JBRA Assist Reprod. 2018;22(4):369–74. https://doi.org/10.5935/1518-0557.20180046.
91. Sharma AP, Sharma G, Kumar R. Systematic review and meta-analysis on effect of carnitine, coenzyme Q10 and selenium on pregnancy and semen parameters in couples with idiopathic male infertility. Urology. 2022;161:4–11. https://doi.org/10.1016/j.urology.2021.10.041. Epub 2021 Dec 4. PMID: 34871624.
92. Showell MG, Mackenzie-Proctor R, Jordan V, Hodgson R, Farquhar C. Inositol for subfertile women with polycystic ovary syndrome. Cochrane Database Syst Rev. 2018;12(12):CD012378. https://doi.org/10.1002/14651858.CD012378.pub2. PMID: 30570133; PMCID: PMC6516980.
93. Showell MG, et al. Antioxidants for female subfertility. Cochrane Database Syst Rev. 2020;8:CD007807.
94. Siristatidis CS, et al. Aspirin for in vitro fertilisation. Cochrane Database Syst Rev. 2016;11:CD004832.
95. Smits RM, Mackenzie-Proctor R, Yazdani A, Stankiewicz MT, Jordan V, Showell MG. Antioxidants for male subfertility. Cochrane Database Syst Rev. 2019;3:CD007411.
96. Society for Assisted Reproductive Technology. IVF success rates. 2022. Accessed December 30, 2024. https://www.sartcorsonline.com/CSR/PublicSnapshotReport?ClinicPKID=&reportingYear=2022.
97. Sood A, Mohiyiddeen G, Ahmad G, Fitzgerald C, Watson A, Mohiyiddeen L. Growth hormone for in vitro fertilization (IVF). Cochrane Database Syst Rev. 2021;11(11):CD000099.

https://doi.org/10.1002/14651858.CD000099.pub4. PMID: 34808697; PMCID: PMC8608438.
98. Steiner AZ, Hansen KR, Barnhart KT, Cedars MI, Legro RS, Diamond MP, Krawetz SA, Usadi R, Baker VL, Coward RM, Huang H, Wild R, Masson P, Smith JF, Santoro N, Eisenberg E, Zhang H, Reproductive Medicine Network. The effect of antioxidants on male factor infertility: the Males, Antioxidants, and Infertility (MOXI) randomized clinical trial. Fertil Steril. 2020;113(3):552–560.e3. https://doi.org/10.1016/j.fertnstert.2019.11.008. Epub 2020 Feb 25. PMID: 32111479; PMCID: PMC7219515.
99. Sunkara SK, Coomarasamy A, Arlt W, Bhattacharya S. Should androgen supplementation be used for poor ovarian response in IVF? Hum Reprod. 2012;27(3):637–40. https://doi.org/10.1093/humrep/der464.
100. Tamblyn JA, Pilarski NSP, Markland AD, Marson EJ, Devall A, Hewison M, Morris RK, Coomarasamy A. Vitamin D and miscarriage: a systematic review and meta-analysis. Fertil Steril. 2022;118(1):111–22. https://doi.org/10.1016/j.fertnstert.2022.04.017. Epub 2022 May 28. PMID: 35637024.
101. Tartagni M, et al. Dehydroepiandrosterone decreases the age-related decline of the in vitro fertilization outcome in women younger than 40 years old. Reprod Biol Endocrinol. 2015a;13:18.
102. Tartagni M, Matteo M, et al. Males with low serum levels of vitamin D have lower pregnancy rates when ovulation induction and timed intercourse are used as a treatment for infertile couples: results from a pilot study. Reprod Biol Endocrinol. 2015b;13:127.
103. Teissier MP, et al. Comparison of follicle steroidogenesis from normal and polycystic ovaries in women undergoing IVF: relationship between steroid concentrations, follicle size, oocyte quality and fecundability. Hum Reprod. 2000;15(12):2471–7.
104. Tirabassi G, Cutini M, et al. Association between vitamin D and sperm parameters: clinical evidence. Endocrine. 2017;58:194–8.
105. Ubaldi F, et al. Low dose prednisolone administration in routine ICSI patients does not improve pregnancy and implantation rates. Hum Reprod. 2002;17(6):1544–7.
106. Unfer V, et al. Myo-inositol rather than D-chiro-inositol is able to improve oocyte quality in intracytoplasmic sperm injection cycles. A prospective, controlled, randomized trial. Eur Rev Med Pharmacol Sci. 2011;15(4):452–7.
107. van de Vijver A, et al. Vitamin D deficiency and pregnancy rates following frozen-thawed embryo transfer: a prospective cohort study. Hum Reprod. 2016;31(8):1749–54.
108. Waldenstrom U, Hellberg D, Nilsson S. Low-dose aspirin in a short regimen as standard treatment in in vitro fertilization: a randomized, prospective study. Fertil Steril. 2004;81(6):1560–4.
109. Wilkinson J, et al. Do a la carte menus serve infertility patients? The ethics and regulation of in vitro fertility addons. Fertil Steril. 2019;112(6):973e.
110. Wiser A, Gonen O, Ghetler Y, Shavit T, Berkovitz A, Shulman A. Addition of dehydroepiandrosterone (DHEA) for poor-responder patients before and during IVF treatment improves the pregnancy rate: A randomized prospective study, Human Reproduction, 2010;25(10):2496–2500. https://doi.org/10.1093/humrep/deq220
111. Xu Y, et al. Pretreatment with coenzyme Q10 improves ovarian response and embryo quality in low-prognosis young women with decreased ovarian reserve: a randomized controlled trial. Reprod Biol Endocrinol. 2018;16(1):29.
112. Xu L, Hu C, Liu Q, Li Y. The Effect of Dehydroepiandrosterone (DHEA) supplementation on IVF or ICSI: a meta-analysis of randomized controlled trials. Geburtshilfe Frauenheilkd. 2019;79(7):705–12. https://doi.org/10.1055/a-0882-3791.
113. Yang B, Sun H, et al. Association between testosterone, bone mineral density, vitamin D and semen quality in fertile and infertile Chinese men. Int J Androl. 2012;35:783–92.
114. Yang P, Wu R, Zhang H. The effect of growth hormone supplementation in poor ovarian responders undergoing IVF or ICSI: a meta-analysis of randomized controlled trials. Reprod Biol Endocrinol. 2020;18(1):76.

115. Yeung TW, et al. A randomized double-blinded placebo-controlled trial on the effect of dehydroepiandrosterone for 16 weeks on ovarian response markers in women with primary ovarian insufficiency. J Clin Endocrinol Metab. 2013;98(1):380–8.
116. Yeung TW, et al. A randomized, controlled, pilot trial on the effect of dehydroepiandrosterone on ovarian response markers, ovarian response, and in vitro fertilization outcomes in poor responders. Fertil Steril. 2014;102(1):108–15.
117. Yoshizawa T, et al. Mice lacking the vitamin D receptor exhibit impaired bone formation, uterine hypoplasia and growth retardation after weaning. Nat Genet. 1997;16(4):391–6.
118. Zhang HH, et al. Dehydroepiandrosterone improves follicular fluid bone morphogenetic protein-15 and accumulated embryo score of infertility patients with diminished ovarian reserve undergoing in vitro fertilization: a randomized controlled trial. J Ovarian Res. 2014;7:93.
119. Zhang M, Niu W, Wang Y, Xu J, Bao X, Wang L, et al. Dehydroepiandrosterone treatment in women with poor ovarian response undergoing IVF or ICSI: a systematic review and meta-analysis. J Assist Reprod Genet. 2016;33(8):981–91.
120. Zheng X, et al. Inositol supplement improves clinical pregnancy rate in infertile women undergoing ovulation induction for ICSI or IVF-ET. Medicine (Baltimore). 2017;96(49):e8842.
121. Zhou P, et al. IGF-I signaling is essential for FSH stimulation of AKT and steroidogenic genes in granulosa cells. Mol Endocrinol. 2013;27(3):511–23.
122. Zhu CI, Xu QF, et al. Investigation of serum vitamin D levels in Chinese infertile men. Andrologia. 2016;48:1261–6.
123. Zhu F, Yin S, Yang B, et al. TEAS, DHEA, CoQ10, and GH for poor ovarian response undergoing IVF-ET: a systematic review and network meta-analysis. Reprod Biol Endocrinol. 2023;21(1):64. Published 2023 Jul 18. https://doi.org/10.1186/s12958-023-01119-0.
124. Zini A, de Lamirande E, Gagnon C. Reactive oxygen species in semen of infertile patients: levels of superoxide dismutase- and catalase-like activities in seminal plasma and spermatozoa. Int J Androl. 1993;16:183–8.

IVF Protocols and Their Rationales

8

Najia Baria

8.1 Introduction

The IVF nurse is the key person who is involved in all the steps of IVF treatment. She serves as a caregiver, educator, and a coordinator helping patients navigate the medical and emotional aspects of IVF. She also contributes to the success of the IVF cycle by educating the patient about their personalized IVF treatment, including medication protocols and procedures, and ensuring the compliance of the patient to the IVF protocol and to the time-sensitive medications.

During this complex IVF journey, the IVF nurse will face many questions from the patients about their treatment protocol, the rationale, and what it is involved in terms of duration, cost, and side effects.

Therefore, it is important to increase the nursing knowledge about the different ovarian stimulation protocols used in IVF and to understand better the rationale behind them. This will help the IVF nurse to gain confidence in providing high quality teaching to the patient and advocate for the patient's needs, ensuring they receive appropriate care and support.

Objectives

In this chapter, the nurse will be able:

A. To know and understand the rationale of the controlled ovarian stimulation process, the ovulation triggering mode, and the luteal support
B. To know, understand, and explain the common protocols used in IVF treatment

N. Baria (✉)
Department of Fertility, Institution: Mc gill University Health Center, Montreal, QC, Canada
e-mail: najia.baria@muhc.mcgill.ca

M. Das, M. H. Dahan (eds.), *A Comprehensive Guide to Reproductive Health and Infertility Medicine for Nurses*, https://doi.org/10.1007/978-3-032-24372-0_8

The chapter will cover the following protocols:

I. The long GnRH agonist protocol (long protocol)
II. The GnRh antagonist protocol (short protocol)
III. Microdose flare agonist protocol (MDF)
IV. Progestin-primed ovarian stimulation protocol (PPOS)

The fertility specialist has the expertise to choose the suitable protocol and the appropriate dose of fertility medications for the patient, to personalize the treatment protocol depending on each patient's individual circumstances.

Generally, the IVF protocol selection and the dose of gonadotrophin stimulation are based on different criteria such as age, body mass index, ovarian reserve (as assessed by the antral follicle count (AFC) and/or anti-Mullerian hormone l (AMH), previous response to stimulation, and the medical history of the patient [1, 2].

The physician's decision is based on the benefits and shortcomings of each treatment and most importantly on the patient's response [3]. The target is to maximize the ovarian response, the implantation rate and pregnancy rate without compromising patient safety. Usually, the chosen protocol will consider these four important elements:

1. Ovarian stimulation and the control of the ovulation
2. The use of the birth control pill
3. The trigger mode for the final maturation and OHSS prevention
4. Luteal support after the egg retrieval

8.2 Ovarian Stimulation and the Ovulation Control

The ovarian stimulation (OS) is one of the key factors in the success of in vitro fertilization-embryo transfer (IVF-ET), by enabling the recruitment of numerous healthy fertilizable oocytes and, thereby, multiple embryos. OS usually includes the co-administration of gonadotropins and gonadotropins-releasing hormone (GnRh) analogues or GnRh antagonists. The two most commonly used protocols are the long GnRh agonist suppressive protocol and the GnRh antagonist protocol [4].

The gonadotropins were first introduced in the early 1960s and have been used in ovarian stimulation cycles to induce multiple follicular development, particularly during the past three decades, in women undergoing in vitro fertilization (IVF) treatment. A major drawback with super-ovulation was the precipitation of a premature LH surge and premature follicular luteinization, which leads to treatment cancellation [5].

Since the early 1980s, gonadotropin-releasing hormone (GnRH) analogues have been developed and employed along with gonadotropins to prevent the occurrence of a surge in luteinizing hormone (LH), which may occur prematurely before the leading follicle reaches the optimum diameter ($\geq$17 mm) for triggering ovulation by human chorionic gonadotropin (hCG) injection. Without the use of GnRH analogs, LH surges would occur in approximately 20% of stimulated IVF patients.

The use of GnRH agonists in ovarian stimulation has greatly improved the success rate of IVF. Preventing LH surges using GnRH analogues improves oocyte yield with more embryos for selection, therefore leading to an increase in pregnancy rates [5, 6].

The GnRH agonist dominated the ovarian stimulation until the early 2000s. At that time, the third generation of GnRh antagonist, free of allergic reactions, was introduced in ovarian stimulation as an alternative in preventing premature LH surges. This was eagerly awaited since the use of GnRh agonists was characterized by several disadvantages, such as an initial unwelcome increase in the secretion of gonadotrophins (flare up effect), a lengthy treatment period until hypophysis desensitization occurred and a frequent occurrence of ovarian hyperstimulation syndrome (OHSS) [6].

Both oral contraceptive pills (OCPs) and progesterone are effective for scheduling IVF treatment cycles.

8.3 The Use of the Birth Control Pill

Although hormonal contraception is frequently used in the management of reproductive issues for women, it is also heavily relied on in the context of fertility treatments. A unique use of hormonal contraception within infertility treatment is hormonal pretreatment for in vitro fertilization (IVF). Hormonal contraceptive pretreatment includes menstrual cycle control, synchronization of the oocyte cohort, modification of the hormonal milieu before controlled ovarian stimulation (COS) for IVF, and suppression of ovarian cyst formation [7]. Additionally, hormonal contraception can be used in third-party reproductive cycles to coordinate the oocyte donor with the oocyte recipient. Hormonal contraception also plays a pivotal role in reducing the risk of cancellation of cycles from unintended pregnancy in the donor [8].

The practice Committee of the American Society for Reproductive Medicine (ASRM) published in 2024 confirmed the following [7]:

- The hormonal contraception pretreatment can be used for scheduling IVF treatments.
- There are inconsistent data that pretreatment with hormonal contraception impacts ovarian stimulation, although it may increase the amount of gonadotropins required.
- There is inconsistent evidence that the formulation of hormonal contraception impacts IVF outcomes.
- The use of hormonal contraception for the suppression of ovarian cyst has not been substantiated.
- Pretreatment with hormonal contraception has been associated with a reduction in the live birth rate in some studies.

- It has also been reported that hormonal contraception administered for 12–30 days with a 5-days washout period does not affect clinical pregnancy, live birth or cumulative live birth in patients undergoing controlled ovarian stimulation for an IVF cycle.
- A 2017 Cochrane Review of 29 RCTs in GnRH agonist and antagonist cycles found no clear evidence of a difference in the pregnancy or live birth rates [8].
- When the use of hormonal contraception is contraindicated, progesterone maybe used as an alternative for scheduling purposes.

8.4 The Trigger Mode for the Final Maturation and OHSS Prevention

8.4.1 HCG Versus GnRh Agonist Trigger

The physiological luteinizing hormone (LH) surge, well-known as the crucial step in ovum meiosis and maturation, as well as in maturation of its supporting cells, has been traditionally replaced by human chorionic gonadotropin (hCG) in artificial reproductive technologies (ART) cycles. The actual event of ovulation is far from simple and involves multiple cascades and processes [9, 10], most of which are still poorly understood [11].

From a clinical perspective, the most troubling issue arising from the use of hCG for final follicular maturation is ovarian hyperstimulation syndrome (OHSS), because of its prolonged clearance. hCG is considered fundamental in triggering OHSS due to its ability to up-regulate VEGF expression in luteinized granulosa cells [12]. VEGF is considered the major driving force in the hyper-permeability characterizing OHSS and is therefore a key player in its pathophysiology [13]. This reason explains why GnRH agonist triggering in a GnRH antagonist cycle has been suggested and used as an option for triggering ovulation. It can be a preventive measure against OHSS, especially when combined with an efficient freeze/thaw system [13].

The superiority of GnRH agonist triggering is clear in oocyte donors, women or units avoiding fresh embryo transfers, and in the context of fertility preservation [14].

8.4.2 Dual Triggering (HCG + GnRh Agonist)

The use of GnRH agonist triggering has raised interest in a new concept: dual triggering, which combines both hCG and endogenous LH/FSH surges. The idea of combining hCG with GnRH agonist triggering was introduced in 2008 in an effort to reduce the increased pregnancy loss rate associated with triggering [15].

It was suggested that its use, even as a "substituting dose," can aid in ovum maturation, provide sustained support and supplement the surge with endogenous LH [15].

8.4.2.1 The Trigger Criteria and Timing

The timing of human chorionic gonadotropin (HCG) for final maturation of targeted follicles is determined by many factors, such as follicle diameter, estradiol (E2) and progesterone level, the ratio of peak E2 to the number of oocytes larger than 14 mm, previous controlled ovarian hyperstimulation (COH) protocols and embryo development. Timing of the onset of luteinization before oocyte retrieval is a terminal act that influences oocyte quality and endometrium receptivity [16].

8.5 Luteal Support After the Egg Retrieval

After ovulation, the luteal phase of the menstrual cycle starts and continues until the next menstruation. Remnants of the ovulated egg in the ovary are known as "corpus luteum," or yellow body. The yellow body produces hormones, including progesterone. Progesterone stimulates proliferation of the lining of the uterus to prepare for implantation.

During assisted reproduction, the woman's pituitary gland is desensitized with medications so that the ovaries can be stimulated in a controlled manner. Hyperstimulation of the ovaries causes a luteal phase defect, as the corpus luteum is unable to produce sufficient progesterone.

As a low progesterone level may lower the chance of implantation, the luteal phase needs to be supported. This may involve oral, vaginal, or intramuscular progesterone, human chorionic gonadotropin (hCG) (which stimulates progesterone production) or gonadotropin-releasing hormone (GnRH) agonists. GnRH agonists stimulate the production of GnRH, a hormone responsible for follicle-stimulating hormone (FSH), and luteinizing hormone (LH), which triggers ovulation and develops the yellow body. GnRH agonists are thought to restore LH levels and support the luteal phase naturally [17].

Initiation of progesterone for luteal phase support should occur in the window between the evening of the day of oocyte retrieval and day 3 post oocyte retrieval [18]. Progesterone for luteal phase support should be administered at least until the day of the pregnancy test [18].

Progesterone can be administered in various forms including micronized vaginal progesterone (gel or oil capsules) [19], subcutaneous progesterone [20] and intramuscular progesterone [17, 18].

8.6 The Common Protocols Used in IVF Treatment

8.6.1 The Gn-RH Agonist Protocol: (Long Protocol)

The GnRh long agonist in vitro fertilization (IVF) protocol (Fig. 8.1) is a commonly used approach to ovarian stimulation. It starts with administration of gonadotropin-releasing hormone (GnRH) agonists (e.g., buserelin 500mcg) in the luteal phase to suppress the body's natural hormonal cycle (*Downregulation*) followed by

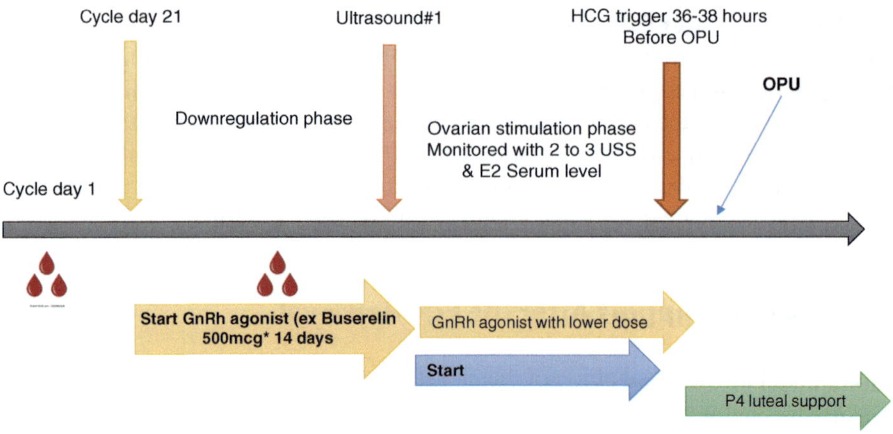

Fig. 8.1 GnRh agonist protocol. Legend: USS Ultrasound, E2 Estradiol, OPU Oocytes pick -up, P4 Progesterone

administration of gonadotropins usually at 150–225 international units (IU) daily starting from day 2 of the cycle to stimulate ovarian follicle development. The adjustment of gonadotropin dose is based on follicular development and E2 level. Continual administration of GnRh agonist and gonadotropin lasts until the start of the human chorionic gonadotropin (HCG) injection, which is approximately 14 days post GnRh agonist regimen or when follicles reached 16–18 millimeters (mm) in size [3].

8.6.1.1 GnRh Agonist Protocol Summary

1. GnRh agonist downregulation
   It suppresses the natural menstrual cycle by desensitizing the pituitary gland to prevent premature ovulation. GnRh (e.g., leuprolide acetate, buserelin, triptorelin) begins in the mid-luteal phase of the previous menstrual cycle (around cycle day 21). The first ultrasound will confirm ovarian suppression (thin endometrial lining and quiet ovaries). Some IVF clinics will use hormonal contraception to "batch" IVF cycles or have several patients complete their IVF cycles at the same time such as donor–recipient cycles
2. FSH/LH start
   Once downregulation is confirmed, the *gonadotropin* injections—follicle-stimulating hormone (FSH) and/or luteinizing hormone (LH) —can be started, and blood tests to track estradiol levels and ultrasound scans to monitor follicle growth are arranged.
3. The trigger
   The trigger is done exclusively by using HCG *never with GnRh agonist* to ensure the final maturation of eggs and preparation for egg retrieval. It is administered approximately 36–38 h before egg retrieval. If the patient has a high risk of OHSS, the physician will decide to freeze all embryos after egg retrieval and will

postpone the embryo transfer. The patient then will later undergo a frozen embryo transfer cycle after her OHSS resolves.

4. Luteal support
   Progesterone supplementation is recommended for luteal support in IVF and is usually started on the evening of the egg retrieval to support the uterine lining and prepare for embryo transfer.

Advantages [5]

- Provides better control over the timing of stimulation
- Reduces the risk of premature ovulation
- May improve outcomes in certain groups of patients, such as those with normal ovarian reserve.

Potential disadvantages [5]

- Extended duration and more injections compared to other protocols.
- Ovarian cyst formation.
- Risk of ovarian hyperstimulation syndrome (OHSS); may not be suitable for women with poor ovarian reserve or certain medical conditions.

8.6.2 GnRh Antagonist Protocol (Short Protocol)

GnRH antagonists cause immediate, rapid gonadotropin suppression by competitively blocking GnRH receptors in the anterior pituitary gland, thereby preventing endogenous GnRH from inducing LH and follicle-stimulating hormone (FSH) release from the pituitary cells. Furthermore, GnRH antagonist suppression of gonadotropin secretion can be quickly reversed [21, 22]. This different pharmacologic mechanism of action makes GnRH antagonists a logical choice to use in IVF for the prevention of premature LH surges [23].

Clinically, stimulation with urinary FSH or recombinant human FSH (rFSH), either alone or in combination with urinary-derived human menopausal gonadotropin (hMG), is started on day 2 or 3 of the menstrual cycle, and the GnRH antagonist is administered in the late follicular phase, from day 5 or 6 of stimulation onward.

The dose of gonadotropins may be adjusted according to individual response. Both gonadotropins are continued daily until two to three follicles reach ≥17 mm in diameter (on ultrasound assessment) at which time hCG is administered to induce final oocyte maturation.

The GnRH antagonist can be planned in two different ways: fixed protocol or flexible protocol.

In the fixed protocol shown in Fig. 8.2, the antagonist is administered on a certain day of stimulation, on which the risk of LH rise is thought to be present in most patients.

In the introductory trials, GnRH antagonist was started on day 6 of follicle-stimulating hormone (FSH) administration [18], while in subsequent studies this was performed on day 5 of stimulation [24].

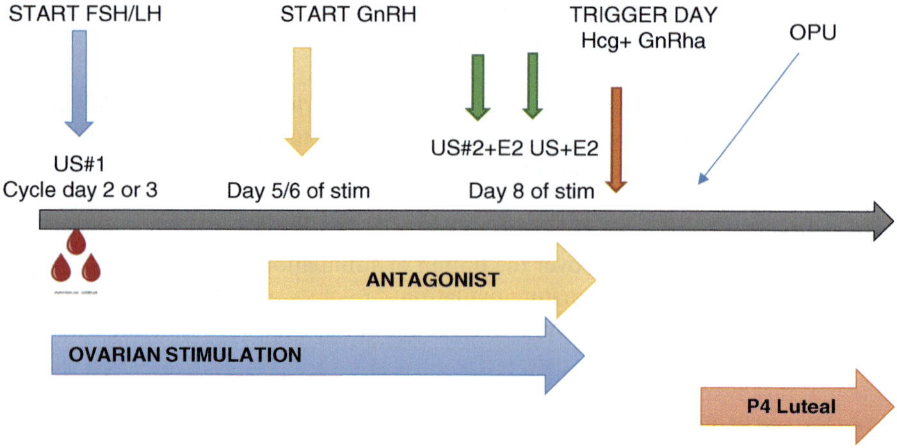

Fig. 8.2 Fixed Gn-RH protocol. Legend: USS Ultrasound, E2 Estradiol, OPU Oocytes pick–up, P4 Progesterone

Table 8.1 Criteria used for GnRH antagonist initiation in the flexible protocol [25]

Ultrasound criteria	Ultrasound and/or hormonal criteria
Follicle ⩾12 mm [21, 22]	Follicle ⩾13 mm or E2 400 pg/mL [23]
Follicle ⩾13 mm [24, 26, 27]	Follicle ⩾14 mm or E2 ⩾ 300 pg/mL [28]
Follicle ⩾14 mm [29–47]	Follicle ⩾14 mm or E2 > 600 pg/mL [48, 49]
Two follicles ⩾14 mm [50]	Follicle >12 mm and/ or LH >10 IU and /or E2 >150 pg/mL [51]
Follicle ⩾15 mm [52]	Follicle >12 mm and/ or LH >10 IU and/or E2 >600 pg/mL [53]
Follicle ⩾12–14 mm [25]	Follicle ⩾14 mm or LH ⩾10 IU or E2⩾200 pg/mL [25]

In the flexible GnRH antagonist protocol, antagonist is administered only after certain sonographic and/or endocrine criteria, indicating a risk for LH rise, are met. A large variation in the criteria used in the flexible protocol is present in the literature (Table 8.1).

Advantages of GnRh antagonist protocol:

There are a number of theoretical advantages of GnRH antagonists versus GnRH agonists [24, 26], including a shorter duration of injectable drug treatment, absence of vasomotor symptoms, less risk of inadvertent administration during early pregnancy, avoidance of ovarian cyst formation, and a significantly smaller dose of gonadotropin per cycle, which translate to improved patient convenience [22, 28]. Due to their increased convenience, GnRH antagonist protocols are often the regimen of choice for oocyte donors. More recently, it has been recommended that treatment guidelines for the prevention of ovarian hyperstimulation syndrome (OHSS) [29] should be updated to incorporate findings from the literature over the past 5 years. The literature shows that GnRH antagonist protocols and GnRH agonist triggering of final oocyte maturation, especially when used in combination, may reduce OHSS and have considerable promise in preventing OHSS [30].

Potential disadvantages of GnRH antagonist protocols:

GnRH antagonist protocols over GnRH agonist protocols include fewer flexible options in terms of cycle programming and early studies suggesting a minor reduction in pregnancy rates per cycle [31].

8.6.2.1 GnRh Antagonist Protocol Summary

1. Ovarian Stimulation:
   The process begins with daily injections of gonadotropins (FSH or FSH/LH combinations) to stimulate the ovaries to produce multiple eggs. The injections usually start on day 2 or 3 of the menstrual cycle. The dose is individualized based on factors like age, ovarian reserve, and response in previous cycles. A GnRH antagonist (e.g., cetrorelix or ganirelix) is introduced midway through the stimulation phase, usually around day 5–6 of stimulation to suppress the body's natural LH surge, which could lead to premature ovulation.
2. Triggering Ovulation:
   Once the follicles reach the desired size (usually 17–20 mm), human chorionic gonadotropin (hCG) or a GnRH agonist or both are administered to trigger final egg maturation. If the patient has a high risk of OHSS, the physician will decide to trigger with *GnRh agonist only* and freeze all embryos after egg retrieval to prevent OHSS. The patient will later undergo a frozen embryo transfer cycle for her embryo transfer.
3. Egg Retrieval:
   It is scheduled 35–38 h post trigger injection.
4. Luteal Support:
   It will start in the evening of the egg retrieval day. In some centers, luteal support is started the day after the egg retrieval.

Advantages: [31]

- Shorter treatment duration compared to other protocols (e.g., long protocol)
- Reduced risk of ovarian hyperstimulation syndrome (OHSS), especially in high responders
- Prevention of OHSS in women with polyendocrine metabolic ovarian syndrome (PMOS) or high ovarian reserve
- Flexibility in scheduling and easier to adjust in case of an unexpected response
- First-time IVF patients seeking a shorter and less intensive protocol

Disadvantages: [31]

- May result in a slightly lower number of retrieved eggs in some cases compared to other protocols
- Risk of cancellation related to asynchronization of the follicle growth

8.6.3 Microdose GnRH Flare Protocol (MDF)

The optimal protocol for poor ovarian responders (POR) undergoing in vitro fertilization (IVF) is still a challenge. Poor response to ovarian stimulation occurs in 9–24% of women undergoing IVF, which results in poor clinical pregnancy rates (CPR), and many of these cycles are cancelled without proceeding to egg collection [32].

For preventing cycle cancellation, several strategies have been suggested such as decreasing the dosage and timing of gonadotropin releasing hormone agonist (GnRHa) [33] or the use of GnRHa flare up regimens [34]. Theoretically, these strategies should eliminate excessive ovarian suppression while capitalizing on the initial stimulatory effect of GnRHa on pituitary gonadotropin release. The overall clinical pregnancy rate (CPR) when using flare protocols in POR has ranged between 12% and 26.3% [35, 36].

A microdose flare-up regimen (Fig. 8.3) has been developed to minimize the ovarian suppression of the GnRHa long protocols while taking the advantage of the initial up-regulatory effect of leuprolide on follicular recruitment which was used successfully in poor ovarian responders [37].

In a recent study, pretreatment with oral contraceptive pills before a GnRh agonist flare protocol suppressed pre-GnRHa FSH levels without blunting FSH flare. It reduced the LH flare responce, which may be beneficial [38].

The GnRHa microdose flare-up protocol has favorable outcomes with respect to the number of oocytes retrieved and implantation rate; nevertheless, the clinical pregnancy rate was found to be similar in comparison to GnRHant protocol in poor responders [39].

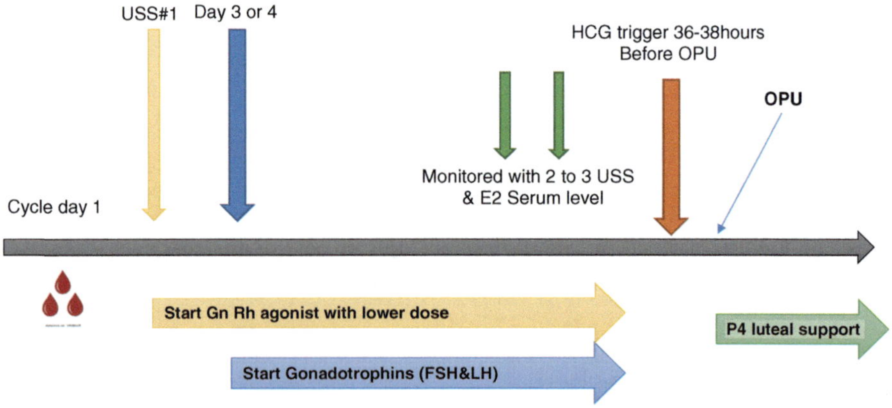

Fig. 8.3 Example of Microdose Flare agonist protocol. Legend: USS Ultrasound, E2 Estradiol, OPU Oocytes pick–up, P4 Progesterone

8.6.3.1 MDF Protocol Steps Summary

1. GnRH Agonist Pre-treatment (Microdose):
   A very low dose (microdose) of a gonadotropin-releasing hormone (GnRH) agonist (e.g., 50 µg twice daily of leuprolide acetate) is administered on day 2 of the cycle or in late luteal phase. This "flare" effect occurs when the agonist initially stimulates the release of follicle-stimulating hormone (FSH) and luteinizing hormone (LH) from the pituitary gland before suppressing them. High doses of gonadotropins (e.g., FSH, LH) are started shortly after the GnRH agonist to stimulate the ovaries to grow multiple follicles. OCP can be used as pretreatment in this protocol [38].
2. The Trigger Shot:
   Once the follicles have reached a mature size, an ovulation trigger injection, with hCG, is given to induce final maturation of the eggs.
3. The Egg Retrieval:
   Occurs 36–38 h after the trigger shot.

MDF advantages:

1. The ovarian suppression is not excessive [40]
2. The initial stimulation effect increases the amount of endogenous FSH and LH available to stimulate the ovaries. Adding "internal production" of FSH to the "external FSH" using the gonadotropins often results in enhanced responsiveness of the ovaries and an increased number of oocytes retrieved. [39, 40].
3. Scott and Navot described the microdose GnRH flare-up protocol for poor responder patients. They reported a higher number of retrieved oocytes, a lower cancellation rate, and higher pregnancy in patients receiving MDF [33]

MDF disadvantages:

- May not be suitable for all patients and success rates can vary depending on individual factors as age and ovarian reserve.
- A criticism of the use of flare protocols is that significantly increased serum progesterone levels may occur during the early follicular phase, which may exert a negative impact on cycle outcome [41].

8.6.4 Progestin Primed Ovarian Stimulation Protocol (PPOS)

Progestin-primed ovarian stimulation (PPOS) is a new ovarian stimulation protocol that can block the luteinizing hormone (LH) surge through progesterone instead of traditional down regulating of GnRH hormone antagonist [42].

Kuang et al. (2015) report the first randomized study with PPOS: they added medroxyprogesterone acetate (MPA) to gonadotrophins in a follicular phase stimulation. MPA was started on day 3 after spontaneous menses at the same time as HMG at 150 or 225 IU, and this protocol was compared with a conventional short protocol and resulted in similar outcomes [43].

Oral administration of exogenous progesterone, such as medroxyprogesterone acetate during early follicular phase of ovarian stimulation, has emerged as an effective alternative to conventional protocols for suppressing the pituitary LH surge. The benefits of progesterone are due to its hypothalamic effect, by which it decreases the production of GnRh [44].

In contrast to GnRh antagonist, progestin inhibits GnRh secretion from the hypothalamus if it is administered during the early part of the cycle before estrogen priming. (32:44–34:45). Several experiments had shown that higher level of progestin from the early follicular phase is able to inhibit follicular growth and LH surge by hindering estrogen's positive feedback on the hypothalamus (35:46, 36:47), thus slowing the LH pulse frequency, increasing its amplitude, and decreasing its plasma content. However, the exact mechanism of action by which it interacts with estradiol to regulate the LH surge remains unclear [49].

Concomitantly, however, the endometrium is not suitable for fresh embryo transfer because early exposure to the progesterone would result in endometrial advancement [50].

In order to overcome the adverse effect of the progesterone on endometrium, one strategy is to freeze all the embryos and defer the embryo-transfer in a future frozen-thawed replacement cycle (FET) [51]

Two major factors encouraged the use of PPOS in ART:

1. The development of cryopreservation techniques, where the quality of embryo or oocyte can be kept the same as fresh, allows the freedom to move away from the standard sequence of ovarian stimulation–retrieval–transfer, to which we were previously bound to provide the best chances of success. Today we are seeing the advent of so-called "freeze all" strategies, that is, freezing of the entire cohort of embryos or oocytes, or a mixture [50].
2. Currently, there is a gradual global increase in the age at which women choose to become mothers and at which they undergo assisted reproductive techniques (ART). This has increased the demand for procedures in which PPOS can play a significant role, namely, any ovarian cycle that is not followed by fresh embryo transfer, such as preimplantation genetic testing (PGT), fertility preservation for all indications, patients at risk of OHSS whose treatment includes freeze-all, or even oocyte donors [51].

Progestin prevents incidence of OHSS in controlled ovarian stimulation at both the follicular phase and luteal phase. Despite the lower dose of hCG triggering and freeze-all strategy, other factors related to the role of the high progestin milieu may also be associated with the low incidence of OHSS. One explanation is that exogenous progestin may exert an autoregulatory positive feedback action to enhance the production of endogenous progestin. However, any benefit of this protocol in such a context needs to be further investigated [52].

In the conventional PPOS protocol (Fig. 8.4) or fixed protocol, progestogens and gonadotropins are administered simultaneously in the early follicular phase and are maintained until the day on which final oocyte maturation is induced [51].

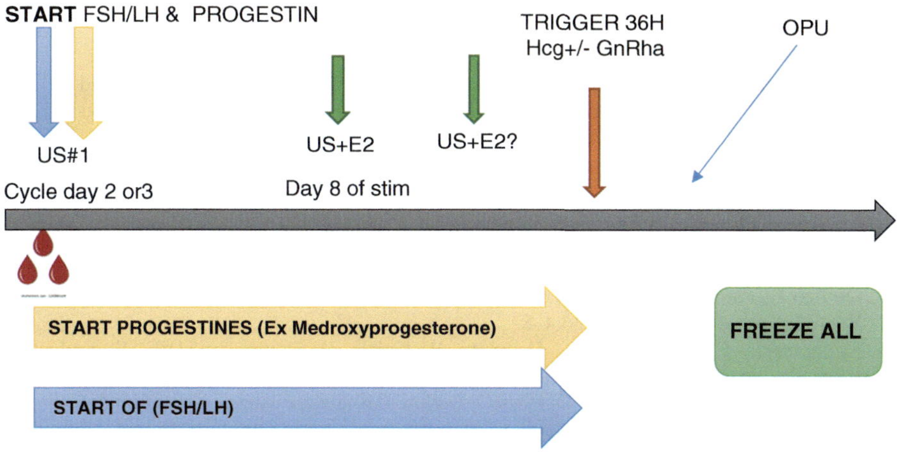

Fig. 8.4 PPOS protocol. Legend: US Ultrasound, E2 Estradiol, OPU Oocytes pick-up

8.6.4.1 PPOS Protocol Summary

1. Cycle Day 2 or 3: Start Stimulation with gonadotropins (FSH with or without LH). At the same time, oral progestin is started (e.g., MPA 10 mg/day or dydrogesterone 20 mg/day).
2. Ultrasounds and hormone levels are checked to monitor follicular development. Both gonadotropin and progestin will continue until follicles reach trigger size (17–20 mm).
3. Trigger ovulation with GnRH agonist or hCG once follicles are ready.
4. Egg retrieval 36 h post-trigger.
5. Freeze-all approach.

PPOS advantages

Progestin primed ovarian stimulation (PPOS) protocols effectively prevent early luteinization [51].

- Progestins have proven their effectiveness as a gonadotropin adjuvant in terms of ovarian response, reproductive outcome, and safety [51].
- Progestins offer the convenience of oral administration and a lower cost than GnRH analogues [51].
- Suitable for women at high risk of OHSS (e.g., PMOS) [50].
- Suitable for cycles and patient preferring a freeze-all approach (e.g., preimplantation genetic testing, fertility preservation, oocytes donors) [51].

PPOS disadvantages

There is no fresh embryo transfer during PPOS; the embryos should be vitrified as it displaces the receptive period with the consequent asynchrony between embryo and endometrium [50, 51].

- It has been less studied in certain populations (e.g., poor responders), although growing evidence supports its use [53].

References

1. Broer SL, Dolleman M, Opmeer BC, Fauser BC, Mol BW, Broekmans FJ. AMH and AFC as predictors of excessive response in controlled ovarian hyperstimulation: a meta-analysis. Hum Reprod Update. 2011;17(1):46e54.
2. Olivennes F, Howles CM, Borini A, Germond M, Trew G, Wikland M, et al. Individualizing FSH dose for assisted reproduction using a novel algorithm: the CONSORT study. Reprod Biomed Online. 2009;18(2):195e2.
3. Deekshy S, Xiaolin L, Huai LF. Comparison of different stimulation protocols used in in vitro fertilization: a review. Ann Transl Med. 2015;3(10):137.
4. Orvieto R, Patrizio P. Agonist versus antagonist in ovarian stimulation: on ongoing debate. Reprod Biomed Online. 2013;26:4–8.
5. Kolibianakis EM, Tarlatzis B, Devrroey P. GnRH atangonists in IVF. Reproductive Biomedecine Online. 2005;10(6):705–12.
6. Forman RG, Frydman R, Egan D, Ross C, Barlow DH. Severe ovarian hyperstimulation syndrome using agonists of gonadotropin-releasing hormone for in vitro fertilization: a European series and a proposal for prevention. Fertil Steril. 1990;53(3):502.
7. 2024 by American Society for Reproductive Medicine. The use of hormonal contraceptives in fertility treatments: a committee opinion. Fertil Steril. 2024;122:243–50.
8. Farquhar C, Rombauts L, Kremer JA, Lethaby A, Ayeleke RO. Oral contraceptive pill, progestogen or oestrogen pretreatment for ovarian stimulation pro tocols for women undergoing assisted reproductive techniques. Cochrane Database Syst Rev. 2017;5:CD006109.
9. De la Iglesia HO, Schwartz WJ. Minireview: timely ovulation: circadian regulation of the female hypothalamo-pituitary-gonadal axis. Endocrinology. 2006;147:1148–53. [CrossRef] [PubMed].
10. Zhang M, Ouyang H, Xia G. The signal pathway of gonadotrophins-induced mammalian oocyte meiotic resumption. Mol Hum Reprod. 2009;15:399–409. [CrossRef] [PubMed].
11. Wissing ML, Kristensen SG, Andersen CY, Mikkelsen AL, Host T, Borup R, Grondahl ML. Identification of new ovulation-related genes in humans by comparing the transcriptome of granulosa cells before and after ovulation triggering in the same controlled ovarian stimulation cycle. Hum Reprod. 2014;29:997–1010. [CrossRef] [PubMed].
12. Roess DA, Jewell MA, Philpott CJ, Barisas BG. The rotational diffusion of LH receptors differs when receptors are occupied by hCG versus LH and is increased by Cytochalasin D. Biochim Biophys Acta. 1997;1357:98–106. [CrossRef].
13. Hershko AK, Adrian S. hCG triggering in ART: an evolutionary concept. J Mol Sci. 2017;18:1075.
14. Youssef MA, van der Veen F, Al-Inany HG, Mochtar MH, Griesinger G, Nagi Mohesen M, Aboulfoutouh I, van Wely M. Gonadotropin-releasing hormone agonist versus hCG for oocyte triggering in antagonist-assisted reproductive technology. Cochrane Database Syst Rev. 2014;2014(10):CD008046. [CrossRef].
15. Shapiro BS, Daneshmand ST, Garner FC, Aguirre M, Thomas S. Gonadotropin-releasing hormone agonist combined with a reduced dose of human chorionic gonadotropin for final oocyte maturation in fresh autologous cycles of in vitro fertilization. Fertil Steril. 2008;90:231–3. [CrossRef] [PubMed].
16. Xiaokun H, Yingyi l, Kejun H, Yubing L, Yanwen X, Canquan Z, Qingyun M. New perspectives on criteria for the determination of HCG trigger timing in GnRH antagonist cycles. Medicine. 2016;95(20):1–8.
17. Van der Linden M, Buckingham K, Farquhar C, Kremer JAM, Metwally M. Cochrane library: luteal phase support for assisted reproduction cycles. Cochrane Database Syst Rev. 2015;2015(7):CD009154.
18. Bosch E, Broer S, Griesinger G, Grynberg M, Humaidan P, et al. ESHRE guideline:ovarian stimulation for IVF/ICSI(dagger). Hum Reprod Open. 2020;2020(2):hoaa009.

19. Feinberg EC, Beltsos AN, Nicolaou E, Marut EL, Uhler ML. Endometrin as luteal phase support in assisted reproduction. Fertil Steril. 2013;99(1):174e178 e1.
20. Baker VL, Jones CA, Doody K, Foulk R, Yee B, Adamson GD, et al. A randomized, controlled trial comparingthe efficacy and safety of aqueous subcutaneous progesterone with vaginal progesterone for luteal phase supportof in vitro fertilization. Hum Reprod. 2014;29(10):2212e20.
21. Gordon k, Hodgen GD. GnRH angonists and antagonists in assisted reproduction. Baillieres Clin Obstet Gynaecol. 1992;6:247–65.
22. Al-Inany H, Aboulghar M. GnRh antagonist is assisted reproduction: a Cochrane review. Hum Rerod. 2022;17:874–85.
23. Huime JA, Homburg R, Lambalk CB. are GnRH antagonists comparable to agonists for use in IVF? Hum Reprod. 2007;22:2805–13.
24. Devroey P, Boostanfar R, Koper NP, Mannaerts BM, Ijzerman-Boon PC, Fauser BC, et al. A double-blind, noninferiority RCT comparing corifollitropin alfa and recombinant FSH during the first seven days of ovarian stimulationusing a GnRH antagonist protocol. Hum Reprod. 2009;24(12):3063e72.
25. Kolibianaki, E, Kolibianakis E. Handbook of Current and Novel Protocols for the Treatment of Infertility. Elsevier Inc p.127
26. Shapiro DB, Mitchell-Leef D, Carter M, Nagy ZP. Ganirelex acetate use in normal-and poor-prognosis patients and the impact of estradiol patterns. Fert Steril. 2005;83:666–70.
27. Shapiro DB, Mitchell-Leef D. GnRh antagonists in in vitro fertilization:where we are now. Minerva Ginecol. 2003;55:373–88.
28. Tarlatzis BC, Kolibianakis EM. GnRH agonists vs anatgonists. Best Pact Res Clin Obstet Gynaecol. 2007;21:57–65.
29. The practice Committee of the American Society for reproductive medicine. Ovarian hyperstimulation syndrome. Fertil Steril. 2008;90:S188–93.
30. Humaidan P, Quartarolo J, Papanikolaou EG. Preventing ovarian hyperstimulation syndrome:guidance for the clinician. Fertile Steril. 2010;94:389–400.
31. Copperman AB, Benadiva C. Optimal usage of GnRH antagonists: a review of the literature. Reprod Biol & Endocrinol. 2013;11:20.
32. Keay SD, Liversedge NH, Mathur RS, Jenkins JM. Assisted conception following poor ovarian response to gonadotrophin stimulation. Br J Obstet Gynaecol. 1997;104(5):521–7.
33. Scott RT, Navot D. Enhancement of ovarian responsiveness with microdoses of gonadotropin-releasing hormone agonist during ovulation induction for in vitro fertilization. Fertil Steril. 1994;61:880–5.
34. Surrey ES, Bower J, Hill DM, Ramsey J, Surrey MW. Clinical and endocrine effects of a microdose GnRH agonist flare regimen administered to poor responders who are undergoing in vitro fertilization. Fertil Steril. 1998;69(3):419–24.
35. Akman MA, Erden HF, Tosun SB, Bayazit N, Aksoy E, Bahceci M. Comparison of agonistic flare up-protocol and antagonistic multiple dose protocol in ovarian stimulation of poor responders: results of a prospective randomized trial. Hum Reprod. 2001;16(5):868–70.
36. Fasouliotis SJ, Laufer N, Sabbagh-Ehrlich S, LewinA, Hurwitz A, Simon A. Gonadotropin-releasing hormone (GnRH)-antagonist versus GnRH-agonist in ovarian stimulation of poor responders undergoing IVF. J Assist Reprod Genet. 2003;20(11):455–60.
37. Toth TL, Awawad JT, Veeck LL, Jones HW Jr, Muasher SJ. Suppression and flare regimens of gonadotropin-releasing hormone agonist. Use in women with different basal gonadotropin values in an in vitro fertilization program. J Reprod Med. 1996;41(5):321–6.
38. Keltz MD, Gera PS, Skorupski J, Stein DE. Comparison of FSH flare with and without pre-treatment with oral contraceptive pills in poor responders undergoing in vitro fertilization. Fert Steril. 2007;88:350–3.
39. Boza A, Cakar E, Boza B, Kayatas S, Sofuoglu K. Microdose flare-up gonadotropin-releasing hormone (GnRH) agonist versus GnRH antagonist protocols in poor ovarian responders undergoing intracytoplasmic sperm injection. J Reprod Infertil. 2016;17(3):163–8.
40. Kahraman K, Berker B, Atabekoglu CS, Sonmezer M, Cetinkaya E, Aytac R, Satiroglu H. Microdose gonadotropin-releasing hormone agonist flare-up protocol versus multiple dose

gonadotropin-releasing hormone antagonist protocol in poor responders undergoing intracytoplasmic sperm injection-embryo transfer cycle. Fertil Steril. 2009;91(6):2437–44.
41. San Roman GA, Surrey ES, Judd HL, Kerin JF. A prospective randomized comparison of luteal phase versus concurrent follicular phase initiation of gonadotropin-releasing hormone agonist for in vitro fertilization. Fertil Steril. 1992;58:744–9. [PubMed: 1426320].
42. Shaogan G, Yuezhi F, Yonghan H, Jia H. Progestin-primed ovarian stimulation for patients in assisted reproductive technologies: a meta-analysis of randomized controlled trails. Front Endocrinol. 2021;12:702558.
43. Kuang Y, Chen Q, Fu Y, Wang Y, Hong Q, Lyu Q, Ai A, Shoham Z. Medroxyprogesterone acetate is an effective oral alternative for preventing premature luteinizing hormone surges in women undergoing controlled ovarian hyperstimulation for in vitro fertilization. Fertil Steril. 2015;104:62–70.e3.
44. Speroff LF. Pituitary gonadotropin secretion. 7th ed. Philadelphia: Lippincott Williams &Willkins; 2005.
45. Dierschke DJ, Yamaji T, Karsch FJ, Weick RF, Weiss G, Knobil E. Progesterone of estrogen-induced LH and FSH release in the RhesusMonkey. Endocrinology. 1973;92:1496–50.
46. Kasa-Vubu JZ, Dahl GE, Evans NP, Thrun LA, Moenter SM, Padmanabhan V, et al. Progesterone blocks the estradiol-induced gonadotropin Dischargein the ewe by inhibiting the surge of gonadotropin-releasing hormone. Endocrinology. 1992;131:208–12.
47. Evans NP, Richter TA, Skinner DC, Robinson JE. Neuroendocrine mechanisms underlying the effects of progesterone on the oestradiol-induced GnRH/LH surge. Reprod Suppl. 2002;Suppl. 59:57–66.
48. Heikinheimo O, Gordon K, Williams RF, Hodgen GD. Inhibition of ovulation by progestin analogs (agonists vs antagonists): preliminary evidence for different sites and mechanisms of actions. Contraception. 1996;53:55–64.
49. Ata B, Capuzzo M, Turkgeldi E, et al. Progestins for pituitary suppression during ovarian stimulation for ART: a comprehensive and systematic review including meta-analyses. Hum Reprod Update. 2021;27:48–66.
50. Massin N. New stimulation regimens: endogenous and exogenous progesterone use to block the LH surge during ovarian stimulation for IVF. Hum Reprod Update. 2017;23(2):211–20.
51. Giles J, Cruz F, Garcia-Velasco JA. Progestin-primed ovarian stimulation. vol. 2024;36(3):165. www.co-obgyn.com.
52. Wang Y, Chen Q, Wang NL, Chen H, Lyu Q, Kuang Y. A double-blind randomized crossover clinical trial.controlled ovarian stimulation using medroxyprogesterone acetate and hMG in patients with polycystic ovary syndrome treated for IVF. Medicine. 2016;95(9):e2939.
53. Ahui L, Jie L, Haofei S, Lili Z, Qiuyuan L, Xuehong Z. progestin-primed ovarian stimulation protocol with or without clomiphene citrate for poor ovarian responders: a retrospective cohort study. Medicine. 2016;95(9):e2939.

Triggering Final Oocyte Maturation

9

Shahad Alharazi and Michael H. Dahan

9.1 Introduction

Triggering is a critical step in the ovarian stimulation process, aimed at inducing final oocyte maturation, which prepares them for fertilization and releasing the oocytes from the follicular wall ultimately preparing for oocyte retrieval. The choice of trigger strategy can significantly impact the number and quality of oocytes retrieved, as well as subsequent fertilization, embryo development, and pregnancy outcomes.

9.2 Related Physiology

In nature, the ovulatory cycle is orchestrated by the hypothalamus, which prompts the pituitary gland to secrete two pivotal hormones: follicle-stimulating hormone (FSH), which causes follicular growth, and luteinizing hormone (LH), which potentiates follicular growth, among other things. Approximately midway through the cycle, an LH surge triggers a cascade of physiological events. This surge induces the disintegration of gap junctions connecting the oocyte (egg) and cumulus cells (supporting cells, feeding the oocyte), facilitating cumulus cell expansion. Concurrently,

S. Alharazi (✉)
Department of Reproductive Endocrinology and Infertility, McGill University, Montreal, QC, Canada

Department of Obstetrics and Gynecology, King Abdulaziz Medical City, Ministry of National Guard Health Affairs, Jeddah, Saudi Arabia

M. H. Dahan
Department of Reproductive Endocrinology and Infertility, McGill University, Montreal, QC, Canada

M. Das, M. H. Dahan (eds.), *A Comprehensive Guide to Reproductive Health and Infertility Medicine for Nurses*, https://doi.org/10.1007/978-3-032-24372-0_9

the oocyte resumes its development, marked by the breakdown of the germinal vesicle and the continuation of meiosis. Up until this point, oocytes were frozen in a state of genetic development, not yet ready to be fertilized. Additionally, luteinization occurs, wherein granulosa cells (the cells surrounding the oocyte) enhance progesterone production.

The initially mildly elevated progesterone levels seen before ovulation occur, amplifying the effects of estradiol, leading to a subsequent peak in FSH production. This peak is crucial for ensuring a sufficient presence of LH receptors on the granulosa cells and promoting the synthesis of hyaluronic acid. This FSH production leads to more expression of the LH receptors so that ovulation can soon occur. LH is then released in a surge 1–2 days before ovulation and aids in the expansion and separation of cumulus cells from the wall of the follicle, enabling the oocyte-cumulus cell complex to float freely within the ovarian fluid, enabling the collection of oocytes or, in nature, the ovulation of the egg [1]. This egg can next be fertilized by sperm in the fallopian tube.

In fertility care we need to precisely time the egg collection or the insemination in the case of ovarian stimulation and intrauterine insemination. To do this, we rely on medicines to either release LH from the patient's pituitary gland or bind to the LH receptor because it is similar in form to LH. Triggering can be mainly divided into hCG triggering, GnRH agonist triggering, and dual triggering.

Overall, the choice of triggering method should be individualized based on patient characteristics, risk of ovarian hyperstimulation syndrome (OHSS), and the specific goals of the IVF cycle.

9.3 HCG Triggering

Human chorionic gonadotropin (HCG) (which is the hormone released in pregnancy by the placenta) triggering is a well-established method for inducing final oocyte maturation in *in vitro* fertilization (IVF) cycles. It mimics the natural luteinizing hormone (LH) surge, promoting the luteinization of granulosa cells, the final maturation of the oocyte, and the resumption of meiosis so that the egg can get ready to be fertilized [2, 3]. The reason it can do this is because it is similar in shape (form) to LH. This similarity is close enough that at high levels, HCG can bind to the LH receptor. In most cases, things can only bind to their own receptors, but this is an exception for HCG in the LH receptor. This injection of HCG will then result in the egg detaching from the wall of the follicle and ovulating. This ovulation occurs about 40 hours after the HCG trigger, and as such, this can be used to time intra-uterine insemination. Pregnancy rates with intra-uterine insemination are the same if the HCG injection is given 12–48 hours before the insemination. This is because the sperm can live in the reproductive tract for up to 4 days while the oocyte (egg) can live for up to 24 hours waiting to be fertilized. To avoid ovulation in the IVF cycle, which would prevent the physician from collecting the egg if it were released into the belly cavity, we do egg collections between 32 and 38 hours after HCG triggering. However, collections 32–34 hours after triggering are less likely to have the egg detached from the wall of the follicle than triggering at 36–38 hours. Studies have shown that more mature eggs are obtained at 38 hours after HCG triggering when compared to 36 hours. However, there may be an increased risk of spontaneous ovulation in the 38-hour triggered group, which is why most centers collect 36 hours after HCG triggering in IVF. Each center will have its own protocols to determine the time of triggering after IVF. In busy centers, if the operating room is running late; it is possible that the patient will ovulate and eggs will not be collected, this will particularly occur as the 40-hour window post-HCG triggering is reached. Older women (38 years of age or older) and women with decreased ovarian reserve are more likely to ovulate less than 38 hours post-HCG trigger.

A typical practice involves administering a single dose of urinary or laboratory-made recombinant HCG (ranging from 5000 to 10,000 units, urinary, and 250 MCG recombinant). The timing of oocyte retrieval is crucial, with evidence suggesting that oocyte aspiration should occur at least 35 hours after the ovulation trigger to maximize the proportion of mature metaphase II (MII) oocytes [4]. Urinary HCG is obtained from the urine of pregnant women and concentrated down. This product could contain infectious agents such as prions, which are a type of disease transmitter. However, contamination has turned out to be rare. However, for safety reasons, recombinant HCG has been developed. This is made by immortalized cells that are programmed to just produce HCG primarily in a laboratory and have almost no risk of infection contamination. The dose of 250 mcg of recombinant HCG is equivalent to about 6500 IU of urinary HCG. Studies have shown that for oocyte trigger 250 mcg recombinant HCG performed as well as 5000 or 10,000 IU of urinary HCG. HCG is usually given as a subcutaneous injection. Although urinary HCG was first indicated as an intramuscular injection, studies have shown equal success rates in injecting urinary HCG subcutaneously or intramuscularly.

However, using hCG for final follicular maturation can increase the risk of ovarian hyperstimulation syndrome (OHSS). This risk arises because hCG has a much longer half-life than natural LH and activates different intracellular signaling pathways, which can affect blood vessel function. Additionally, hCG is associated with greater systemic inflammation and higher expression of vasoactive peptides when compared to LH. When we perform ovarian stimulation, we develop many follicles in the ovaries. The more follicles that are developed, the more hormones and blood vessels affect the products that they make. While natural LH lasts about 24 hours in spontaneous ovulation, HCG effects can last up to 7 days. This long duration of action, combined with many follicles being stimulated, can result in a complication called ovarian hyperstimulation syndrome. This syndrome will be discussed in a different chapter. Suffice it to say that women who develop OHSS can get very ill. When at risk, it is preferential to avoid the injection of HCG. In the past, we used to try to give lower doses of HCG 3300 IU to prevent the development of OHSS, but better options exist today. Even with lower doses, it is unclear if the risk of OHSS is decreased.

9.4 GnRH Agonist Triggering

Gonadotropin-releasing hormone agonist (GnRHa)-only triggering is primarily used to reduce the risk of ovarian hyperstimulation syndrome (OHSS), and it is particularly beneficial in high responders. GnRH agonists resemble gonadotropin-releasing hormone, which is made in the hypothalamus of the brain and triggers the LH and FSH surge from the pituitary gland. GnRHa induces a shorter LH surge than occurs in nature, lasting about 12 instead of 24 hours. This short duration of action results in rapid luteolysis, which means that the hormones and products favoring the development of OHSS stop being produced rapidly. However, this means that all the embryos must be frozen and cannot be put back in the uterus as part of the fresh IVF cycle because GnRHa triggering leads to luteal phase insufficiency and affects endometrial receptivity (the ability of the embryo to attach and stay attached to the uterus); this can lead to lower live birth rates in fresh cycles. However, GnRHa triggering causes luteal-phase insufficiency and may impair endometrial receptivity without appropriate luteal support. When a fresh embryo transfer is planned, modified luteal-phase support is required; freeze-all is commonly used in patients at high risk of OHSS [2, 3, 5]. One option to perform a fresh transfer in a cycle triggered with GnRHa was to introduce an injection of 1500 IU of HCG on the day of egg collection. However, severe OHSS still occurs with this mechanism, and as such, most centers prefer to freeze all the embryos in cases of GnRHa triggering.

The effects of using a gonadotropin-releasing hormone agonist (GnRHa) trigger alone compared to human chorionic gonadotropin (hCG)-only triggering in *in vitro* fertilization (IVF) cycles have been explored in various studies, particularly focusing on outcomes such as oocyte maturation, oocyte count, embryo quality, and live birth rates.

Oocyte Maturation and Count: The use of a GnRHa trigger alone is generally associated with effective oocyte maturation, similar to hCG-only triggering. However, the number of oocytes retrieved may vary depending on the specific patient population and protocol used. For instance, in high responders, a GnRHa trigger alone can effectively mature oocytes while reducing the risk of ovarian hyperstimulation syndrome (OHSS) [6].

Embryo Quality: The quality of embryos, including the number of good-quality embryos, can be comparable between GnRHa-only and hCG-only triggers. Some studies suggest that dual triggering (which will be discussed subsequently) (GnRHa combined with hCG) may improve embryo quality compared to either trigger alone, but this is not the case when comparing single triggers directly [7].

Live Birth Rates: The live birth rate (LBR) is a critical outcome in IVF. Studies have shown that the LBR can be similar between GnRHa-only and hCG-only triggers, particularly when considering specific patient populations such as high responders or those undergoing a freeze-all strategy.

Overall, while both GnRHa-only and hCG-only triggers are effective for final oocyte maturation, the choice between them may depend on individual patient characteristics and the specific IVF protocol being used.

In contrast, GnRHa-only triggering may be more suitable for high responders or in freeze-all strategies to minimize OHSS risk despite a potentially lower oocyte retrieval rate compared to dual triggering. GnRHa triggering can be given intramuscular, subcutaneously, or as an intranasal spray. In the case of intranasal spray, excessive mucus production, such as in viral infections, can affect the absorption and efficacy. Some centers give two injects of GNRHa 12 hours apart to more closely mimic the duration of the spontaneous LH surge. To verify the GnRHa induced an LH surge, a blood's LH level can be drawn about 10 hours after injection, and it should be at least 14.0 IU/L. If the level is lower than this, eggs may not be collected at the time of the IVF pick-up procedure. GnRHa triggering should not be used for insemination cycles due to inadequate luteal support, resulting in low pregnancy rates and little progesterone being produced in the luteal phase. Progesterone is the hormone that helps keep and nurture the growth of the pregnancy. Without adequate progesterone, pregnancies would not develop or miscarry. The timing of GnRHa triggering is similar to that of HCG.

9.5 Dual Triggering

Dual triggering, consisting of a standard hCG dose combined with the GnRHa dose.

This approach leverages the benefits of both an LH and follicle-stimulating hormone (FSH) surge and the LH analogue HCG. Dual triggering has been shown to improve outcomes in certain patient populations. For instance, dual triggering can enhance oocyte maturity, increase the number of good-quality embryos, and improve live birth rates compared to hCG-only triggering, particularly in normal responders and in fresh embryo transfer cycles without significantly increasing the risk of OHSS [8–10]. Other specific patient populations that may benefit from dual triggering include advanced-age women; dual triggering has been associated with a higher number of good-quality embryos compared to both hCG-only and GnRHa-only triggers, although the live birth rate was not significantly superior to hCG-only triggering [8, 10]. In light of these findings, the combination of GnRHa and hCG triggers for final follicular maturation has been adopted in many clinical settings. The timing and methods of administration can be tailored to meet the specific needs of different IVF patient subgroups.

"Dual trigger refers to the concomitant administration of a GnRH agonist (GnRHa) and hCG for final oocyte maturation. In a standard dual-trigger regimen, both agents are administered 35–37 hours before oocyte retrieval. This should be distinguished from sequential 'double-trigger' protocols, in which GnRHa and hCG are administered 40 hours and 34 hours before oocyte retrieval, respectively [1]."

Other timing strategies have been implemented for poor responders with a high prevalence of premature ovulation, including shortening the period between triggering and OPU [1].

Several studies and meta-analyses have evaluated the efficacy of dual triggering. A systematic review and meta-analysis by He et al. found that dual triggering significantly increased the number of oocytes retrieved, mature oocytes, and good-quality embryos in normal responders undergoing IVF/ICSI cycles with a GnRH-antagonist protocol when compared to single triggering [10]. Similarly, Hsia et al. reported that dual triggering was associated with a higher number of retrieved oocytes and mature oocytes compared to hCG alone, along with improved clinical pregnancy rates and live birth rates in fresh embryo transfer cycles [8].

Zhang et al. also demonstrated that dual triggering resulted in a higher number of retrieved cumulus-oocyte complexes and mature oocytes compared to hCG alone, although the impact on pregnancy rates was not significant. Additionally, Haas et al. found that dual triggering increased the number of oocytes, mature oocytes, and blastocysts, as well as improved clinical pregnancy and live birth rates [11].

Moreover, the benefits of dual triggering may vary depending on patient characteristics. For instance, for poor responders (those who developed four or fewer follicles with ovarian stimulation), dual triggering has demonstrated improved live birth rates and embryo quality compared to hCG-only triggering [13, 14]. Poor response occurs with aging or can affect young women less than 35 years of age with decreased ovarian reserve. Besides aging, decreased ovarian reserve can be genetic, unexplained, due to chemotherapy, radiation, or other gonadotoxic drugs; antibodies against the ovary causing an autoimmune state; or due to surgical damage to the ovary.

These benefits seen in dual trigger are likely due to the enhanced oocyte maturation and luteal phase support provided by the combined hormonal surge. Chen et al. observed that dual triggering increased the number of oocytes retrieved in women with diminished ovarian reserve but did not significantly affect clinical pregnancy rates or live birth rates [15]. Similarly, Zhou et al. found that while dual triggering improved the number of good-quality embryos in advanced-age women, it did not significantly increase the number of oocytes retrieved compared to hCG alone [7]. However, another study by Tulek et al. demonstrated that dual triggering significantly enhances live birth rates in POSEIDON group 3 and 4 patients, who are characterized as expected poor responders [13]. This improvement is attributed to the increased number of retrieved oocytes, mature oocytes, and higher quality embryos observed with dual triggering compared to hCG-only triggering. Dual trigger in general should be avoided in women at risk for ovarian hyperstimulation syndrome.

Overall, the evidence supports the use of dual triggering to enhance oocyte retrieval and potentially improve pregnancy outcomes in certain patient populations, particularly in normal responders and those undergoing fresh embryo transfer [12].

In conclusion, there are different options for triggering the final oocyte maturation; some can be used for insemination and IVF fresh embryo transfer, while others cannot. The trigger used will depend on the need to minimize the risk of ovarian hyperstimulation syndrome if a freeze-all cycle is planned or if a pregnancy is planned within the current IVF or ovarian stimulation cycle.

References

1. Orvieto R. Triggering final oocyte maturation: the role of human chorionic gonadotropin, gonadotropin-releasing hormone agonist, and dual trigger. In: Handbook of current and novel protocols for the treatment of infertility. Elsevier; 2023. p. 189–96.
2. Beebeejaun Y, Copeland T, Duffy JMN, et al. Triggering oocyte maturation in in vitro fertilization treatment in healthy responders: a systematic review and network meta-analysis. Fertil Steril. 2024;S0015-0282(24):02389–6. https://doi.org/10.1016/j.fertnstert.2024.11.011.
3. Zhang Y, Guo X, Guo L, et al. Outcomes comparison of IVF/ICSI among different trigger methods for final oocyte maturation: a systematic review and meta-analysis. FASEB J. 2021;35(7):e21696. https://doi.org/10.1096/fj.202100406R.
4. Weiss A, Neril R, Geslevich J, et al. Lag time from ovulation trigger to oocyte aspiration and oocyte maturity in assisted reproductive technology cycles: a retrospective study. Fertil Steril. 2014;102(2):419–23. https://doi.org/10.1016/j.fertnstert.2014.04.041.
5. Practice Committee of the American Society for Reproductive Medicine. Prevention of Moderate and Severe Ovarian Hyperstimulation Syndrome: A Guideline. Fertil Steril. 2024;121(2):230–45. https://doi.org/10.1016/j.fertnstert.2023.11.013.
6. He Y, Tang Y, Chen S, Liu J, Liu H. Effect of GnRH agonist alone or combined with different low-dose hCG on cumulative live birth rate for high responders in GnRH antagonist cycles: a retrospective study. BMC Pregnancy Childbirth. 2022;22(1):172. https://doi.org/10.1186/s12884-022-04499-0.
7. Zhou C, Yang X, Wang Y, et al. Ovulation triggering with hCG alone, GnRH agonist alone or in combination? A randomized controlled trial in advanced-age women undergoing IVF/ICSI cycles. Hum Reprod. 2022;37(8):1795–805. https://doi.org/10.1093/humrep/deac114.
8. Hsia LH, Lee TH, Lin YH, et al. Dual trigger improves the pregnancy rate in fresh in vitro fertilization (IVF) cycles compared with the human chorionic gonadotropin (hCG) trigger: a systematic review and meta-analysis of randomized trials. J Assist Reprod Genet. 2023;40(9):2063–77. https://doi.org/10.1007/s10815-023-02888-8.
9. Hu KL, Wang S, Ye X, Zhang D, Hunt S. GnRH agonist and hCG (dual trigger) versus hCG trigger for follicular maturation: a systematic review and meta-analysis of randomized trials. Reprod Biol Endocrinol. 2021;19(1):78. https://doi.org/10.1186/s12958-021-00766-5.
10. He FF, Hu W, Yong L, Li YM. Triggering of ovulation for GnRH-antagonist cycles in normal and low ovarian responders undergoing IVF/ICSI: a systematic review and meta-analysis of randomized trials. Eur J Obstet Gynecol Reprod Biol. 2023;289:65–73. https://doi.org/10.1016/j.ejogrb.2023.08.014.
11. Haas J, Bassil R, Samara N, et al. GnRH agonist and hCG (dual trigger) versus hCG trigger for final follicular maturation: a double-blinded, randomized controlled study. Hum Reprod. 2020;35(7):1648–54. https://doi.org/10.1093/humrep/deaa107.
12. Li Q, Li X, Li T, et al. Comparison of an HCG-only trigger versus dual trigger for final oocyte maturation in a progestin-primed ovarian stimulation protocol. Reprod Biomed Online. 2022;45(6):1176–81. https://doi.org/10.1016/j.rbmo.2022.08.101.
13. Tulek F, Kahraman A, Demirel LC. Dual trigger with gonadotropin releasing hormone agonist and human chorionic gonadotropin improves live birth rates in POSEIDON group 3 and 4 expected poor responders. Gynecol Endocrinol. 2022;38(9):731–5. https://doi.org/10.1080/09513590.2022.2101635.
14. Chern CU, Li JY, Tsui KH, et al. Dual-trigger improves the outcomes of in vitro fertilization cycles in older patients with diminished ovarian reserve: a retrospective cohort study. PLoS One. 2020;15(7):e0235707. https://doi.org/10.1371/journal.pone.0235707.
15. Chen K, Zhang C, Chen L, et al. Reproductive outcomes of dual trigger therapy with GnRH agonist and hCG versus hCG trigger in women with diminished ovarian reserve: a retrospective study. Reprod Biol Endocrinol. 2024;22:35. https://doi.org/10.1186/s12958-024-01211-z.

10 The Oocyte Collection, Embryo Transfer, and Sperm Collection Procedures for Nurses

Tiffany Tseng and Catty Chien Ju Yang

10.1 Oocyte Retrieval

Historically, oocyte retrievals were done via laparoscopy or laparotomy under general anesthesia. Eventually, transabdominal-transvesical ultrasound-guided oocyte aspiration was shown to be less invasive [1]. After the invention of the vaginal ultrasound probe, the transvaginal ultrasound-guided oocyte retrieval technique provides an even more precise method for oocyte aspiration and comparatively poses the least issues [2]. Some advantages of the transvaginal approach include more anesthesia options, better visualization of the ovaries, shorter distance between the transducer and ovary access, and a relatively uncomplicated recovery period [3]. While transabdominal-transvesical access may still be used for certain circumstances, transvaginal-guided oocyte retrieval technique has now become the most common method, perhaps the gold standard, of oocyte aspiration.

10.2 Preoperative Preparations

Prior to the procedure, the nurse should collect relevant patient information:

- Medical History: It is important to screen for medical comorbidities, history of anesthesia, current medications taken, and medication allergies. Relevant gynecological history, such as past pelvic inflammatory disease, endometriosis, surgeries, and bleeding disorders, should be noted.

T. Tseng (✉) · C. C. J. Yang
HRC Fertility, Pasadena, CA, USA
e-mail: tiffanyt@havingbabies.com; chienjuy@havingbabies.com

M. Das, M. H. Dahan (eds.), *A Comprehensive Guide to Reproductive Health and Infertility Medicine for Nurses*, https://doi.org/10.1007/978-3-032-24372-0_10

- Physical exam: A baseline ultrasound examination assessing the uterus and ovaries' position and accessibility should be documented. Prior transvaginal ultrasounds during the treatment cycle may detect the gynecological anatomical anomalies (such as endometrioma, uterine fibroids, and hydrosalpinx) that may impact the retrieval technique.
- Laboratory screening: Infectious disease screening status should be noted, along with a complete blood count and blood type. Any other laboratory screening and baseline value pertaining to existing medical conditions should be obtained.
- Informed consent: Informed consent with the patient outlining the risks and alternatives of the procedure should be discussed.
- Pain relief consultation: Various pain relief options may be available depending on the oocyte retrieval facility and may include general anesthesia, local anesthesia, or conscious sedation [4]. Depending on the form of pain relief, additional preoperative and postoperative side effects should also be reviewed and implemented (such as overnight fasting prior to general anesthesia, or nausea during the postoperative time frame).

10.3 Oocyte Retrieval Procedure

The procedure is typically done in an outpatient setting, usually in a facility that has proper surgical setup and equipment. The patient will first lie on a table in a lithotomy position with her legs adducted and supported. Sterile technique will be used by the surgical operator and physician with a sterile surgical field created. The vulva, and sometimes vagina, will be washed with normal saline or sterile water. A speculum will then be introduced to note the cervix and vagina for anatomic issues. If applicable, local anesthesia such as paracervical blocks can be introduced and administered during this time. A vaginal probe, equipped with a sterile cover, ultrasound gel, and needle with its guide attached, is introduced into the vagina and held firmly to the vaginal wall, against the ovary. With the ultrasound as guidance, the physician will carefully use the needle to puncture the vaginal wall, ovary, then the follicle. The needle, which is attached to a suction device, will then aspirate follicular fluid containing the mature egg via negative pressure. This process will be repeated until all follicles of the ovary are aspirated. Transabdominal pressure on the patient's torso may be applied by an assistant to stabilize the ovary during aspiration. At the end of the procedure, pressure is applied to the puncture sites of the vaginal wall to stop any residual bleeding [5].

10.4 Postoperative Expectations and Complications

Although severe complications postaspiration are rare, it is important to educate the patient on recovery expectations and postprocedure care. The most common side effects are vaginal bleeding and pain [3]. Vaginal bleeding usually presents as spotting. Pain may present as soreness or cramping and may be more present in women who had more oocytes aspirated than those with less. Hence, postoperative pain relief is commonly prescribed for the patient to take home. In the days following the procedure, over-the-counter pain relief may be sufficient for any discomfort.

Infection is a rare complication as antibiotics are commonly administered before or during the oocyte aspiration. Other rare complications of egg retrieval may include injury to adjacent pelvic organs, such as the ureter, bowel, intestines, or appendix [3].

Patients should also be educated for signs and symptoms of ovarian hyperstimulation syndrome (OHSS), which may happen in the days after the procedure. OHSS is a self-limiting disease characterized by a shift of fluid from the intravascular to the third space, along with cystic enlargement of the ovaries, due to increased capillary permeability from the use of human chorionic gonadotropin (hCG) during the stimulation cycle [6]. While OHSS is usually mild, it can become severe in rare cases, especially if conception ensues. Patients are encouraged to monitor for signs and symptoms of OHSS and report to the clinic if moderate-to-severe symptoms are present.

Mild OHSS symptoms may include abdominal distention and discomfort, nausea, vomiting, and diarrhea. Management is largely supportive, and resolution usually happens in 10–14 after initial onset, or until menstrual bleeding occurs if no subsequent embryo transfer takes place.

Postoperative recovery education for patients includes:

- Bed rest for 24 h after the procedure.
- Pantyliner for vaginal spotting.
- Nausea relief may be found by increasing fluid intake and a bland diet.
- Over-the-counter acetaminophen and a heating pack placed over the pelvis may alleviate discomfort associated with postoperative distention.
- Refrain from exercise and heavy lifting during this time.
- Abstinence until the presence of menstrual bleeding or pregnancy confirmation after the embryo transfer procedure.

Patients should be instructed to inform the clinic for further evaluation if the following symptoms are present:

- Vaginal bleeding that is heavier than a period.
- Foul-smelling vaginal discharge.
- Fever.
- Nausea and/or vomiting that persists after 24 h.
- Inability to urinate regularly.
- Persistent pelvic pain not resolved by prescribed pain relief.
- Shortness of breath.
- Weight gain more than 3 lb in a day.

10.5 Embryo Transfer

Embryo transfer is the determining step in assisted reproductive technology (ART), particularly for patients undergoing in vitro fertilization (IVF). The procedure involves the placement of one or more embryos into the uterus to achieve a viable pregnancy. After fertilization of oocytes, the best quality embryo is selected for transfer. With recent ART advancements, the 2012 Practice Committees of American Society for Reproductive Technology (ASRM) acknowledged improved implantation rates, thus recommending single-embryo transfers. In 2016, elective single-embryo transfer (eSET) accounted for 50.1% of embryo transfers [7]. Additional ART progress involving cryopreservation of embryos, namely, vitrification, has propelled frozen embryo transfer (FET) to become mainstream. Vitrification eliminates the formation of ice crystals between the extra- and intracellular spaces, to avoid cell deformation, and has shown improved postwarming survival rate [8]. This "freeze-all" strategy with subsequent FET decreases the risk for ovarian hyperstimulation syndrome, allows for preimplantation genetic testing (PGT), and avoids embryo-endometrial asynchrony [9].

10.6 Pre-operative Preparations

Prior to the procedure, the nurse should ensure all prerequisites are complete:

- Uterine Evaluation: A recent uterine evaluation via hysterosalpinogram, sonohysterogram, or hysteroscopy to rule out uterine cavity abnormality, i.e., myomas, polyps, adhesions, or other morphological anomalies [10]. Mock embryo transfers are routinely performed beforehand to assess endometrial cavity length and uterine cavity angle, as to decrease the risk of encountering difficulties at the live transfer [11].
- Laboratory Screening: Up-to-date serological screenings, pap smear, and other routine prenatal testing, i.e., complete blood count (CBC), blood type, Rh factor, Vitamin D, and immunity to viral infections. Age-related screening considerations, including mammograms may also be applicable [10].
- Informed Consent: Patients must understand all associated risk factors with embryo transfer, including side effects of medicated protocols. Common hormone replacement therapy (HRT) stimulates endometrium proliferation with Estradiol via oral tablet, vaginal inserts, transdermal patch, or intramuscular injections. Progesterone supplementation routes of administration also comprise intramuscular, oral, or vaginal. Corticosteroid to decrease risk of embryo rejection can sometimes be used for HRT protocols. Some studies have shown that FET may contribute to higher risk for pregnancy-related hypertensive disorders, particularly for HRT, leading to a recent shift for natural protocol with minimal hormone supplementations [9]. Nurse should also verify availability of selected embryo to transfer, developmental stage, and any other applicable specification as indicated by the informed consents.

- Adjunct Therapy: Alternative treatment interventions may be incorporated with embryo transfers to increase success rate, i.e., acupuncture, analgesics, and anesthesia. Routine acupuncture regimen may comprise sessions pre- and postprocedure. Oral valium before transfer aims to prevent uterine contraction, and the use of conscious sedation may decrease anxiety or alleviate discomfort in cases of difficult embryo transfers. These interventions provide theoretical benefits of hormone modulation, enhancing uterine circulation, and stress reduction. However, there is currently insufficient evidence for or against any supplemental methodologies to optimize embryo implantation potential [12].

10.7 Embryo Transfer Procedure

Starting with the patient in a lithotomy position, a bivalve speculum is placed intravaginally to visualize the cervix. The cervix is first cleansed with culture medium, and an outer transfer catheter, typically thin and flexible, is inserted through the cervix to about 10–15 mm from the uterine fundus. The procedure is commonly guided by transabdominal or transvaginal ultrasound for precision of embryo placement. A comfortably full bladder will be required with transabdominal ultrasound to aid in visualization of the uterus. Once catheter placement is confirmed, the embryologist is notified to transport the embryo from the lab, revalidating the embryo selection with proper identifiers, the embryologist will place the embryo within the catheter. The patient is able to visualize the embryo being transferred on the ultrasound screen. The embryologist will confirm under a microscope that the catheter is empty, to rule out embryo retention. Embryo retention incidence ranges from 1% to 8% [13]. However, retransferring of retained embryos does not appear to have significant adverse impact on reproductive outcomes, particularly with single-blastocyst transfer, mitigating risk as compared to double-blastocyst transfer [14]. In some clinics, the patient is advised to remain supine for about 15–20 min postprocedure prior to discharge.

10.8 Postoperative Expectations and Complications

Risk for significant complications following embryo transfer occurs rarely. Although patients may experience spotting and cramping on day of placement, primarily related to catheter instrumentation. Patients should be reassured that pink and clear vaginal discharge postprocedure may also be common. Pregnancy test is performed by determining serum β-hCG 11–12 days after embryo transfer in most IVF settings. Under physiological conditions, a positive pregnancy is generally indicated at β-hCG levels of 25mIU/ml 10 days postconception. Similarly for β-hCG tracking to determine pregnancy viability in common IVF practices, level increases exponentially, doubling approximately every 48–72 h. In contrast, β-hCG below 5mIU/ml excludes pregnancy, and slower than expected increases indicate abnormal outcomes, i.e., biochemical or ectopic pregnancy [15]. The waiting period for confirmatory pregnancy test can pose significant emotional stressors, and nurses should provide sufficient expectant management, offering open communication for questions and support.

Postoperative Patient Education:

- Day post embryo transfer, bedrest with feet elevation as much as possible. Patients may use the restroom or sit up to eat as necessary but to maintain pelvic rest whenever allowed.
- Light activity may resume after 24 h.
- Avoid strenuous activity or heavy lifting for 2 weeks post-transfer.
- Avoid douching and sexual intercourse. Nothing per vagina except for medications as prescribed.
- For HRT protocols, continue all medications until serum β-hCG test, regardless of spotting or cramping.
- Notify the office if complaints of heavy menstrual bleeding, soaking through a pad per hour, fever, or malodorous vaginal discharge.

10.9 Sperm Retrieval Procedures

If there is no sperm found in the semen, the physician may recommend surgical sperm extraction procedures. Anatomical issues may be presented as obstructive azoospermia (OA) or non-obstructive azoospermia (NOA). Documented azoospermia, along with medical history, physical exam, and laboratory testing, NOA or OA can be diagnosed. In OA, sperm is usually harvested from the epididymis, while testicular sperm extraction is reserved for when epididymal sperm extraction fails and for patients who are diagnosed with NOA [16]. Surgically extracted sperm from TESA & TESE should be done in conjunction with IVF/ICSI.

10.10 Pre-operative Preparation

- Documentation of azoospermia: Azoospermia, defined by normal ejaculate volume but absence of spermatozoa after centrifugation, should be confirmed by two consecutive semen analyses [17].
- Medical history: It is important to note any medical comorbidities, allergies, and current or recent medications taken.
- Physical examination: An assessment of testicular volume and the choice of aspiration side can be determined during this time. Any anatomical anomalies of the testis and epididymis that may impact the procedure should be noted.
- Laboratory testing: infectious disease screening status, a complete blood count, and blood type should be obtained. Other prior diagnostic results should also be noted, including follicle stimulating hormone, serum testosterone, and relevant genetic testing (such as karyotype, y-microdeletion, relevant single gene testing).

- Pain relief consultation: Depending on the type of sperm extraction procedure, different pain relief and anesthesia options may be available. Additional preoperative and postoperative side effects pertaining to pain relief should also be reviewed.
- Informed consent for the specific procedure: Informed consent with the patient outlining the risks and alternatives should be discussed.

10.11 Testicular Sperm Aspiration (TESA)

Testicular sperm aspiration (TESA) is a percutaneous technique and can be performed as an outpatient procedure under local or regional anesthesia. The skin is prepared with a non-betadine solution, then a spermatic cord block with 1% lidocaine will be administered in the scrotal skin, dartos muscle above the testis, and directly into the testis. A 16-gauge needle with an angiocatheter is directed through the scrotal skin into the testis, with the catheter kept in place and the needle drawn. A syringe with sperm buffer is attached to the angiocatheter on the outside, so when negative pressure is created, testicular fluid and tissue will be aspirated. After several passes, the needle is removed and flushed. As the aspirated tissue emerges and is rescued by forceps, it is placed into a sterile dish and immediately examined under the microscope to confirm the presence of spermatozoa. After spermatozoa are confirmed, the procedure concludes; the angiocatheter needle is removed, and gentle pressure is applied to the puncture site to minimize bleeding [18]. Each TESA sampling may yield enough tissue for pathology or multiple egg retrieval cycles.

10.12 Percutaneous Epididymal Sperm Aspiration (PESA)

PESA is a noninvasive method of sperm recovery. The technique is relatively simple, often performed under light IV sedation or local anesthesia, and the patient is able to return to work the following day without significant risk of complications. The procedure starts with immobilization of the testicle as the surgeon stabilizes between the thumb and index finger and is able to palpate the epididymis distinctively. A butterfly needle connected to a syringe enters the head of the epididymis, and suction is applied. Steady, negative pressure is maintained until fluid from the epididymis ceases to flow, and the needle is withdrawn. The embryologist will then inspect the aspirate for the presence of sperm. This procedure can be performed repeatedly if indicated, and often so, because some tubules entered may have less favorable sperm than others. The procedure usually will be repeated on the other testis to maximize the amount and quality of sperm retrieved for microinjection. Harvested sperm will be utilized for intracytoplasmic sperm injection (ICSI) of the oocytes [19].

10.13 Testicular Sperm Extraction (TESE)

Testicular sperm extraction (TESE) may be considered for NOA patients, or patients who had a failed TESA [20]. This process, considered an open biopsy, can yield significant amounts of testicular tissue, as it allows for multiple sampling. TESE can be performed as an outpatient under local or regional anesthesia, although some providers may opt to use general anesthesia in a surgical setting due to its more invasive nature.

For certain patient populations (such as men with prior scrotal surgery, or with hematoma risk), perioperative antibiotics may be used. The scrotum is shaved and prepared with a non-betadine scrub, and sterile surgical field are created with drapes. A median raphe incision is created and extended through the dartos fibers to the tunica to give access to both sides of the scrotum. The incision will reveal the epididymis and testicle. An incision (or incisions, if obtaining multiple biopsy samples) is created in avascular regions of the tunica albuginea. As the testes are gently squeezed, seminiferous tubules protrude and can be transected and excised. The seminiferous tubule biopsy sample is placed in sperm wash medium, and a microscope is used to confirm the presence of spermatozoa. Once sperm is confirmed, the tunica albuginea can be closed with suture, and the procedure concludes [16].

10.14 Microdissection Testicular Sperm Extraction (MicroTESE)

MicroTESE is the gold standard for surgical sperm retrieval in patients with NOA. It evolved from conventional TESE, due to the advantage of magnification provided by an operating microscope. In 1999, Dr. Peter Schlegel observed heterogeneity among seminiferous tubules within the testicle and noted focal areas of dilated tubules demonstrated more active spermatogenesis. Medical optimization may be considered prior to surgery if indicated based upon medical history and lab testing. Common medication classes include gonadotropins and aromatase inhibitors. Sperm mapping via TESA in a systematic grid-like fashion, also known as FNA mapping, may be performed beforehand. MicroTESE, routinely performed under general anesthesia, starts with an incision to allow easy access to both testes. The larger of the two testicles is examined first under the operating microscope. Using a microknife, the surgeon incised transversely to avoid testicular vessels and visualize the seminiferous tubules. Once visualization is achieved, the entire length of the tubule is removed with tissue microforceps and placed in a small petri dish. The embryologist will examine and remove testicular tissue for sperm. If sperm is identified, dissection of the contralateral testicle will be unnecessary. MicroTESE has proven to be 1.5-fold more effective at sperm retrieval than conventional TESE [21].

10.15 Postoperative Complications and Precautions

- Epididymal or vascular injury may result from needle punctures. Incidence of injury is higher in men with a history of scrotal surgery and scar tissue.
- Testicular hematoma and postretrieval fibrosis are also possible complications.
- TESE or microTESE may lead to compromise of testicular blood flow from interference of the vascular supply or from bleeding enclosed within the tissue, leading to an increased intratesticular pressure.
- Functional evaluation of the testicles after TESE and microTESE demonstrated structural changes on ultrasound up to 6 months and decrease in serum testosterone [16].
- Localized scrotal swelling or discoloration may be common for 2–3 days post-procedural; compression, ice packs, and athletic support are recommended.
- Refrain from sexual activity for 1–2 weeks.
- Keep the area dry by avoiding a bath or submergence in water until the incision has healed.
- Avoid strenuous activity or heavy lifting for 2–3 weeks.
- Prevent constipation by increasing hydration, fiber-rich diet, or use over-the-counter stool softener as needed.

References

1. Lenz S. Ultrasonically guided aspiration of human oocytes. Ultrasound Med Biol. 1984;10(5):625–8. https://doi.org/10.1016/0301-5629(84)90077-2. PMID: 6531823
2. Feichtinger W, Kemeter P. Transvaginal sector scan sonography for needle guided transvaginal follicle aspiration and other applications in gynecologic routine and research. Fertil Steril. 1986;45(5):722–5. https://doi.org/10.1016/s0015-0282(16)49349-0. PMID: 3516731
3. Ludwig AK, Glawatz M, Griesinger G, Diedrich K, Ludwig M. Perioperative and post-operative complications of transvaginal ultrasound-guided oocyte retrieval: prospective study of >1000 oocyte retrievals. Hum Reprod. 2006;21(12):3235–40. https://doi.org/10.1093/humrep/del278. Epub 2006 Jul 27. PMID: 16877373
4. Kwan I, Wang R, Pearce E, Bhattacharya S. Pain relief for women undergoing oocyte retrieval for assisted reproduction. Cochrane Database Syst Rev. 2018;5(5):CD004829. https://doi.org/10.1002/14651858.CD004829.pub4. PMID: 29761478; PMCID: PMC6953349
5. Jančar N, Ban Frangež H. Oocyte retrieval. In: Guglielmino A, Lagana AS, editors. Management of infertility: a practical approach. Philadelphia: Elsevier; 2023. p. 205–9.
6. Kumar P, Sait SF, Sharma A, Kumar M. Ovarian hyperstimulation syndrome. J Hum Reprod Sci. 2011;4(2):70–5. https://doi.org/10.4103/0974-1208.86080. PMID: 22065820; PMCID: PMC3205536
7. Kim H, Matevossian K. Are two better than one? Two sequential transfers of a single embryo may be better than a double-embryo transfer. Fertil Steril. 2020;114(2):267–8. https://doi.org/10.1016/j.fertnstert.2020.04.064. PMID: 32741464
8. Valojerdi MR, Eftekhari-Yazdi P, Karimian L, Hassni F, Movaghar B. Vitrification versus slow freezing gives excellent survival, post warming embryo morphology and pregnancy outcomes for human cleaved embryos. J Assist Reprod Genet. 2009;26(6):347–54. https://doi.org/10.1007/s10815-009-9318-6. Epub 2009 Jun 10. PMID: 19513822

9. Zhang Y, Xiao F, Gao S, Gao S, Gao S, Ma J, Chen Z. Preparation of the endometrium for frozen embryo transfer: an update on clinical practices. Reprod Biol Endocrinol. 2023;21(1):52. https://doi.org/10.1186/s12958-023-01106-5. PMID: 37291605
10. Buzzaccarini G, Vitagliano A, Lagana A. Management of infertility a practical approach book. Elsevier; 2023. p. 31–9. https://doi.org/10.1016/B978-0-323-89907-9.00024-7.
11. Inaudi P, Scarselli B. Management of infertility a practical approach book. Elsevier; 2023. p. 269–73. https://doi.org/10.1016/B978-0-323-89907-9.00039-9
12. Alan, Penzias Kristin, Bendikson Samantha, Butts Christos, Coutifaris Tommaso, Falcone Gregory, Fossum Susan, Gitlin Clarisa, Gracia Karl, Hansen Andrew, La Barbera Jennifer, Mersereau Randall, Odem Richard, Paulson Samantha, Pfeifer Margareta, Pisarska Robert, Rebar Richard, Reindollar Mitchell, Rosen Jay, Sandlow Michael, Vernon (2017) Performing the embryo transfer: a guideline Fertility and Sterility 107(4) 882-896 10.1016/j.fertnstert.2017.01.025
13. Kadour-Peero E, Tulandi T, Feferkorn I, Hiszkiahu R, Buckett W. Effects of embryo retention during embryo transfer on IVF outcomes. J Assist Reprod Genet. 2022;39(5):1065–8. https://doi.org/10.1007/s10815-022-02450-y. PMID: 35243568
14. Yi HJ, Koo HS, Cha SH, Kim HO, Park CW, Song IO. Reproductive outcomes of transferring retained embryos in blastocyst transfer cycles. Clin Exp Reprod Med. 2016;43(2):133–8. https://doi.org/10.5653/cerm.2016.43.2.133. PMID: 27358833
15. Yadid IM, Criscuolo TS, Santos JF, Giordano LA. Can biochemical pregnancy be determined 5 days after frozen-thawed embryo transfer? JBRA Assist Reprod. 2022;26(1):62–7. https://doi.org/10.5935/1518-0557.20210054. PMID: 34415123
16. Janosek-Albright KJC, Schlegel PN, Dabaja AA. Testis sperm extraction. Asian J Urol. 2015;2(2):79–84. https://doi.org/10.1016/j.ajur.2015.04.018. Epub 2015 Apr 16. PMID: 29264124; PMCID: PMC5730746
17. Boeri L, Pozzi E, Salonia A. Work-up of male infertility. In: Guglielmino A, Lagana AS, editors. Management of Infertility: a practical approach. Philadelphia: Elsevier; 2023. p. 41–53.
18. Al-Malki AH, Alrabeeah K, Mondou E, Brochu-Lafontaine V, Phillips S, Zini A. Andrology. 2017;5(2):226–31. https://doi.org/10.1111/andr.12317. Epub 2017 Feb 10. PMID: 28187532
19. Craft I, Khalifa Y, Sirigotis M, Hogewind G, Bennet V, Nicholson N, Taranissi M. Percutaneous epididymal sperm aspiration and intracytoplasmic sperm injection in the management of infertility due to obstructive azoospermia. Fertil Steril. 1995;63(5):1038–42. https://doi.org/10.1016/s0015-0282(16)57544-x. PMID: 7720914
20. Malhotra J, Devi MG, Patil M. Best practice recommendations for infertility management. J Hum Reprod Sci. 2024;17(Suppl 1):S1–S240. https://doi.org/10.4103/jhrs.JHRS_ISAR_IFS. Epub 2024 Feb 15. PMID: 38495807; PMCID: PMC10942128
21. Flannigan R, Bach P, Schlegel P. Microdissection testicular sperm extraction. Transl Androl Urol. 2017;6(4):745–52. https://doi.org/10.21037/tau.2017.07.07. PMID: 28904907

Assisted Reproductive Technologies 11

Marta Jansa Perez and Eilis Moody

11.1 In Vitro Fertilization: IVF

11.1.1 Who It Is Used For

IVF was originally developed for the use of patients whose fallopian tubes were damaged or blocked. The first birth from IVF was reported in the UK by the group of Steptoe, Edwards and Purdy in 1978 after many years of research in the field. Today, millions of births from IVF have occurred through IVF worldwide, and it is routinely used to overcome other causes of infertility for heterosexual couples but also to help same sex couples and single people to conceive.

Initially IVF was carried out during the natural menstrual cycle of the patient, but later FSH stimulation protocols were developed that allowed for the development and retrieval of multiple eggs and also gave the fertility service team the ability to control the time of ovulation by reversibly suppressing the pituitary secretion of LH.

IVF is used when the initial sperm parameters are within the normal range, the preparation fulfils the requirements of the fertility service where treatment is received, and the patients have not had a previous IVF cycle with very low or no fertilisation [4].

M. J. Perez (✉)
Bourn Hall Fertility Clinic, Bourn Hall, Wickford, UK
e-mail: mjansaperez@gmail.com

E. Moody
Newcastle Fertility Centre, Newcastle upon Tyne Hospitals NHS Foundation Trust, Newcastle upon Tyne, UK
e-mail: e.moody1@nhs.net

M. Das, M. H. Dahan (eds.), *A Comprehensive Guide to Reproductive Health and Infertility Medicine for Nurses*, https://doi.org/10.1007/978-3-032-24372-0_11

11.1.2 Egg Collection

During IVF, the eggs are collected from the ovaries just before ovulation, transvaginally using ultrasound guidance [10], see Fig. 11.1. Usually the patient is sedated, either using conscious sedation or with deeper sedation, but occasionally only local anaesthetics or no analgesia at all are used.

Using an ultrasound probe with a needle attached, the follicular fluid is collected into test tubes kept at 37 °C in a heated tube block and is examined under the stereo microscope for the presence of eggs. These will be washed to remove follicular fluid, blood and blood clots and placed in culture dishes in an incubator at 37 °C with controlled CO_2 and oxygen levels.

11.1.3 Sperm

The eggs need to be placed together with sperm on the day of egg collection. The semen is prepared in the laboratory in order to select the sperm that are alive and motile in the semen sample. Fresh or frozen sperm can be used for IVF insemination as long as the final preparation reaches the minimum thresholds of concentration, motility and morphology established by the embryology laboratory [4].

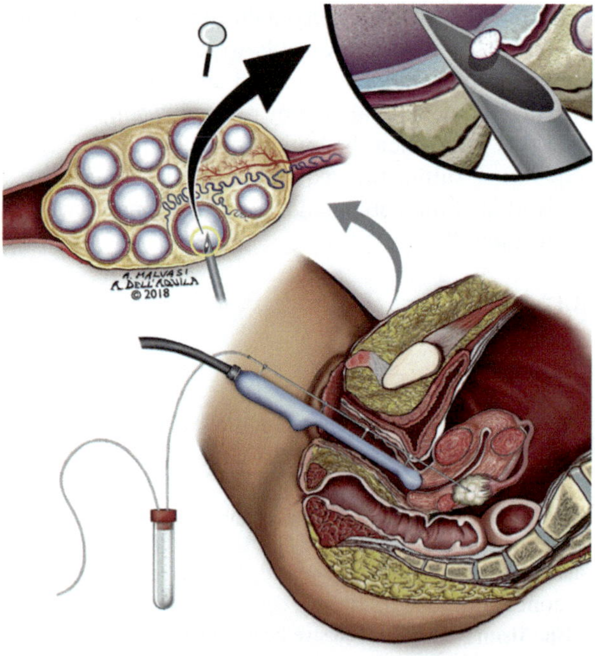

Fig. 11.1 Egg collection procedure (with permission Baldini et al. [2])

11.1.3.1 Fresh Sperm

If the patient has a male partner, the sperm for IVF is usually obtained from the ejaculate produced in the clinic by masturbation. After the sperm is visualised and analysed down the microscope as shown in Fig. 11.2, it is usually prepared using a density gradient centrifugation. This enables the motile sperm to accumulate in the pellet of a conical tube, whilst the immotile ones, cells, cell debris and seminal plasma remain in the interfaces of the gradient. The solution used for the gradient is then removed by subsequent washes with culture media with final resuspension in the same culture media that the eggs have been placed in culture after the egg collection.

11.1.3.2 Frozen Sperm

Sometimes the use of previously frozen sperm is required in IVF. This may occur if the partner has previously frozen sperm for fertility preservation (e.g. due to cancer treatment, gender transitioning or other treatments), if they will be absent on the day of egg collection, or if they anticipate some difficulty producing a sperm sample on demand on that day.

Frozen sperm is also used when the sperm has been donated to the patient. Donor sperm, which may be a from known or anonymous donor, is always used frozen, as it needs to be quarantined to ensure safety for both the recipients and the baby [5]. It is used for heterosexual couples where the male partner is azoospermic (has no sperm in their ejaculate) or does not wish to pass a genetic condition, in same-sex female couples or in single women seeking fertility treatment.

Frozen-thawed sperm is prepared like fresh sperm and needs to fulfil the same parameters as fresh sperm to be suitable for IVF.

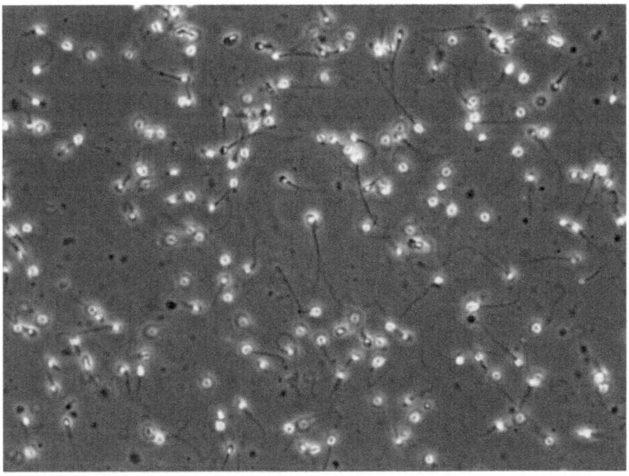

Fig. 11.2 Image of a wet preparation (400 × magnification) of a fresh semen sample. (Published in: Hicks et al. [12], under a Creative Commons Attribution 4.0 International License http://creativecommons.org/licenses/by/4.0/)

11.1.4 Insemination

During the process of insemination, usually 100,000 motile sperm are added to 3–5 eggs in culture and left overnight in the same incubator where the eggs were placed after egg collection to fertilise. This process is carried out whilst visualising under the microscope the moving sperm being placed next to the eggs.

11.1.5 Fertilisation Check

The inseminated eggs are checked for fertilisation typically 16–18 hours post insemination (early in the morning after egg collection) [6]. To check for fertilisation, the embryologists need to mechanically remove all the cumulus cells around the eggs. Usually, the bonds between those cells will have been disrupted by the action of the sperm overnight. A pipette with a diameter slightly larger than the average egg at 135–145 um is used to denude or strip the eggs under the microscope.

11.1.5.1 Fertilisation Rates

The normal fertilisation rate (i.e. the proportion of inseminated oocytes with two pronuclei at the time of the fertilisation check on Day 1) is expected to be around 67%. Normally fertilised eggs are called zygotes. Only the eggs that are mature (a median of 75% of the collected eggs) can be fertilised.

Abnormal Fertilisation The presence of three or more pronuclei is indicative of an abnormal fertilisation, arising from either failure to extrude the second polar body or polyspermy. From the literature, the incidence of ≥3PN is 4–7% in IVF [15]. Eggs with a single pronucleus after insemination by IVF, which occurs in 1–5% of cases, can be indicative of fertilisation and fusion of the two pronuclei, asynchronous appearance of pronuclei (an extremely rare event, as evidenced by the use of time-lapse microscopy) or parthenogenetic activation [17].

Failed Fertilisation The incidence of failed fertilisation in IVF whereby none of the collected eggs fertilise is between 4% and 6% of the cases. This is a difficult event for patients as most of the time it means that they won't reach the embryo transfer stage in their treatment. However, in a very small proportion of the cases, the eggs will show signs of late normal fertilisation. Additionally, in some cases, rescue ICSI can be offered to patients with failed IVF fertilisation, with a much lower chance of success.

11.2 ICSI (Intra-Cytoplasmic Sperm Injection)

11.2.1 Who It Is Used For

ICSI is a modification of IVF whereby a single sperm is injected into each mature egg. The procedure itself was first performed in 1987. The first successful birth by ICSI took place on January 14, 1992 [22]. The process of ovarian stimulation and egg collection is the same for ICSI as it is for IVF.

ICSI is usually performed when the sperm parameters of the partner or the donor are below the normal range and/or the sperm preparation on the day of egg collection is below the threshold parameters specific to the fertility service where the patient is having treatment [4].

ICSI is also often used when patients have had IVF before where none or a small proportion of the mature eggs fertilised. It is also used as the only way to attempt fertilisation in all the cases where either testicular or epididymal sperm is used, as these samples often contain a high proportion of immature, abnormal and immotile sperm in concentrations far below the normal ranges (see Section 11.3 below on TESA, micro-TESA and PESA sperm).

ICSI is also routinely carried out when the sperm is obtained from the urine of patients who present to the clinic with retrograde ejaculation.

Occasionally frozen sperm from either partner or donor, which are within the normal range at the time of production, might have a survival rate below expectation, and therefore, on the day of egg collection, a conversion of treatment from IVF to ICSI might be necessary if the preparation does not reach the minimum threshold for IVF to be performed.

11.2.2 How It Works

ICSI requires the use of very specialised equipment in the IVF laboratory in the form of a high-magnification inverted microscope and micromanipulators (Fig. 11.3) that are used to hold the egg on one side and to catch and inject the sperm at the point of injection on the other side [9].

On the day of egg collection, all the eggs are denuded (also referred to as stripped) with the use of an enzyme called cumulase or hyaluronidase, which will disrupt the bonds between the cumulus cells just as the sperm does when IVF insemination is carried out. A combination of the enzymatic and mechanical activities by pipetting the eggs through tips of decreasing diameter down to 135–145 uM will remove enough cumulus cells around the zona pellucida in order to assess the maturity of each egg. Only eggs that are at the Metaphase II stage and characterised by the presence of one polar body next to the egg can fertilise and can therefore be injected. Occasionally eggs that are at the stage of Metaphase I at the point of stripping will mature in vitro and become Metaphase II later on in the day and therefore can also be injected.

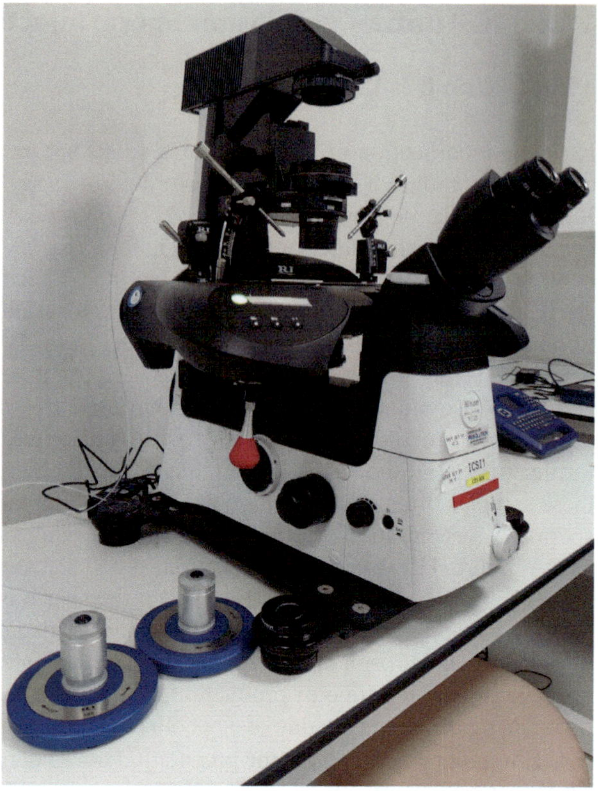

Fig. 11.3 ICSI microscope and micromanipulators

An ICSI dish is prepared with a few drops of culture media, in which the denuded eggs are placed, along with a drop or a pool of culture medium for sperm and one or two drops with polyvinylpyrrolidone (PVP) where the sperm tail will be slashed with the injection pipette prior to its aspiration into the pipette and injection into one of the eggs, as shown in Fig. 11.4. PVP is a synthetic copolymer that is used to help with the handling and immobilisation of sperm during ICSI.

11.2.3 Fertilisation Rate

The fertilisation rates are very similar for ICSI and IVF, and therefore, they are different technical approaches to minimise the chances of failed fertilisation whilst providing patients with the best chance of a successful pregnancy. For ICSI, the expectation is that on average 65% of the mature eggs will fertilise. From the zygote stage, embryo development is the same for IVF and for ICSI embryos.

Abnormal Fertilisation A proportion of the injected eggs will show abnormal fertilisation 1.4% for 1PN and 0.8% for ≥3PN [11]. The rate of ≥3PN is higher in

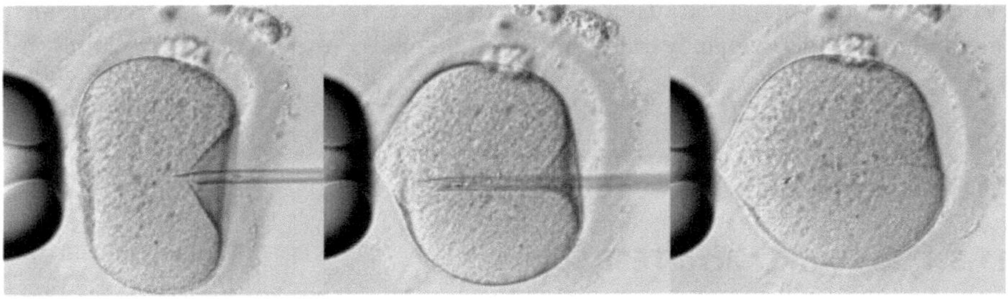

Fig. 11.4 The process of injection of the sperm into an egg. Initially the injection pipette is passed through the zona pellucida and into the cytoplasm of the egg. A gentle aspiration force is applied to ensure that the egg membrane is broken before inserting the sperm into the egg with a minimum quantity of media, removing the injection pipette and releasing the egg from the holding pipette [16]

IVF as more than one sperm can penetrate the egg during the time that eggs and sperm are together in culture.

11.2.4 Lysis/Damage Rate

This is one of the risks of ICSI, and patients should be counselled about this when making decisions between IVF and ICSI as possible approaches to fertilise their eggs and before consenting for either treatment. The lysis rate should be below 10% of the eggs injected.

11.2.5 ICSI Conversion from IVF

On rare occasions, patients may plan to have their eggs inseminated via IVF, but on the day of egg collection, the sperm sample may either be below the normal range or fail to meet the minimum threshold required for IVF. Sometimes this happens when frozen sperm is used, when the survival rate or the yield of sperm after preparation is below expectation, and to minimise the risk of failed fertilisation using IVF, it is recommended to patients that ICSI is used in an attempt to fertilise their eggs.

11.2.6 Rescue ICSI

Rescue ICSI can be attempted in the UK in cases of fertilisation failure with IVF. This can be offered to patients on the understanding that the chances of normal fertilisation will be much lower than with ICSI performed on the day of egg collection and that any embryos developed as a result of rescue ICSI, if they are of suitable quality, will have to be vitrified and transferred in a frozen embryo cycle as they will be 24 hours delayed and therefore out of synchrony with the endometrium in a fresh

IVF/ICSI cycle [4]. The transfer of cryopreserved rescue ICSI embryos yielded implantation and pregnancy rates of 18% and 36%, respectively, in a study by Paffoni et al. in [21].

11.3 Surgically Retrieved Sperm

11.3.1 TESE and Micro-TESE Sperm

Some patients who do not produce sperm in the ejaculate might require the surgical extraction of sperm from the testis. Testicular sperm extraction (TESE) and microsurgical testicular sperm extraction (micro-TESE) are both procedures used to retrieve sperm from the testis, but they differ in the techniques used. These are usually performed in advance of the start of ovarian stimulation in order to assess for the presence of sperm. If sperm is identified, then it will be frozen with a view to thawing and using it for ICSI on the day of egg collection.

11.3.1.1 TESE (Testicular Sperm Extraction)

A minimally invasive procedure that involves making a small incision in the testicle to extract one or several tissue samples. This is passed on to the clinical scientists in the laboratory, who will dissect the tissue and disrupt the microtubules before examining an aliquot of the sample under the microscope for the presence of sperm. Often, the sperm retrieved with this procedure is of low quality, and it can always only be used for ICSI, which can be technically challenging as it will involve searching for motile sperm under the microscope in a tissue sample that contains other cell types.

11.3.1.2 Micro-TESE

This is an open surgical procedure that uses an operating microscope to identify and extract testicular tubules that are most likely to contain sperm. Micro-TESE is considered the best option for patients with non-obstructive azoospermia, as several areas of the testis can be examined in this way. It requires the use of highly specialised equipment and the presence of urologists, nurses and clinical scientists in the operating theatre as it is shown in Fig. 11.5. Micro-TESE is 1.5 times more likely to be successful at retrieving sperm than conventional TESE [8].

The fertilisation rates of testicular sperm by ICSI have been reported to be about 57% [1], so slightly lower than the ones reported with the use of ejaculated sperm at 65%, and this is most likely related to the quality of the sperm used for the injections.

11.3.2 PESA (Percutaneous Epididymal Sperm Aspiration)

PESA is a surgical procedure that involves using a fine needle to extract sperm from the epididymis, the sperm reservoir located above the testicle. This is shown in Fig. 11.6. It is a quick, relatively painless procedure that is usually performed under

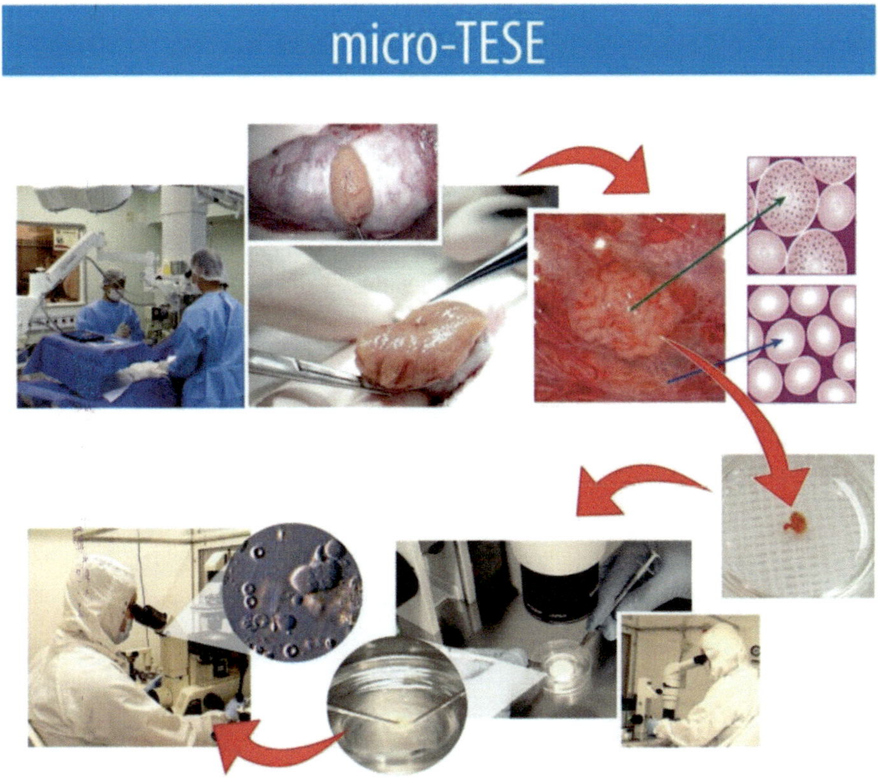

Fig. 11.5 The testicle is opened to reveal the seminiferous tubules which are then dissected under the microscope to isolate the sperm [19]

local anaesthetic. PESA is used to retrieve sperm for patients with obstructive azoospermia, which can be caused by a vasectomy, infection or congenital absence of the vas deferens.

The sample obtained through aspiration is quickly examined under a microscope in the laboratory to see if it contains motile sperm and to estimate the concentration. This can be repeated until an adequate number of motile sperm are recovered. Like with TESE and micro-TESE, the sperm obtained are usually frozen and kept in storage until the day of egg collection when, if the survival is sufficient, they can only be used for ICSI. The fertilisation rates with ICSI using PESA sperm are very similar to those achieved when using ejaculated sperm [14].

This is the least invasive method of obtaining sperm from the epididymis. If no sperm are recovered with this approach, a TESE or a micro-TESE might be necessary.

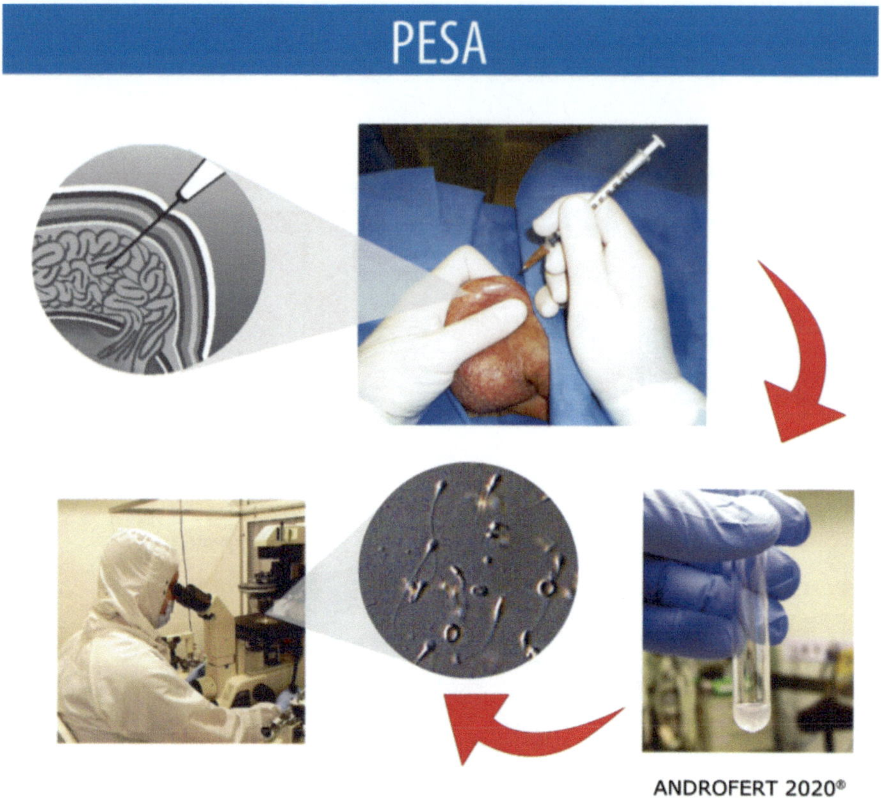

Fig. 11.6 The needle is inserted through the upper part of the scrotum to reach the head of the epididymis and aspirate the sperm [19]

11.4 Embryo Development

Figure 11.7 shows how human embryos develop in vitro from the day after egg collection, when embryologists will check for fertilisation, until day 5 of embryo development, usually the day of embryo transfer [18]. With current time-lapse technology available in most embryology laboratories, it is now possible to observe all stages of embryo development without disruption of culture conditions.

On average, 50% of the embryos will reach the blastocyst stage on days 5 or 6 of embryo development [6]. The number of normally fertilised eggs is therefore relevant as not all of them will usually become blastocysts, and the best chances of pregnancy will be provided to those patients who have more and better quality blastocysts on days 5 and 6. The aim is usually to transfer the best blastocyst fresh and vitrify any surplus blastocysts of suitable quality for later use, either after a successful pregnancy in order to conceive a sibling or after a failed fresh embryo transfer.

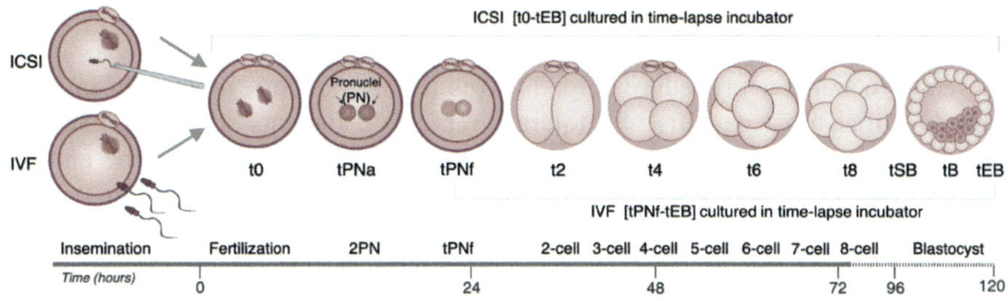

Fig. 11.7 Morphological changes over time during early embryonic development. The zygote undergoes three divisions to reach the 8-cell stage, at which time the embryo undergoes compaction and polarisation. The blastomeres then differentiate into the Inner Cell Mass and Trophectoderm and form a cavity. (Published in: Wiegel et al. [23], under a Creative Commons Attribution 4.0 International License http://creativecommons.org/licenses/by/4.0/)

11.5 Fresh Embryo Transfer

A fresh embryo transfer is the placement of one or more embryos into the uterus in the days following the egg retrieval. The fresh embryo transfer can occur on any day up to Day 6 of embryo development, but it is now widely accepted that embryo transfer should be carried out on Day 5 to aid the selection of the best available embryo. Nurses should be aware that not all patients will have a viable embryo to transfer. Those patients who fail to reach embryo transfer should be offered support and counselling to protect their emotional wellbeing and an early opportunity for a discussion regarding their future options.

11.5.1 Pre-procedure

Prior to embryo transfer, the fertility team should explain the number and quality of available embryos and make a recommendation for the number and selection of embryo(s) to be transferred. A shared decision-making approach with the patient should be taken ensuring that the patient understands their chances of pregnancy and the risks of a multiple pregnancy in relation to the quality and number of embryos to be transferred. The discussion should reflect on both the healthcare professionals' good clinical judgement and the patients' values and personal context.

To maximise the chance of success as well as to reduce the risk of a multiple pregnancy, the number of embryos recommended for transfer should be based on the egg provider's age, treatment cycle history and the quality of the embryos available. For most patients, a single embryo transfer is preferred as this will offer a good chance of a live birth and reduce the multiple pregnancy rate and the associated risks. However, patients aged 37 years and older, patients with poor quality embryos or patients with repeated IVF failures may opt for the transfer of more than one embryo [20]. Local policies and national regulations regarding the allowed number of embryos to be transferred must be followed.

11.5.2 Procedure

The embryo transfer procedure (Fig. 11.8) is usually a short, minimally invasive procedure that most patients will tolerate very well. Patients should be asked to attend with a partially full bladder to aid ultrasound visualisation of the embryo transfer catheter. A policy should be in place to confirm the identity of the patient, thus ensuring the correct embryo(s) are transferred into the patient. In some clinics, embryos can be shown to the patient on a monitor prior to the embryo transfer.

The embryo transfer procedure is done using a non-touch aseptic technique protecting the sterility of the tip of the catheter. The procedure begins with the gentle placement of a Cusco's vaginal speculum to centralise the cervix. Once the patient and the embryo transfer operator are comfortable with the position of the speculum, the operator should gently clean around the cervix removing any cervical mucus before beginning to place the embryo transfer catheter in the uterine cavity.

The embryologist will load the embryo(s) into the embryo transfer catheter in a very small volume of culture media and pass the loaded catheter to the operator. Abdominal ultrasound guidance is used to visualise the movement of the embryo transfer catheter through the cervical canal into the uterus. The tip of the catheter is placed 1–2 cm from the uterine fundus. When the operator is confident with the placement of the embryo transfer catheter, they can gently depress the plunger of the syringe attached to the catheter to expel the fluid containing the embryo(s) into the uterus. This can be viewed on ultrasound and shown to the patient. When the operator is confident that the embryo(s) has been transferred into the uterus, they should slowly remove the catheter from the uterus, maintaining pressure on the plunger of the syringe, and pass the catheter back to the embryologist to ensure that the embryo(s) has left the catheter successfully.

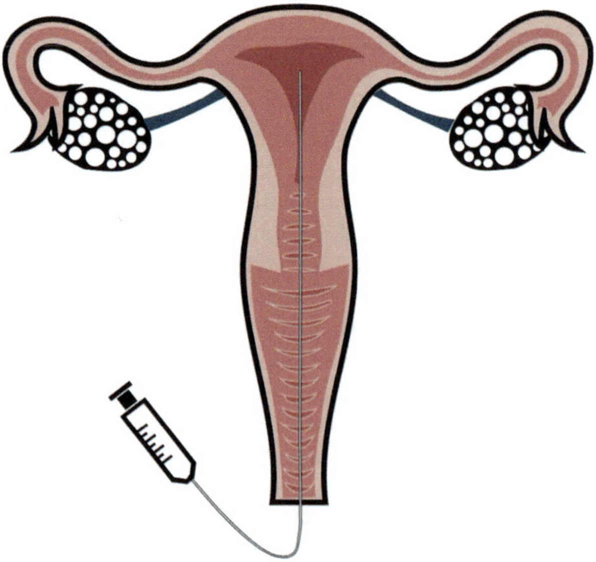

Fig. 11.8 Embryo transfer procedure (Kindly shared by Dr. Matthew Prior)

The speculum can be removed when it is confirmed that the embryo(s) has left the catheter and entered the uterus. Occasionally embryos fail to leave the catheter. In this situation, the embryologist will recheck the viability of the embryo(s), reload the catheter and pass the reloaded catheter to the operator to repeat the procedure detailed above.

Most embryo transfers are conducted quickly and easily with a smooth transfer of embryo(s) from the incubator to the patient. On occasion, it can be difficult to negotiate the cervical canal with a soft catheter, requiring the use of a stylet with the catheter. This allows the embryo transfer catheter to be shaped to negotiate the contours of the cervical canal. More rarely, the use of a tenaculum or vulsellum can help pull the cervical canal into a straighter position. These difficulties can often be avoided by identifying the patients who are more likely to have a difficult embryo transfer before the start of their treatment. This can include patients who have had previous treatment to their cervix such as loop excision, patients with uterine fibroids, patients with congenital abnormalities of the uterus and patients who had previous difficult cannulation of their cervix, for example, during intrauterine insemination treatment or cannulation of the cervix for the purpose of tubal patency testing. These patients should be offered a mock embryo transfer, using an empty embryo transfer catheter, prior to the start of their IVF treatment. This can help identify the best approach to the embryo transfer procedure, including the best catheter to suit that patient.

Occasionally, an embryo transfer might unexpectedly be difficult, and it may not be possible to pass the catheter successfully into the uterus despite multiple attempts. In this circumstance, it is possible to abandon the intended treatment cycle and freeze the embryo(s) intended for fresh transfer until a suitable approach is found to pass the catheter successfully. It might be necessary for the patient to undergo dilatation of the cervix before a further attempt at embryo transfer, or in extremely difficult situations, there is an option for trans-myometrial embryo transfer.

11.5.3 Post-procedure

Once the speculum is removed, the patient should be slowly returned to a seated position and when ready, aided to stand. They can then be escorted to the changing area and advised they can empty their bladder. Patients should be advised that extended bed rest has no beneficial effect on outcomes [20] and encouraged to remain gently mobile in the days following embryo transfer. They may return to work if they feel physically and emotionally able to do so.

Patients should be advised of the date for pregnancy test. They are advised to continue luteal support, usually in the form of progesterone pessaries or subcutaneous injections, until pregnancy test, which is typically done 9–11 days following embryo transfer. Patients should be advised that it is normal to experience some vaginal spotting for 1–2 days after embryo transfer. This is particularly relevant if the cervical canal has been difficult to negotiate or if there is an ectropion of the cervix.

Patients with surplus good quality blastocysts can be offered vitrification of the surplus blastocysts.

11.5.4 Nursing Role

For most nurses, their role during embryo transfer will be that of assistant, guiding the abdominal scan probe to aid visualisation of the uterus, making the correct equipment available to the operator and supporting the patient physically and emotionally during the procedure. However, there are nurses trained to perform embryo transfer with this first described by Barber et al. in 1996. This can be done safely and effectively, without detriment to patient outcomes, if a competency-based training and assessment process is used with monitoring of key performance indicators and regular peer reviews of performance against the clinic's embryo transfer standard operating procedure.

Care should be taken to maintain the patient's physical dignity during the procedure. Reassurance should be offered throughout the procedure and time allocated post-procedure for the patient (and their partner if applicable) to ask any questions. They should be given a point of contact between embryo transfer and pregnancy test in case they have any concerns.

Sadly, not all patients will have an embryo to transfer. This might be due to no eggs collected, failed fertilisation of the eggs or arrested development of the embryos prior to the date of embryo transfer. Although this only occurs in less than 10% of IVF cases, these risks should be discussed with patients prior to starting their IVF treatment. Patients who fail to reach embryo transfer will need additional emotional support. They should be offered counselling support and signposted to any patient support groups that could offer them peer support. An early opportunity to discuss their future options is useful.

11.6 Frozen Embryo Transfer

A frozen embryo transfer cycle (FET) is the warming and transfer of previously vitrified embryos into the uterus. An FET can be offered to patients who have previously undergone a freeze-all cycle, patients with remaining frozen embryos from a previous failed cycle or patients returning to try for a sibling using their remaining frozen embryos.

Freezing and warming of embryos is stressful to the cells of an embryo. For some embryos, all of the cells remain intact, while in others all of the cells break up and are no longer viable. Poor quality embryos very rarely survive the freezing and warming process so only embryos considered robust enough to survive these processes should be frozen. Advances in embryo freezing techniques with the use of vitrification have improved embryo warming survival rates with most clinics using vitrification as their preferred freezing method.

11.6.1 Pre-procedure

A discussion should take place before the cycle to explain the stages of the treatment cycle to the patient, gain their written consent for the treatment cycle and explain the risks involved including the side effects of any medication used and the possibility that the embryo/s may not survive warming. Patients should be advised of their likelihood of successful outcome prior to the cycle. The patient's obstetric history and previous IVF/FET cycle outcomes should be reviewed when deciding how many embryos to warm and transfer, and consideration should also be given to the number of children they hope to have in their family. It might be that a patient who conceived following a previous multiple embryo transfer prefers to limit the number of embryos transferred in their frozen cycle to reduce their chance of a multiple pregnancy and adding more than one child to their existing family.

Patients can be prepared for an FET cycle using a medicated cycle approach using hormonal preparation to prepare the endometrium or a natural cycle approach, with the transfer timed according to the patient's naturally occurring ovulation.

11.6.2 Medicated Cycle

A medicated FET cycle involves hormonal preparation of the endometrium prior to the embryo warming. Oral oestrogen can be started at the beginning of the menstrual cycle and a scan organised for 10–12 days later to review the thickness and appearance of the endometrium. Once the endometrium is deemed ready, typically achieving a thickness of 7 mm + with a trilaminar appearance on ultrasound, progesterone support is added and a date is scheduled for embryo warming, typically 5 days after the commencement of progesterone. Local protocols may vary slightly though each medicated FET cycle will aim to prepare the endometrium appropriately before setting a date for embryo warming.

11.6.3 Natural Cycle

Patients can be monitored using ultrasound to monitor follicle growth and trigger or detect ovulation, or patients can use ovulation kits to detect their LH surge from home. Once the date of ovulation is confirmed, a date is set for embryo warming depending on the stage the embryo was stored at. Blastocysts are typically warmed in preparation for same-day transfer 5 days after ovulation so that the endometrium is in synchrony with the embryo(s). Local protocols may vary slightly though each natural-cycle FET protocol will aim to detect or trigger ovulation before setting a date for embryo warming.

11.6.4 Embryo Warming

On the set date of embryo warming, it is a good practice to confirm that the patient is well and fit to proceed with the transfer before warming the embryo. Once this has been confirmed, the embryology team will remove the required number of embryos from storage and begin the embryo warming process. Patients should be advised prior to their FET cycle that there is a risk that their embryos will not survive the warming process though this is unusual, and most patients proceed to having at least one embryo to transfer.

Once the embryo has been confirmed as surviving the warming process (usually at least after one hour in culture), the patient is asked to attend the same day for embryo transfer. Patients whose embryos fail to survive the warming process should be offered counselling support and signposted to any patient support groups. An early opportunity to discuss their future options is helpful.

11.6.5 Procedure

The embryo transfer process is followed, as detailed for the fresh embryo transfer.

11.6.6 Post-procedure

The pregnancy test is typically performed 9–11 days following the embryo transfer. Patients who opt for a medicated cycle must continue their medication until their pregnancy test. Patients who have a positive pregnancy test in a medicated cycle must then continue their medication throughout their first trimester.

11.7 Egg Freezing

Egg freezing allows for the storage of mature eggs following ovarian stimulation and egg retrieval. There are several reasons why patients might want to freeze their eggs. These will include patients of reproductive age (including adolescents), who are preparing for medical treatment for cancer or other conditions that are likely to make them infertile, patients who are transitioning from female to male, patients at high risk of premature ovarian insufficiency, patients at risk of the surgical removal of their ovaries and single women or women in relationships who want to delay childbearing.

Patients who wish to freeze their eggs will undergo ovarian stimulation and egg retrieval as described in the section regarding IVF. Mature eggs collected on the day of egg retrieval are vitrified and stored on the same day. Patients may need multiple cycles of egg freezing to store enough eggs to allow them a good chance of pregnancy should they return to use them. However, multiple cycles are not always possible especially if medical constraints such as waiting to start chemotherapy are in place. Patients who are self-funding egg freezing may not also have the financial resources available for multiple cycles. This should be considered when deciding the ovarian stimulation protocol for patients storing eggs as a higher-than-usual ovarian stimulation dose could be used to maximise the number of eggs available for storage in one cycle. While the risk of ovarian hyperstimulation syndrome (OHSS) must always be considered during ovarian stimulation, the risk of OHSS can be minimised by following an antagonist stimulation protocol and using an agonist to trigger oocyte maturation, allowing for a higher-than-usual dose of ovarian stimulation if needed.

Patients planning egg freezing should be counselled prior to the start of a stimulation cycle and given information about the likelihood of a successful egg freeze cycle and the chance of a live birth should they return to use the stored eggs. They should also be counselled about the risks of ovarian stimulation and egg retrieval. Local and national policies should be followed regarding consent for egg storage and use.

Egg freezing is often an emotionally significant decision, and nurses should approach patient care with empathy and understanding. For patients storing eggs prior to urgent medical or surgical treatment, the egg-freezing process can add additional emotional stress, so care must be taken to ensure these women are supported emotionally throughout the egg-freezing cycle.

11.8 Witnessing

All the laboratory procedures that require the entrance of eggs, sperm or embryos into the laboratory, the movement of eggs, sperm or embryos between tubes or culture dishes, the mixing of eggs and sperm or the exit of eggs, sperm or embryos from the lab require documented double witnessing. This can be manual—with two professionals checking three patient identifiers—or electronic, where the vessels are electronically tagged and assigned to a specific patient. In the UK, this is an HFEA requirement and includes processes such as egg collection, embryo transfer, insemination, ICSI, fertilisation check, embryo, egg or sperm freezing and thawing (HFEA Code of Practice).

References

1. Achermann APP, Pereira TA, Esteves SC. Microdissection testicular sperm extraction (micro-TESE) in men with infertility due to nonobstructive azoospermia: summary of current literature. Int Urol Nephrol. 2021;53(11):2193–210. https://doi.org/10.1007/s11255-021-02979-4. Epub 2021 Aug 19. PMID: 34410586.
2. Baldini D, Lavopa C, Matteo M, Malvasi A. Oocyte Retrieval. In: Malvasi A, Baldini D, editors. Pick up and oocyte management. Cham: Springer; 2020. https://doi.org/10.1007/978-3-030-28741-2_10.

3. Barber D, Egan D, Ross C, Evans B, Barlow D. Nurses performing embryo transfer: successful outcome of in-vitro fertilization. Hum Reprod. 1996;11:105–8. https://doi.org/10.1093/oxfordjournals.humrep.a018999.
4. Bolton VN, Perez MJ, Hughes G, Moodley T, Dean M, Fernandez-Ponce A, Southall-Brown G, Kasraie J. The use of ICSI in ART: evidence for practice. Hum Fertil (Camb). 2023;26(3):414–32. https://doi.org/10.1080/14647273.2023.2243071. Epub 2023 Aug 23. PMID: 37609991
5. Clarke H, Harrison S, Perez MJ, Kirkman-Brown J. UK guidelines for the medical and laboratory procurement and use of sperm, oocyte and embryo donors (2019). Hum Fertil (Camb). 2021;24(1):3–13. https://doi.org/10.1080/14647273.2019.1622040. Epub 2019 Jun 6. PMID: 31169420. https://portal.hfea.gov.uk/media/yrkn55xa/2024-10-01-hfea-code-of-practice-v9-4.pdf
6. ESHRE Special Interest Group of Embryology and Alpha Scientists in Reproductive Medicine. Electronic address: coticchio.biogenesi@grupposandonato.it. The Vienna consensus: report of an expert meeting on the development of ART laboratory performance indicators. Reprod Biomed Online. 2017;35(5):494–510. https://doi.org/10.1016/j.rbmo.2017.06.015. Epub 2017 Aug 4. PMID: 28784335
7. Esteves S, Agarwal A. What is new in the clinical assessment and treatment of the infertile male. The Open Reproductive Science Journal. 2011;3:16–26. https://doi.org/10.2174/1874255601103010016.
8. Esteves SC. Microdissection TESE versus conventional TESE for men with nonobstructive azoospermia undergoing sperm retrieval. Int Braz J Urol. 2022;48(3):569–78. https://doi.org/10.1590/S1677-5538.IBJU.2022.99.14. PMID: 35333489; PMCID: PMC9060172
9. Fleming SD. Micromanipulation, micro-injection microscopes and systems for ICSI. In: Palermo GD, Nagy ZP, editors. Manual of intracytoplasmic sperm injection in human assisted reproduction: with other advanced micromanipulation techniques to edit the genetic and cytoplasmic content of the oocyte. Cambridge University Press; 2021. p. 114–28.
10. Girsh E, editor. A Textbook of Clinical Embryology. Cambridge University Press; 2021. p. i–ii.
11. Hanson B, et al. The relationship between age and rates of abnormal fertilization following intracytoplasmic sperm injection (ICSI). Reprod Biomed Online. 2020;41:e8.
12. Hicks SA, et al. Machine learning-based analysis of sperm videos and participant data for male fertility prediction. Sci Rep. 2019;9:16–770.
13. Invitra. What is epididymal sperm aspiration? Procedure & Techniques; 2021.
14. Javed A, Ramaiah MK, Talkad MS. ICSI using fresh and frozen PESA-TESA spermatozoa to examine assisted reproductive outcome retrospectively. Obstet Gynecol Sci. 2019;62(6):429–37. https://doi.org/10.5468/ogs.2019.62.6.429. Epub 2019 Oct 28. PMID: 31777739; PMCID: PMC6856474
15. Joergensen MW, Labouriau R, Hindkjaer J, Stougaard M, Kolevraa S, Bolund L, Agerholm IE, Sunde L. The parental origin correlates with the karyotype of human embryos developing from tripronuclear zygotes. Clin Exp Reprod Med. 2015;42(1):14–21. https://doi.org/10.5653/cerm.2015.42.1.14. Epub 2015 Mar 31. PMID: 25874169; PMCID: PMC4390676
16. Kocur OM, Xie P, Cheung S, et al. The intricate "ART" of ICSI. J Assist Reprod Genet. 2025;42:349–65. https://doi.org/10.1007/s10815-024-03322-3.
17. Levron J, Munné S, Willadsen S, Rosenwaks Z, Cohen J. Male and female genomes associated in a single pronucleus in human zygotes. Biol Reprod. 1995;52(3):653–7. https://doi.org/10.1095/biolreprod52.3.653. PMID: 7756458
18. Mu J, Zhou Z, Sang Q, Wang L. The physiological and pathological mechanisms of early embryonic development. Fundam Res. 2022;2(6):859–72., ISSN 2667-3258. https://doi.org/10.1016/j.fmre.2022.08.011.
19. Miyaoka R, Esteves SC. Sperm retrieval techniques. In: Parekattil S, Esteves S, Agarwal A, editors. Male infertility. Cham: Springer; 2020. https://doi.org/10.1007/978-3-030-32300-4_50.
20. National Institute for Health and Care Excellence (2013) Fertility Problems: assessment and treatment. Available at www.nice.org.uk/guidance/cg156

21. Paffoni A, Reschini M, Pisaturo V, Guarneri C, Palini S, Viganò P. Should rescue ICSI be re-evaluated considering the deferred transfer of cryopreserved embryos in in-vitro fertilization cycles? A systematic review and meta-analysis. Reprod Biol Endocrinol. 2021;19(1):121. https://doi.org/10.1186/s12958-021-00784-3. PMID: 34348713; PMCID: PMC8336078
22. Palermo G, Joris H, Devroey P, Van Steirteghem AC. Pregnancies after intracytoplasmic injection of single spermatozoon into an oocyte. Lancet. 1992;340(8810):17–8. https://doi.org/10.1016/0140-6736(92)92425-f. PMID: 1351601
23. Wiegel RE, et al. Human oocyte area is associated with preimplantation embryo usage and early embryo development: the Rotterdam Periconception Cohort. J Assist Reprod Genet. 2023;40:1495–506.

Embryology

12

Sara Henderson and Heather E. Fice

12.1 Introduction

Embryonic development begins with each of the individual gametes, the oocyte and the spermatozoa. The oocyte provides the developing zygote with maternal DNA and large cellular mass including the cell membrane, the cytoplasm, various organelles, growth factors, and the mitochondria. The oocyte is also responsible for the meiotic spindle formation (which separates the two copies of the maternal DNA into the single copy needed by the egg) and provides sperm-activating factors for DNA decondensation allowing the genetic code contained in the DNA to be opened and read to make the child. The sperm in turn provides the paternal DNA, oocyte activating factors, and the centrosome required for the final stages of meiosis and formation of the second polar body. When the two copies of the maternal DNA are separated, the other copy is put into the polar body. It is only with the correct fusion of the two gametes that successful fertilization may occur. The fertilized egg transitions to a zygote after its first cell division, called cleavage. After subsequent cell divisions, the cleavage embryo has an increasing number of blastomeres until they become so small and tightly bound to one another that they form a morula and individual cells are hard to differentiate. The morula then undergoes differentiation giving rise to the blastocyst (Fig. 12.1), a fluid-filled cavity.

S. Henderson (✉) · H. E. Fice
McGill University Health Centre Reproductive Centre, Montreal, QC, Canada
e-mail: sara.henderson@muhc.mcgill.ca; heather.fice@mail.mcgill.ca

M. Das, M. H. Dahan (eds.), *A Comprehensive Guide to Reproductive Health and Infertility Medicine for Nurses*, https://doi.org/10.1007/978-3-032-24372-0_12

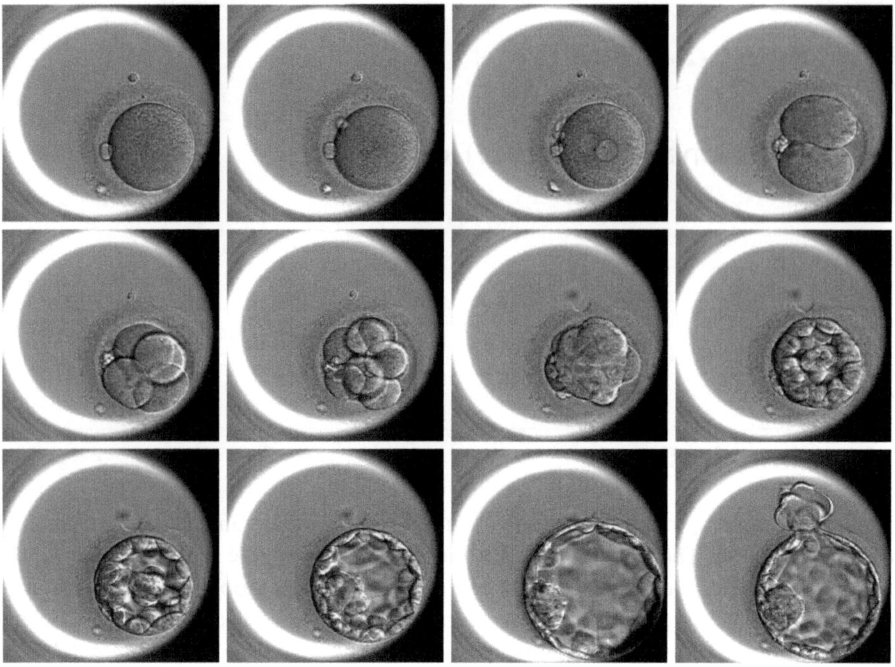

Fig. 12.1 Embryonic development—from metaphase II oocyte to hatching blastocyst

12.2 Fertilization

An embryologist will check for fertilization 16–18 h after insemination. Normal fertilization appears as two separate pronuclei (PN) within the center of the oocyte, with one pronucleus forming from each of the parental genomes (Fig. 12.2b, c). When abnormal fertilization occurs, there may be 1 PN (Fig. 12.2d), 3 PN (Fig. 12.2e, f), or multiple PN. A single pronucleus may be genetically normal and be a result of the fusion of the two parental pronuclei; however, more commonly eggs with 1 PN after fertilization are abnormal and do not result in a baby. An embryo with three pronuclei is genetically abnormal, having three copies of each chromosome, and may be a result of the oocyte failing to extrude the second polar body, two sperm entering the egg, sperm with multiple nuclei, or failed cytokinesis. After the two pronuclei form, they go through a process called juxtaposition where the maternal PN moves towards the paternal PN. The two pronuclei then fuse, a process called syngamy, to form a euploid (genetically normal) nucleus, and embryonic genome.

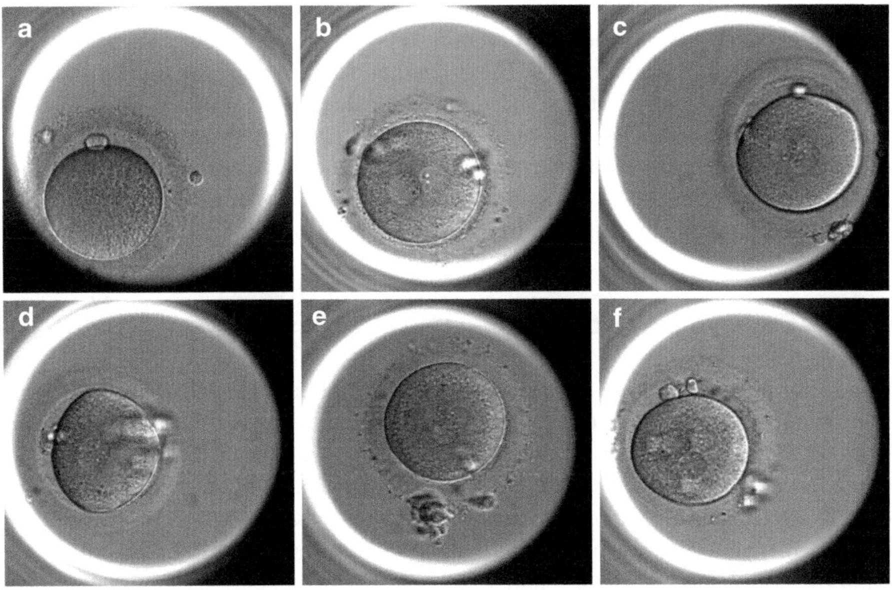

Fig. 12.2 Fertilization. (**a**) Unfertilized Metaphase II oocyte. (**b**, **c**) Normally fertilized 2PN. (**d**) Abnormal fertilization of 1 PN. (**e**, **f**) Abnormal fertilization of 3 PN

12.3 Fertilization Failure

It is possible that during the fertilization check, no PN are observed; this signifies that either fertilization was missed or that fertilization may have failed (Fig. 12.2a). Failed fertilization typically indicates an issue with one or both of the gametes. The oocyte may contribute to failure due to factors such as abnormal morphology, maturity, activation, and poor ovarian response. Failure can also be related to the sperm motility and progression, origin, maturity, morphology, DNA damage, and premature chromosome decondensation. It remains challenging to ascertain the exact cause of fertilization failure as any combination of factors may contribute. When doing conventional IVF, the fertilization failure rate may range anywhere from 5% to 20% [3]. As the issue with fertilization during conventional IVF is likely related to the early events of fertilization (sperm-egg binding, zona penetration, etc.), it is possible that an embryologist may be able to perform rescue ICSI upon observation of failed fertilization. Rescue ICSI, typically performed on day one, has generally lower success rates, likely due to the time-dependent decrease in oocyte quality, and competence, however, is not without merit in cases of failed fertilization.

It is also possible that when performing the fertilization check after 16–18 h, there are no apparent PN as the pronuclei may have appeared earlier or later than anticipated. An important element of embryology is the inherent timing to each developmental window, where certain milestones are used to gauge the quality and potential success of each embryo. Embryos that develop after the missed fertilization check are typically not optimal for transfer due to the aberrant timing of this milestone and the inability to confirm normal fertilization; however, these zygotes are kept for further observation to monitor subsequent development. This phenomenon occurs more frequently in static observation, as a lack of PN when using time-lapse observation is more likely a true failed fertilization.

12.4 Embryo Development

Following fertilization, the embryo begins a series of cellular divisions resulting in a growing number of blastomeres (cells) that decrease in size with each division (Fig. 12.3). A cleavage embryo will maintain its size within the zona pellucida, while its cells undergo division. On day 2, the embryo should have between 2 and 4 cells (Fig. 12.3a–d). Evidence suggests that embryos with four cells on day 2 are optimal for good-quality blastocyst development (Fig. 12.3c, d). On day 3, the embryo should have between 6 and 9 cells, with 8 cells being the optimal number (Fig. 12.3e, f). Day 3 is also when the activation of the embryonic genome occurs, as a result, there are typically embryos that arrest at this stage and do not form

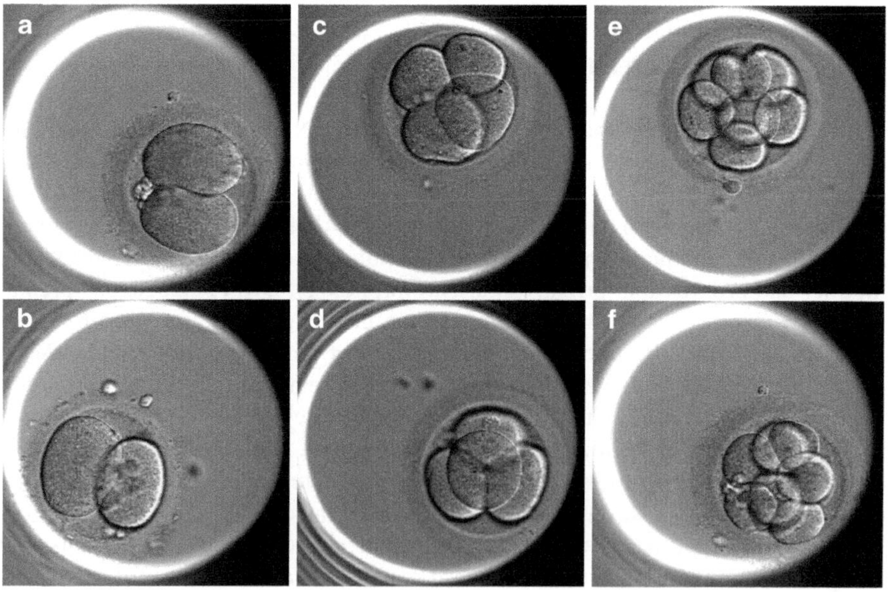

Fig. 12.3 Cleavage stage embryo. (**a**, **b**) Two-cell grade 2. (**c**, **d**) Four-cell grade 2. (**e**) Eight-cell grade 1. (**f**) Eight-cell grade 2

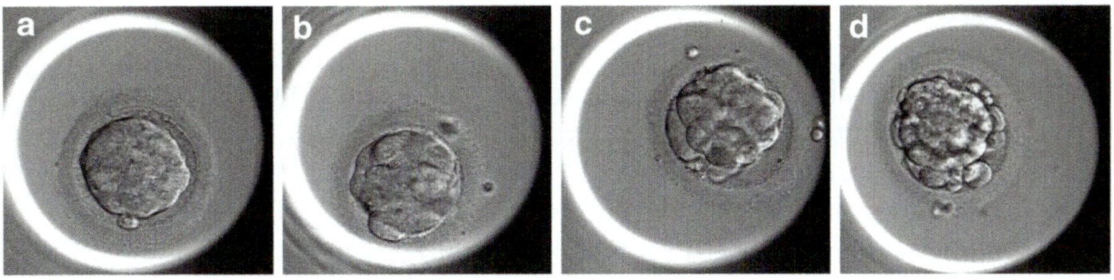

Fig. 12.4 Compaction—Morula stage embryo. (**a**, **b**) Compacting grade 2. (**c**) Compacting grade 3. (**d**) Compacting grade 4

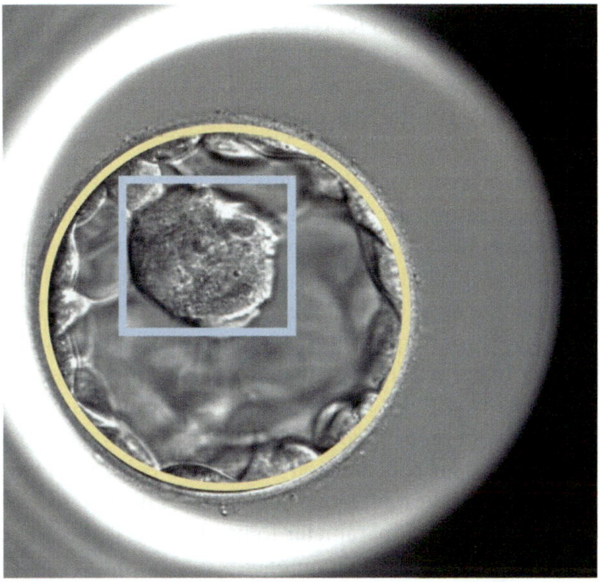

Fig. 12.5 Fully expanded good-quality blastocyst. Inner cell mass outlined in blue square, trophectoderm cells outlined in yellow. Grade 4AA per Gardner grading

blastocysts. As the number of blastomeres increases, there are an increasing number of both tight and adherens junctions. The increase in junctions between cells leads to the tight compaction and merging of cells forming the morula stage embryo (Fig. 12.4a–d). The compaction of the embryo can begin anywhere from the 8–16 cell stage on day 3 and continue into day 4 of development. Once the cells are compacted, typically by days 5–6, they begin to differentiate into the inner cell mass (ICM) and the trophectoderm (TE) (Fig. 12.5). The blastomeres forming the ICM will eventually give rise to the fetus, and the TE cells will aid in implantation of the embryo leading to the placenta. The number of blastocysts that form depends primarily on the embryonic genome; however, this may also be impacted by the culture media composition and potentially the environmental conditions of the laboratory. The environmental vulnerability of the developing embryos results in each laboratory having blastocyst formation rates that may differ slightly.

12.5 Grading

The frequency of embryo grading is dependent on the clinic, though common practice is to check embryo development each day, some groups do not, to minimize handling and temperature shifts. Typically, the embryos are checked using microscope examination at the same time each day in the morning. There are several different grading systems that exist for embryos including but not limited to: ASEBIR in Spain, BFS and ACE in the UK, SART in the USA, but the most commonly used systems are The Istanbul Consensus from 2011 for cleavage embryos and the Gardner grading system for blastocysts. Within this text, The Istanbul Consensus and Gardner system will be used to describe the process of embryo grading and discuss high-quality embryos.

12.5.1 Cleavage Stage

At the cleavage stage, the embryo is graded based on: blastomere number and size, multinucleation, vacuoles, and the degree of fragmentation. The first parameter assessed is blastomere number and size, which is a simple count of the number of cells present within the embryo. When assessing the number of blastomeres, it is important to consider that the embryo may either be between divisions or some cells may divide more quickly than others, and an embryologist may observe an uneven number of cells. When an uneven number of cells is observed, it is expected that the blastomeres will not be of equal size as some may have undergone more divisions. This does not reflect poor quality. Occasionally, an uneven number of cells is indicative of aberrant cell division where one cell may give rise to three daughter cells after mitosis. Normally, one cell should give rise to two daughter cells, not more at one time. The next parameter to be checked is the degree of fragmentation present. Fragmentation is small components of cytoplasm left after incomplete cell division, sometimes enclosed by a membrane. When fragmentation is present, it is incorporated into the grade based on the percentage of fragmentation [6]. Higher levels of fragmentation are generally associated with less chance of pregnancy.

The Istanbul Consensus method of grading for cleavage embryos includes the number of blastomeres in the embryo followed by a numerical grade based on the percentage of fragmentation. The numerical grades are as follows: grade 1 < 10% mild fragmentation, grade 2 10–25% moderate fragmentation, and grade 3 > 25% severe fragmentation (Fig. 12.6). A high degree of fragmentation is associated with poor-quality embryos and has shown a negative correlation on later embryo development and ultimately live birth rates [1, 2, 11].

As briefly mentioned, at this stage, aberrant cleavage may become apparent. Methods have been developed to more closely monitor embryo development, allowing for the direct observation of potentially harmful events. For example, time-lapse observation allows for analysis of cleaving patterns to assess abnormal divisions such as direct cleavage, reverse cleavage, and chaotic division. Direct cleavage is observed when the embryo will divide from one cell directly to three. Reverse

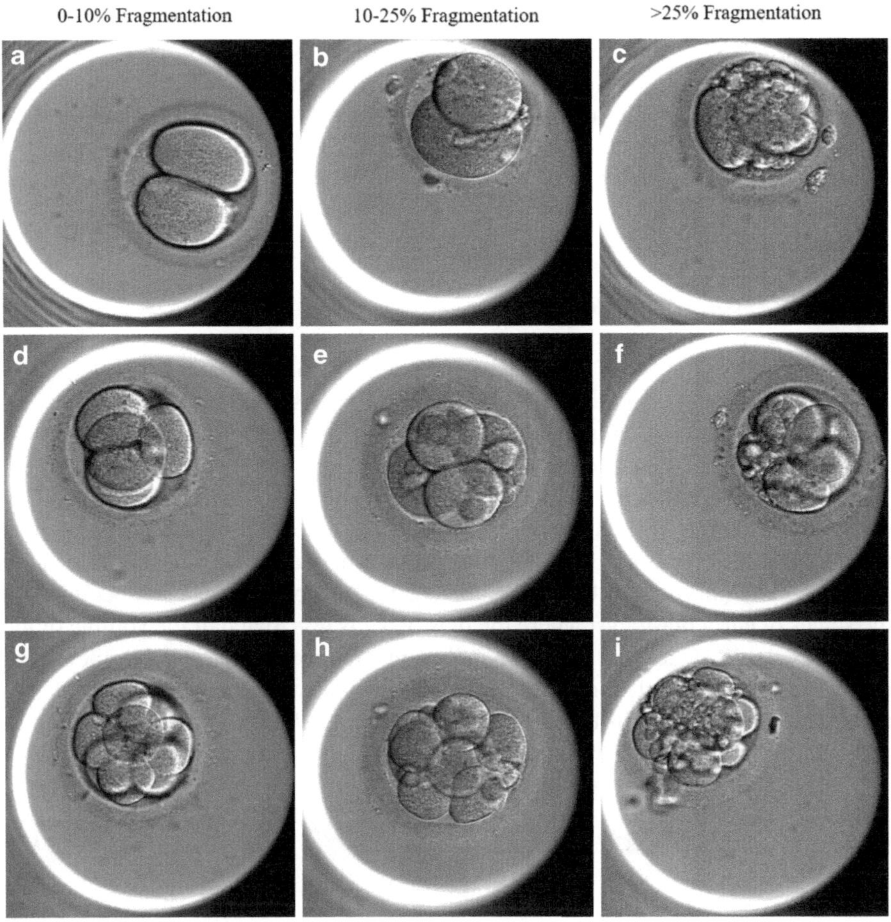

Fig. 12.6 Cleavage embryo grading per Istanbul Consensus. (**a**–**c**) Two cell. (**d**–**f**) Four cell. (**g**–**i**) Eight cell

cleavage is when the embryo will divide, most probably with errors, and will therefore reabsorb the division in an attempt to correct the error before dividing again. These division patterns would normally be missed in static observation. Aberrant cleavage or abnormal division has been associated with lower live birth rate and higher incidence of aneuploidy [7, 9, 10, 12].

12.5.2 Compacting Stage

As the embryos begin compaction, it becomes harder to assign a grade to the embryo due to the cellular complexity and the tight connecting junctions between cells. Evaluating the number of cells becomes increasingly difficult as the cells decrease in size, and it is challenging to differentiate between blastomeres and potential fragmentation. When grading a morula, the focus remains on the proportion of cells involved in the compaction. An increase in blastomere inclusion during compaction will be graded as a good quality embryo, and the more blastomere exclusion and fragmentation, the lower the grade. This is often denoted simply as a compacting embryo, with a grade taking into consideration blastomere inclusion and fragmentation (Fig. 12.4a–d).

12.5.3 Blastocyst Stage

Following compaction, cell differentiation and blastocoel cavitation begin typically around day 5 or 6. At this stage, the Gardner grading system remains the most commonly used system [5]. This grading system provides a grade with three characters in the format #XX. The number provided is between 1 and 6 and represents the expansion of the blastocoel cavity, the letters A-C represent the quality of the ICM (first letter) and the TE cells (second letter). The numbers provided do not denote the quality of the embryo, simply the expansion of the blastocoel, the fluid-filled cavity in the embryo (Fig. 12.7 and Table 12.1). Blastocyst expansion begins with the stages of early blastocyst where the blastocoel is less than half the volume of the embryo; at this stage, we focus on inclusion of blastomeres and fragmentation (Fig. 12.8). As the blastocoel cavity expands, the blastocyst becomes a full blastocyst where the embryo fills the zona pellucida (Fig. 12.9). The expansion continues, and when the volume of the blastocoel is larger than the early embryo and the ZP is

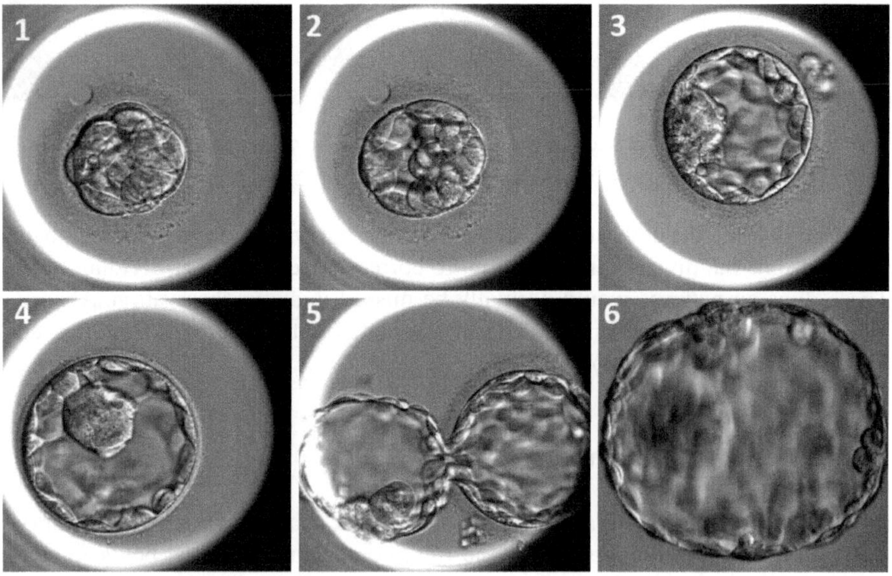

Fig. 12.7 Gardner grading stages of blastocyst expansion

Table 12.1 Gardner grade descriptions for blastocyst expansion

Numerical Gardner grade for embryo expansion	Blastocyst stage	Description
1	Early	Blastocoel is less than half the volume of the embryo
2	Blastocyst	Blastocoel is greater than half the volume of the embryo
3	Full	Blastocoel completely fills the embryo
4	Expanded	Blastocoel volume is now larger than that of the early embryo and the zona pellucida is thinning
5	Hatching	Trophectoderm has started to herniate through the zona
6	Hatched	Blastocyst has completely escaped from the zona pellucida

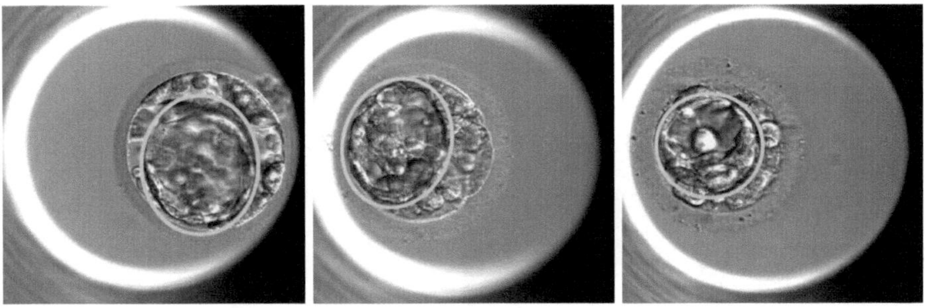

Fig. 12.8 Early blastocyst (Gardner Stage 1–2). Blastocyst circled in blue to highlight cellular debris and fragmentation that is not being included in blastocyst development

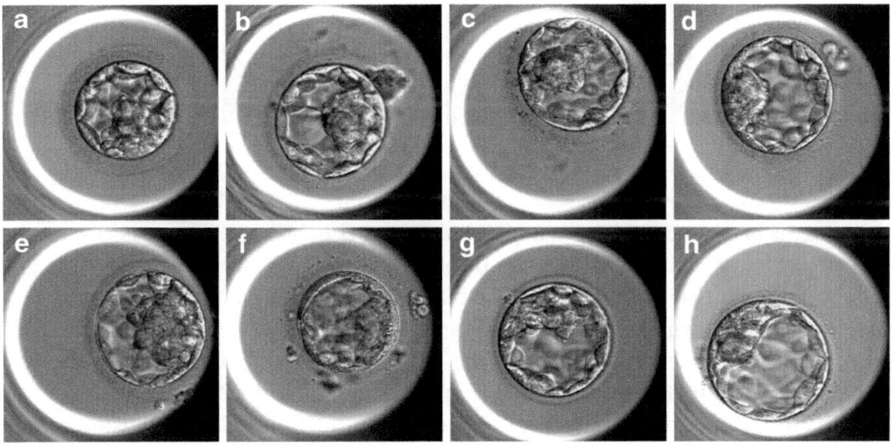

Fig. 12.9 Full blastocyst (Gardner Stage 3). (**a–d**) 3AA (**e**) 3AB (**f**) 3CC (**g**) 3BA (**h**) 3BB

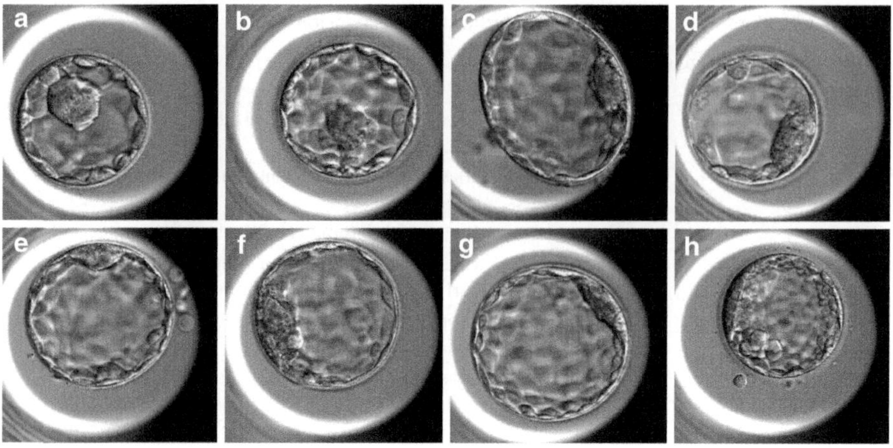

Fig. 12.10 Expanded blastocyst (Gardner Stage 4). (**a–c**) 4AA (**d**) 4 AC (**e**) 4BA (**f**) 4AB (**g**) 4BA (**h**) 4CC

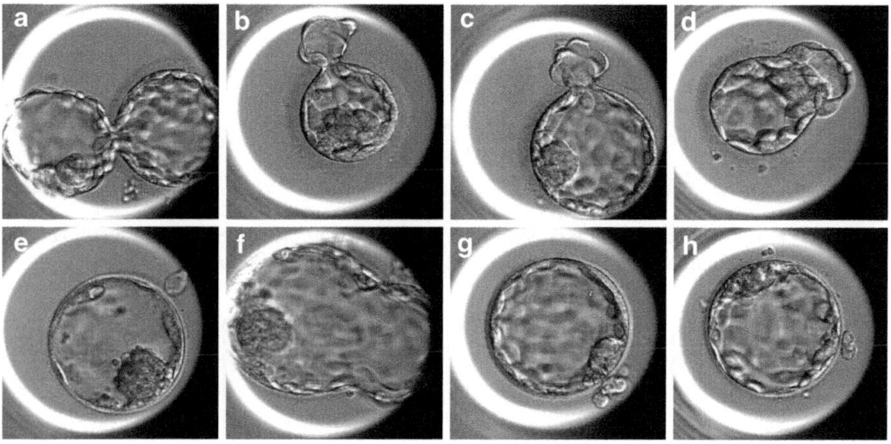

Fig. 12.11 Hatching blastocyst (Gardner Stage 5). (**a–d**) 5AA (**e**) 5CC (**f**) 5CB (**g**, **h**) 5BB

thinning, it is denoted as an expanded blastocyst (Fig. 12.10). The pressure on the zona pellucida eventually causes the trophectoderm to break through the zona and is now hatching (Fig. 12.11). Once the blastocyst has completely left the zona pellucida, this is known as a hatched blastocyst (Fig. 12.12). At every stage of expansion, the letters reflect the quality of the ICM and TE cells, with A being the best quality and C being the least optimal (Fig. 12.5 and Table 12.2).

The trophectoderm cells control the regulation of fluid into the blastocyst and thus regulate the expansion of the embryo blastocoel cavity and eventual hatching through the zona pellucida. During blastocyst expansion, cytoplasmic strings may be visible between the ICM and TE cells (Fig. 12.13). The cytoplasmic strings are involved in cellular communication and are positively associated with successful

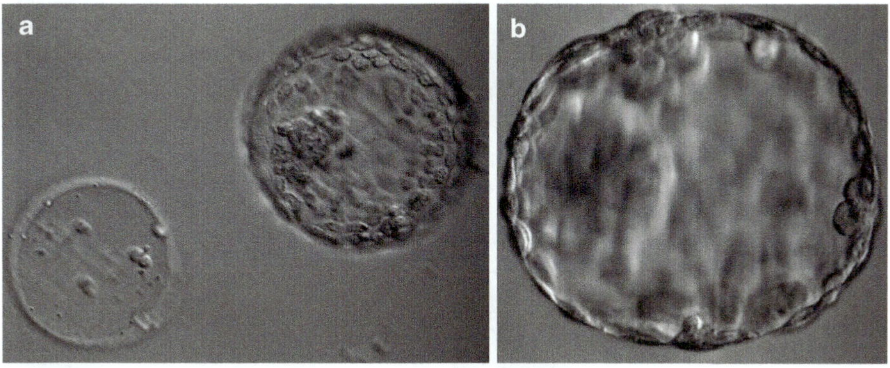

Fig. 12.12 Hatched blastocyst (Gardner Stage 6). (**a**) Hatched blastocyst (right) next to its empty zona pellucida (Grade 6BA). (**b**) Hatched blastocyst (Grade 6AA)

Table 12.2 Gardner grade descriptions for blastocyst quality

Letter grade for Gardner blastocyst quality	Inner cell mass	Trophectoderm cells
A	Tightly packed, many cells	Many cells of equal size forming a cohesive epithelium
B	Loosely grouped, several cells	Few cells forming a loose epithelium
C	Little clear grouping, very few cells	Very few cells forming a sparse epithelium

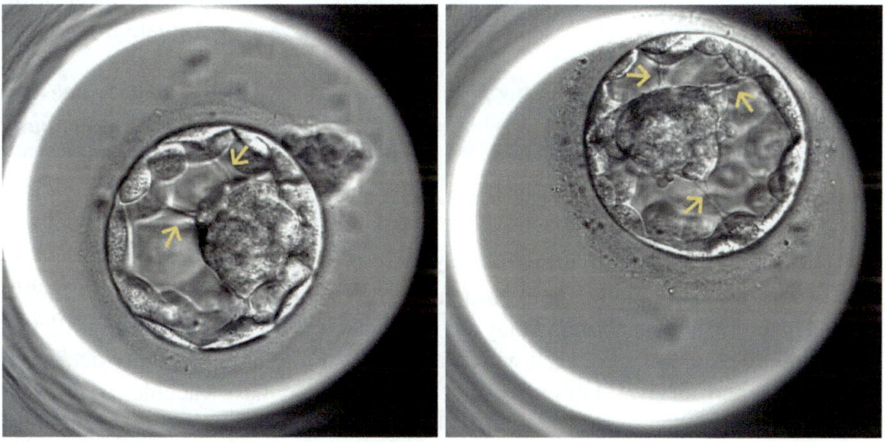

Fig. 12.13 Cytoplasmic strings in expanding blastocyst connecting the ICM and TE cells

implantation [4]. A series of spontaneous collapse and re-expansion cycles will allow the embryo to break the zona pellucida and hatch out naturally (Figs. 12.12 and 12.14). If grading a collapsed blastocyst during static observation, it is best to

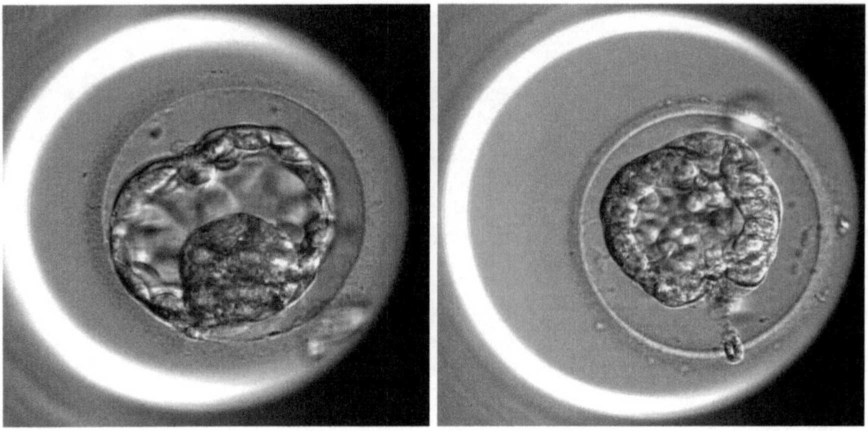

Fig. 12.14 Blastocyst shrinking within the zona pellucida

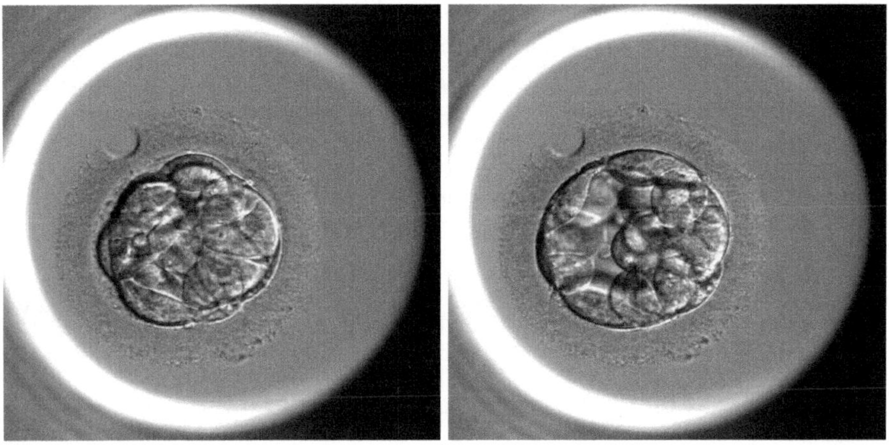

Fig. 12.15 Blastocyst with artificial hole in the zona pellucida created using laser

wait 1–4 h for the embryo to properly re-expand in order to observe all the cells. In cases where the zona pellucida is hardened, such as after egg freezing, artificial/assisted hatching or zona thinning may aid in the hatching of the embryo (Fig. 12.15).

Additional elements may exist within a blastocyst that are potentially detrimental to quality and survival. For example, a blastocyst may have vacuoles or arrested and potentially degenerated blastomeres (Fig. 12.16). Vacuoles are fluid-filled cytoplasmic inclusions bound by a membrane that often result due to stress at any stage during oocyte or embryo development. Blastocysts with at least one vacuole have been negatively correlated with pregnancy outcomes [8]. In addition to the presence of vacuoles, cells may arrest at any point during development; these cells may degenerate and appear dark and grainy relative to other cells within the blastocyst. They may be isolated outside of the trophectoderm, meaning they are not truly part

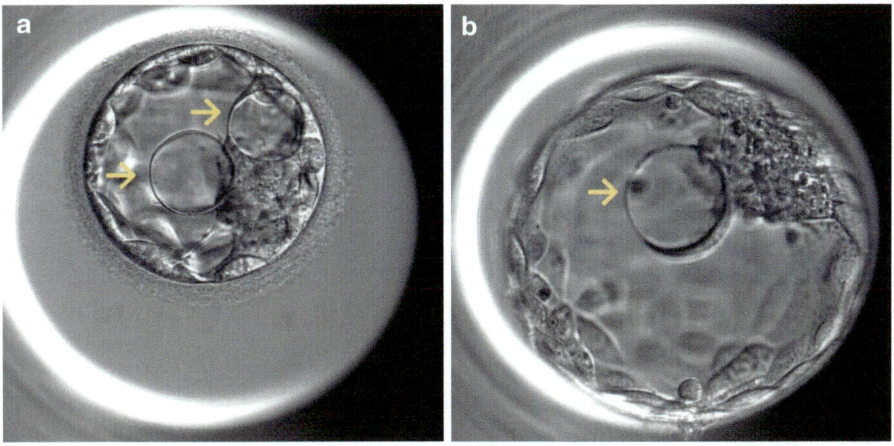

Fig. 12.16 Blastocysts with present vacuoles. (**a**) 4BA blastocyst with two vacuoles. (**b**) 5BA Blastocyst with one vacuole. Vacuoles indicated by yellow arrow

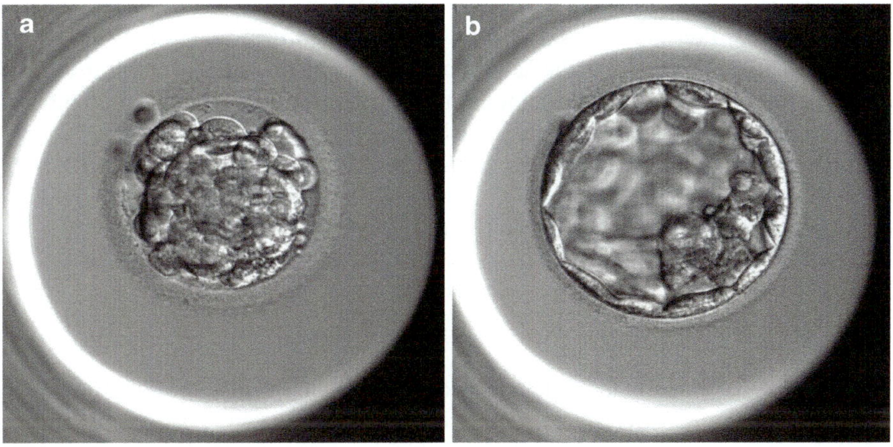

Fig. 12.17 Embryo quality improving after blastocyst expansion. (**a**) Poor quality compacting stage embryo with grade 3 fragmentation. (**b**) Good quality expanded blastocyst of quality 4BA

of the blastocyst and will not contribute to the development, or they may be integrated into the blastocyst. If cells arrest or begin to degenerate prior to blastocyst formation or compaction, those cells would be excluded and pushed out of the embryo toward the zona. Thus, in some cases, "poor"-quality compacting embryos may result in good quality blastocysts after exclusion of degenerated cells and debris (Fig. 12.17). If cells arrest or begin to degenerate later in development, they will remain inactive and are instead pushed toward the blastocoel cavity.

Blastocyst quality has been correlated with many clinical outcomes including the rates of clinical pregnancy, implantation, miscarriage, and live birth. It is the general consensus among all studies that the likelihood of clinical pregnancy, implantation, and live birth is higher with good quality blastocysts, while miscarriage risk is higher with poor quality blastocysts. Generally, good quality blastocysts are those with letter grades AA, AB, BA, and poor-quality blastocysts are those with a C letter grade for either the ICM or TE. It is often the case that embryos that reach the blastocyst stage on day 5 are higher quality, as this is optimal timing for embryonic development. In most embryology labs, the embryos are kept in culture for six days following the egg retrieval/thaw on day zero. Some groups culture embryos until day 7; however, at this time-point, blastocysts are likely of poorer quality and have correspondingly low potential for pregnancy. Although live birth rates with good quality day 7 blastocysts are in the 15% range and slightly higher if the embryo is genetically tested and euploid.

12.6 Embryo Environment

One of the goals during ART treatment in the lab is to provide the embryo with an environment that is most similar to an in vivo environment for embryonic development. The in vivo environment of course comprises the fallopian tubes and uterus. In an attempt to ensure optimal development, a great deal of research has been performed to optimize both the laboratory environment and the embryo culture environment. The general environment includes the physical room, light, temperature, humidity, air quality, incubators, dishes, handling pipettes, microscopes, vitrification carriers, cryogenic tanks for storage, and culture media. In most ART labs, all aspects of the environment are continuously monitored, and reagents making direct contact with embryos undergo rigorous quality control assessment.

12.6.1 Laboratory

An ART lab is a semi-sterile lab. To control the air quality, the lab should be equipped with high-efficiency particulate air (HEPA) filters and positive pressure to minimize air contamination and volatile organic compounds (VOC). It is important to reduce contamination and VOCs as they have been shown to negatively impact embryo development and quality. VOCs are present not only in ambient air but also in inks, cleaning supplies, and many personal products including perfume, hair and skin products, and nail polish. Patients and people working in the IVF center should avoid using products containing VOCs. The temperature and humidity of the lab must also be controlled to avoid large fluctuations, maintaining ambient air quality. Many labs also use reduced light, through either limited number or filtered lights, as during an embryo's in vivo development, it would not be exposed to light.

All equipment (workstations, microscopes, incubators, etc.) must be validated, calibrated, and maintained for proper function. The temperature of incubators and workstations must be maintained at 37 °C, as this is the optimal temperature for embryos, unless otherwise indicated for activities such as vitrification. Workstations and equipment must be easy to disinfect and kept clean to avoid contamination by infectious disease or particulate matter. The number of incubators must reflect the number of cycles performed by the given clinic, and the number of workstations, laminar-flow hoods, and microscopes must reflect the workload of the laboratory. In addition to embryo handling, cryostorage tanks filled with liquid nitrogen are used in ART lab practice to preserve gametes or embryos for future use. The tank integrity must be validated prior to use, with consistent monitoring of adequate liquid nitrogen levels and tank integrity.

The laboratory staff must adhere to certain guidelines in order to maintain the semi-sterile and protected ART lab environment. They are required to wear lab-specific clothing and footwear, practice proper hand hygiene, and use hairnets and masks where applicable (illness, during genetic testing, etc.). Outside materials, such as food and drinks, are strictly forbidden.

12.6.2 Embryo Culture

All consumables, media, and reagents that will be interacting with gametes must be embryo culture grade and approved for use by the governing body of the specific ART lab (i.e, FDA, Health Canada). Quality control testing must be supplied by the company if purchased commercially, in addition to the quality control testing performed by the lab. The embryo culture media must always be maintained at appropriate temperature, pH, and osmolality depending on the composition of the various types of media. To reduce embryo stress, time outside of incubators should be minimized to reduce fluctuations in the direct media environment. Laminar flow hoods and microscope stations are equipped with heated stages to maintain temperature. However, room temperature stable buffered media should be used if the embryos will be exposed to ambient surroundings for a more extended period to maintain pH. Additionally, by reducing time outside of the incubator, this minimizes exposure to light and ambient air.

Incubators have evolved and are becoming much smaller than the large "box" ones once used. This ensures a quicker recovery after opening the incubator doors, which should be kept to a minimum. It has been shown that lower oxygen levels are ideal for blastocyst culture. This is created using a mix of gases at the concentrations of 5% oxygen, 6% carbon dioxide, and approximately 90% nitrogen gas, similar to the inner reproductive tract. The temperature of the incubator is set to ensure the medium holding the embryos is maintained around 37 °C. Appropriate pH and osmolality are equally important to ensure proper development and avoid media evaporating during culture. All these components are measured regularly as part of the lab quality control and corrected as needed. When preparing culture media dishes for patient use, it must be done hours in advance to allow time for the media to equilibrate in the incubator before use. Oil overlay of culture dishes is beneficial to minimize changes in temperature, pH, and osmolality.

12.6.3 Lab Safety and Emergency Situations

Gas cylinders supplying the incubators must be kept outside the laboratory and include an automatic changeover system and an alarm to indicate when these tanks are empty and needs to be replaced. Uninterrupted power supply (UPS) systems or generators should be in place for critical equipment to ensure continuous power to incubators during potential outages. All critical equipment and cryostorage units should be equipped with an alarm to ensure proper functioning and maintenance of temperature. The alarm system should be available to personnel both in and outside of the lab, 24 h a day, 7 days a week, 365 days a year. Cryopreservation storage should be located outside of the main lab. For safety reasons, the interior of the cryostorage room should be visible to the outside and must have adequate ventilation. While filling cryostorage units, liquid nitrogen used may displace and decrease oxygen levels in the room; thus, there should be oxygen monitors in spaces with abundant liquid nitrogen. For critical equipment in the lab, it is recommended that back-ups are available in the event of emergency or equipment failure; this includes incubators, refrigerator, freezer, and cryostorage tanks/units.

12.7 Final Words

In this chapter, we have given a brief overview of the six days of embryo development in the embryology laboratory, beginning first with the union of individual gametes through various methods, to form a fertilized egg and early zygote. The embryo develops, with its blastomeres dividing to form a cleavage embryo, a morula, and eventually a blastocyst. At each step of the process, an embryologist is able to grade and assess quality of the embryo, selecting those of highest quality for future reproductive use. Since the inception of human-assisted reproductive therapies, there have been many evolutions in laboratory practice and embryo-handling optimization, which have greatly improved the safety and efficacy of embryology practice and ultimately improved patient outcomes.

References

1. Ahlstrom A, Park H, Bergh C, Selleskog U, Lundin K. Conventional morphology performs better than morphokinetics for prediction of live birth after day 2 transfer. Reprod Biomed Online. 2016;33:61–70.
2. Awadalla MS, Ho JR, McGinnis LK, Ahmady A, Cortessis VK, Paulson RJ. Embryo morphology and live birth in the United States. F&S reports. 2022;3:131–7.
3. Combelles CM, Morozumi K, Yanagimachi R, Zhu L, Fox JH, Racowsky C. Diagnosing cellular defects in an unexplained case of total fertilization failure. Hum Reprod. 2010;25(7):1666–71.
4. Eastick J, Venetis C, Cooke S, Chapman M. The presence of cytoplasmic strings in human blastocysts is associated with the probability of clinical pregnancy with fetal heart. J Assist Reprod Genet. 2021;38:2139–49.

5. Gardner DK, Schoolcraft WB. In-vitro culture of human blastocysts. In: Jansen R, Mortimer D, editors. Towards reproductive certainty: fertility and genetics beyond 1999. 1641; 1999. p. 378–88.
6. Keltz MD, Shorupski JC, Bradlye K, Stein D. Predictors of embryo fragmentation and outcome after fragment removal in in vitro fertilization. Fertil Steril. 2006;86:321–4.
7. Liu Z, Jiang M, He L, Liu Y. Cell number considerations for blastocyst transfer in younger patients. J Assist Reprod Genet. 2020;37:619–27.
8. Mayer RB, Shebl O, Oppelt P, Reiter E, Altmann R, Enengl S, Allerstorfer C, Ebner T. Good-quality blastocysts derived from vacuolized morulas show reduced viability. Fertil Steril. 2018;109(6):1025–9.
9. Meseguer M, Herrero J, Tejera A, Hilligsøe KM, Ramsing NB, Remohí J. The use of morphokinetics as a predictor of embryo implantation. Hum Reprod. 2011;26:2658–71.
10. Petersen BM, Boel M, Montag M, Gardner DK. Development of a generally applicable morphokinetic algorithm capable of predicting the implantation potential of embryos transferred on day 3. Hum Reprod. 2016;31:2231–44.
11. Rhenman A, Berglund L, Brodin T, Olovsson M, Milton K, Hadziosmanovic N, Holte J. Which set of embryo variables is most predictive for live birth? A prospective study in 6252 single embryo transfers to construct an embryo score for the ranking and selection of embryos. Hum Reprod. 2015;30:28–36.
12. Zhan Q, Ye Z, Clarke R, Rosenwaks Z, Zaninovic N. Direct unequal cleavages: embryo developmental competence, genetic constitution and 2122 clinical outcome. PLoS One. 2016;11:e0166398.

13 Embryo Transfers

Israel Ortega Sánchez, Carlos Alonso,
and J. A. García Velasco

13.1 Introduction

The first human pregnancy following transfer of cryopreserved embryos occurred in 1983 [1], and since then, it has become a crucial component of assisted reproduction technology. Surplus embryos derived from IVF-ICSI procedures can be stored and transferred at a later stage, yielding similar clinical outcomes compared to those of fresh embryo transfer. In recent years, the use of frozen embryo transfers (FET) cycles has surpassed the number of fresh IVF cycles due to single embryo transfer policies and improved laboratory techniques, such as advances in cryopreservation. However, the most effective method to prepare the endometrium prior to FET is still a matter of debate.

13.2 Fresh Embryo Transfer

Normal luteal function is an essential component for pregnancy maintenance. In IVF cycles, either with gonadotropin-releasing hormone (GnRH) agonist or antagonist protocols, there are several endocrine disorders in the luteal phase that might induce a luteal phase dysfunction leading to lower clinical outcomes. To counteract these effects, luteal phase support (LPS) is a well-known intervention for almost all

I. O. Sánchez (✉) · C. Alonso
IVI-Madrid, Madrid, Spain
e-mail: israel.ortega@ivirma.com; Carlos.Alonso@ivirma.com

J. A. G. Velasco
IVI-Madrid, Madrid, Spain

Department of Gynecology, Rey Juan Carlos University of Medical Sciences, Madrid, Spain
e-mail: Juan.Garcia.Velasco@ivirma.com

M. Das, M. H. Dahan (eds.), *A Comprehensive Guide to Reproductive Health and Infertility Medicine for Nurses*, https://doi.org/10.1007/978-3-032-24372-0_13

Table 13.1 Routes of administration of progesterone for LPS

Route	Advantages	Disadvantages
Vaginal	Well-tolerated Gold standard	Vaginal discharge
Intramuscular	Well-tolerated	Skin inflammation Sterile abscesses
Subcutaneous	Well-tolerated alternative to the vaginal and IM routes	Local reaction at the injection site
Oral	No vaginal discharge	Dizziness and gastrointestinal side effects
Rectal	Patient friendly	Nausea, constipation

stimulated assisted reproductive technology (ART) cycles [2]. Progesterone is a key element for endometrial development and subsequent embryo implantation and has become the most common exogenously supplemented compound employed as support of the luteal phase. Previously, a meta-analysis [3] and two Cochrane systematic reviews [4] have shown that LPS improves the IVF pregnancy outcome. However, LPS does not offer so many options as the individualized controlled ovarian stimulation protocols and endometrium preparation protocols.

Nowadays, there is still no consensus about the ideal LPS method and the duration of progesterone supplementation. Five formulations of progesterone are currently available for assisted reproduction, including vaginal, intramuscular (IM), subcutaneous (SC), oral and rectal preparations (Table 13.1). A Cochrane meta-analysis that compared several routes of progesterone administration in fresh embryo transfer settings demonstrated no statistically significant differences between IM treatment vs oral, or between IM vs vaginal/rectal [4]. Similarly, two recently published retrospective studies compared combined IM and vaginal progesterone vs either IM or vaginal progesterone only LPS, showing similar outcomes for all study arms [5, 6]. Likewise, no significant differences were found between low-dose vs high-dose vaginal agents, short vs long protocol, micronized vs synthetic formulation, or other administration forms [4].

Whereas there is global agreement on supplementing the luteal phase, there is no such agreement on either the initiation or the duration of LPS. An inaccurate timing of LPS introduction may have relevant clinical implications: firstly, a premature exposure to progesterone may perturb the window of implantation, leading to impaired endometrial receptivity; secondly, a delayed LPS might not prevent a premature drop in progesterone and, consequently, endometrial shedding. To date, many studies have addressed this issue, concluding that initiation of LPS from the evening of ovum pickup (OPU) until three days post OPU was associated with optimal chances of pregnancy [7, 8]. According to the currently available data, cessation of progesterone administration may occur on or near the day of a positive β-hCG test [9], on the day of the first ultrasound (5–7 weeks) [10], or as late as the end of the first trimester of pregnancy [11, 12]. A recent meta-analysis that included up to 1201 randomized participants concluded that progesterone supplementation beyond the first positive β-hCG test after IVF/ICSI might generally be unnecessary [13].

Therefore, there is growing evidence demonstrating the lack of efficacy of extending progesterone supplementation beyond the first positive β-hCG test in fresh IVF cycles.

13.3 Frozen Embryo Transfer

After a failed fresh embryo transfer cycle or as part of the "freeze-all" strategy, a FET can be performed when there are surplus frozen embryos. Current data indicate that the use of FET has surpassed the number of fresh embryo transfers over the past decade [14]. The continuing expansion of FET is mainly due to improvement in laboratory techniques (vitrification) and use of the freeze-all strategy, mainly for genetic testing and for ovarian hyper-stimulation prevention [15].

In order to optimize clinical outcomes in FET, the development of embryo and the endometrium should be synchronized to facilitate implantation. In physiological conditions, the secretion of progesterone by the corpus luteum after ovulation plays a crucial role in completing the endometrial preparation after a sufficient estrogenic priming during the proliferative phase. If pregnancy is achieved, both hormones should be administered until the placenta takes over progesterone production.

Different modalities regarding endometrial preparation for controlled FET have been described in the last decade [16]. However, the most common approaches nowadays to prepare the endometrium and to time the FET are represented by natural cycle (NC-FET) and artificial cycle (AC-FET). In the former, there is a natural build-up of the endometrium using the detection of the luteinizing hormone (LH) surge to time the embryo transfer. In the latter, the endometrium is developed by exogenous estrogen and progesterone administration. In spite of the presence of controversial results regarding the efficacy of the different methods in FET cycles, a recent Cochrane review could not draw any conclusions on the superiority of any regimen with regard to ongoing pregnancy rate [16].

13.4 Natural vs Artificial FET

13.4.1 NC-FET

This approach relies on accurate timing of the natural ovulation, which dictates FET timing. Nowadays it is becoming the treatment of choice for women with normal ovulatory menstrual cycles, due to avoidance of exogenous hormonal medication and the shortening of the time taken to complete embryo transfer. Moreover, young women with normal body mass index and without the diagnosis of polyendocrine metabolic ovarian syndrome or other endocrinopathies could also benefit from this approach.

Frozen-thawed embryo transfer in a natural cycle may be programmed following two different protocols. In "true NC-FET" (tNC-FET), there is no pharmacological intervention; it is necessary to identify the onset of LH surge and ovulation that follows. Although there is no consensus as to the clinical approach to pinpoint the onset of LH surge, LH levels are regularly monitored by using daily blood or urine tests twice a day once the leading follicle reaches a mean diameter of 16 mm. This approach requires less ultrasound monitoring, reducing the number of visits to the clinic and, hence, the patient burden. However, LH determinations may be challenging since there is a broad variation in timing of detection of spontaneous LH surges due to a significant inter-cycle and inter-individual variability. Indeed, individual LH surges have shown extremely variable configuration, existing three LH surge patterns: spike, biphasic, and plateau [17]. Moreover, conventional LH urine kits have different thresholds, leading to false-negative results.

In the "modified NC-FET" (mNC-FET), urinary or recombinant human chorionic gonadotropin (hCG) is administered during a natural cycle to stimulate LH surge, enabling proper synchronization between embryo thawing and receptive endometrium. In both true and modified natural cycles, thawing and transfer of the embryo should be performed 3–5 days after ovulation depending on the stage of the embryo when frozen. Classically, the standard mean diameter necessary for triggering hCG has been established as 17 mm, mimicking cycles aiming to obtain a mature oocyte in IVF ovarian stimulation. However, the presence of a mature oocyte is not needed for FET; what is necessary is a functional corpus luteum that produces estrogens, progesterone and other vasoactive substances, like relaxin and vascular endothelial growth factor, with a prominent role in embryo implantation and placenta development. Based on this, a recent study showed that recombinant hCG could be flexibly administered with a mean follicle size ranging between 13 and 22 mm as long as adequate endometrial characteristics are met, and serum progesterone is <1.5 ng/ml. Bearing in mind the follicular growth rate of 1–1.5 mm/day, this strategy might improve the flexibility for FET scheduling of 6–7 days, thus helping to reduce the workload during the weekends [18].

Currently, there is no consensus regarding the potential benefit of luteal phase progesterone supplementation in women undergoing a NC-FET. Endogenous production of progesterone in ovulatory women might be enough to support implantation in a natural cycle. However, there is a specific subset of patients characterized by a defective production of progesterone from the corpus luteum, in terms of both quantity and duration, which might benefit from LPS [19]. Based on the literature, the estimated frequency of luteal phase deficiency (LPD) in infertile patients ranges from 5% to 32.5% [20, 21], being approximately 8.1% in natural cycles in normovulatory patients with primary or secondary infertility [22]. Consequently, women undergoing NC-FET might present a subnormal endometrium due to the presence of a LPD, yielding lower implantation and pregnancy rates.

13.5 Artificial FET

In artificial cycle FET (AC-FET), estrogen and progesterone are sequentially administered aimed to mimic the endocrine exposure of the endometrium in the normal cycle. Estrogen treatment, either orally or transdermal, usually begins on day 2 or 3 of cycle after confirming ovarian quiescence. This induces endometrial proliferation while suppressing the development of the dominant follicle. Around 10–14 days later, the endometrium reaches the optimal endometrial thickness (>7 mm) and its triple-line pattern is confirmed on ultrasound, a blood test is performed to rule out the potential risk of premature ovulation, which might impair the endometrial receptivity during treatment. Although the presence of a dominant follicle is rare during the endometrial preparation, it might be totally avoided with GnRH agonist treatment administered one week before the onset of the treatment.

LPS is usually added in artificial FET cycles to induce endometrial transformation 3–5 days before embryo transfer depending on the age of the embryo. Although the preferred route of administration for progesterone is still a matter of debate, vaginal and intramuscular are the most commonly ones used in the routine clinical practice. To address this issue, a retrospective study analyzing 920 FET cycles concluded that there were no significant differences in the main clinical outcomes when comparing intramuscular and vaginal progesterone administration [23]. These results, consistent with the solid clinical evidence, confirm that vaginal and intramuscular regimens have similar efficacy in providing LPS in FET. However, due to the side effects associated with daily intramuscular administration, such as severe discomfort and, rarely, sterile abscesses and risk of secondary infection, vaginal progesterone administration has become the gold standard in our group.

Over the past decade, several studies have focused on the "optimal luteal" serum progesterone concentration to ensure a successful implantation and early pregnancy in an artificial cycle [24, 25]. However, most studies on the relationship between serum progesterone and pregnancy outcome are retrospective. To clarify the relevance of serum progesterone levels on the day of the embryo transfer during an artificial cycle, *Labarta* et al. carried out a prospective cohort study that enrolled 1205 patients scheduled for embryo transfer after an artificial endometrial preparation cycle with estradiol valerate and micronized vaginal progesterone (400 mg twice daily). This group observed that women with serum progesterone levels <8.8 ng/ml on the day of the embryo transfer had a significantly lower ongoing pregnancy rate and live birth rate (35.5% vs 52%) than the rest of the patients [26], confirming the relevance of serum progesterone levels not only in oocyte donation cycles but also in cycles with own oocytes. However, the optimal duration of progesterone remains controversial. Although progesterone treatment may be withdrawn at luteal placental shift (7 weeks gestational age), it commonly continues up to week 12 in the routine clinical practice. However, the hypothesis that prolonging the duration of progesterone treatment might increase the clinical outcomes has not yet been confirmed [27, 28].

In summary, the artificial FET cycle is advantageous in that it requires minimal monitoring of these cycles and a satisfactory endometrial thickness can be achieved. In addition, the timing of embryo thawing and transfer is more flexible than in the natural cycle, allowing clinic and embryological staff to program treatment cycles according to the moment of progesterone supplementation. Moreover, in postmenopausal women, FET cannot be based on ovulation; therefore, the artificial FET protocol is the only valid approach, being the preferred protocol for women with irregular cycles and women without ovarian function. However, this strategy falls

Table 13.2 Clinical variables that influence the choice of optimal endometrial preparation for FET

Variable	Favors NC-FET	Favors AC-FET
Age	<37	>37
Menstrual cycle	Regular	Irregular/absent
PMOS or other endocrinopathy	Absence	Present
Weight	Normal	Overweight/obesity
Distance from the clinic	Near	Far
Need of scheduling	No	Yes
Obstetric history	Unfavorable	Favorable
Estrogen-dependent condition	Present	Absent
Economic limitation	Yes	No
Previous preeclampsia	Yes	No

short in securing best obstetric and perinatal outcomes. A recent meta-analysis showed poorer obstetric and neonatal outcomes with AC-FET when compared to NC-FET, making the latter the preferred option of treatment in women with ovulatory cycles undergoing FET [29]. However, because of many uncertainties, future studies are needed on efficacy and safety of luteal phase support and clinical recommendations should be made with caution.

To conclude, the choice for endometrial preparation method in FET should be individualized based on clinical variables prior to FET, such as the age, convenience, flexibility, and cost efficiency of the procedure, since current strategies for LPS yield similar reproductive outcomes (Table 13.2).

13.6 Optimizing Uterine Environment

13.6.1 Add Ons, Do They Have a Role?

Patients undergoing IVF treatment are highly motivated to achieve a successful pregnancy, and new technologies are constantly being developed with the intent to improve treatment outcomes. While the basic steps of IVF are relatively consistent, there are many "add-on" technologies that might be incorporated to standard treatments to increase the success rate. However, physicians should be reluctant to recommend these techniques during the FET due to lack of robust clinical evidence and their costs. Here, we aim to provide an overview of the evidence associated with several common FET add-ons and discuss future directions.

13.7 ERA and Endometrial Biopsy

Endometrial receptivity refers to the state in which the endometrium allows embryo attachment and placentation, a process that typically occurs 8–10 days after ovulation as a result of the coordinated action of ovarian hormones, growth factors, transcription factors, cytokines, and other signaling molecules [30]. Despite its importance, clinical diagnosis of the window of implantation (WOI) remains imprecise.

Advances in transcriptomics have enabled the use of DNA microarray techniques when studding endometrial receptivity by biopsy. As a result of that, the endometrial transcriptome has been characterized, providing a "transcriptomic signature" at a specific moment [31]. Using these findings, Díaz-Gimeno et al. developed the Endometrial Receptivity Array (ERA) test, which analyzes the expression of 238 genes to determine the WOI and detect its potential displacements related to progesterone exposure or ovulation [32]. This test aimed to provide a personalized timing for embryo transfer (pET) informing on optimal duration of progesterone exposure before embryo transfer. This would be of particular interest in patients experimenting recurrent implantation failure (RIF). Ruiz-Alonso et al. [33] observed that 25.9% of RIF patients had a displaced WOI compared with 12% of controls. After adjusting endometrial preparation based on ERA results, 15 previously non-receptive patients became receptive, and only three remained non-receptive [33]. However, although the ERA test initially seemed promising, the effectiveness of pET guided by ERA is debated. Some studies report improved implantation and pregnancy rates in RIF patients [34, 35], while others do not [36–38].

A recent randomized controlled trial involving 767 participants undergoing euploid embryo transfers found no improvement in ongoing pregnancy rates (OPR) with ERA-guided pET compared to the standard progesterone protocol [39]. Furthermore, of those patients in the control group, all of which received an embryo transfer regardless of the ERA result, no difference was found on live birth rates (LBR) between those with a receptive result and those with a non-receptive one (61.2% in receptive vs 62.5% in non-receptive, $p = 0.8$). From these findings, it can be concluded that pET guided by ERA test is not associated with better reproductive outcomes, and furthermore, an initial displacement on the WOI is not associated with a worse prognosis.

In a recent multicenter cohort study on patients with a single previous failed transfer, LBR and cumulative LBR were lower after pET, for both autologous and donor transfers [40]. Similarly, women with adenomyosis, who often exhibit dysregulated receptivity, showed no significant differences in early reproductive outcomes after pET [41].

In conclusion, the ERA test lacks robust evidence of benefit in the general population or RIF patients and should be not recommended.

13.8 Endometrial Scratch or Endometrial Injury

Endometrial scratch or endometrial injury (EI) in the cycle prior to IVF has been suggested to prepare the endometrium for implantation by increasing the local cytokines involved in both wound healing and implantation processes [42].

It has been performed by hysteroscopy or by Pipelle biopsy; in follicular phase, the day of the pickup or in mid luteal phase of the previous menstrual cycle; once or even several times in the same cycle. It has even been studied prior to an intrauterine insemination cycle and timed intercourse cycles, but evidence suggests it is not useful in these scenarios [43, 44].

Meta-analyses of randomized controlled trials regarding the benefit of this method in women with RIF have either been unable to extract results due to the between-study clinical heterogeneity or have led to inconsistent conclusions.

Probably the most well designed study has been the Endoscratch trial [45], a RCT that included only egg donor recipients of single embryos from day 3 to 5 in a fresh transfer with hormonal replacement therapy endometrial preparation protocol. They included 352 patients that were randomized into group A, which received an EI by Pipelle biopsy in the luteal phase of the cycle preceding the embryo transfer, and group B, which did not receive any intervention. The results showed no beneficial role of EI.

Although the role of endometrial injury is still controverted after 20 years of its initial description, nowadays evidence supporting its use is insufficient and it should not be recommended.

13.9 Assisted Hatching

The inability of the blastocyst to escape from its zona pellucida is considered a factor leading to unsuccessful ART.

At blastocyst stage, the zona pellucida becomes progressively thinner until it finally breaks. This is triggered by a rise in internal pressure caused by the expansion of the blastocele and the proliferation of trophectoderm cells. The breakage (hatching) is completed by a series of proteases released by uterine and trophectoderm cells.

There are some factors, such as structural anomalies of zona pellucida (double zona pellucida; darkening; thickening >15 μm) that may difficult hatching. These kinds of anomalies are more frequent at advanced maternal age.

Assisted hatching (AH), the artificial manipulation of zona pellucida, has been related to increased CPR, yet also to raised multiple pregnancies in RIF patients receiving fresh embryos [46, 47]. However, the small sample sizes of available studies cannot lead to safe conclusions.

A systematic review, including one RCT and one observational study, evaluated assisted hatching on ART outcomes in patients with RIF after at least three ETs [48]. Assisted hatching did not increase CPR or LBR.

A Cochrane meta-analysis [49] included 39 RCTs. AH did not improve live birth rates compared to no AH, with a slight increase in multiple pregnancy rates. When all the included studies are pooled, the clinical pregnancy rate in women who underwent AH may improve slightly in comparison with no AH (OR 1.20, 95% CI 1.09 to 1.33; 39 RCTs, N = 7249; $I^2 = 55\%$; low-quality evidence). However, when a random-effects model is used due to high heterogeneity, there may be little to no difference in clinical pregnancy rate ($P = 0.04$).

AH should not be recommended routinely. The group of patients that could benefit the most are the ones presenting abnormalities at zona pellucida, specially with advanced maternal age (>38 years) and patients with RIF.

13.10 EmbryoGlue

The composition of the culture medium that surrounds the embryo at time of transfer is important for implantation. Much research has been done on the effect of adding a specific adherence compound, hyaluronic acid (HA), to the medium in which the embryo is transferred into the uterus.

HA is one of the major macromolecules present in the female reproductive tract, including the endometrium. Its expression in the endometrium peaks around the mid-proliferative phase and then in the mid-to-late secretory phase [50], suggesting that it is a key molecule in embryo implantation. It produces a viscous solution that may enhance embryo transfer process and prevent expulsion from the uterine cavity.

A Cochrane meta-analysis of 10 RCTs [51] concluded that the use of HA-enriched transfer medium at a concentration of 0.5 mg/mL improved live birth rates in IVF when compared with low or no HA with a degree of moderate-quality evidence and a number needed to treat of 14. However, most of the embryo transfers included were conducted in the fresh cycle, and subgroup analysis of the three studies that included only frozen embryo transfer (FET) showed no evidence of benefit. This was supported by a later double-blinded RCT that found no improvement in LBR with 0.5 mg/mL HA compared to standard transfer medium for FET [52].

Current data indicate that addition of HA as an adherence compound in ET media in IVF treatment increases LBR following fresh transfers but not after FET.

13.11 Time-Lapse Systems

A time-lapse system (TLS) offers several advantages over static, basic morphological observations. These enclosed incubation systems reduce the need to remove embryos from optimum atmospheric culture conditions by taking microscopic, multiplanar images at regular intervals. This technology facilitates continuous, noninvasive observation and analysis of embryonic morphokinetics while maintaining optimal culture conditions.

Although a 2018 Cochrane review found insufficient data to confirm an impact on live birth rates [53], more recent evidence suggests TLSs improve IVF outcomes, such as ongoing pregnancy and live birth rates [54, 55],

Furthermore, the study of these morphokinetic parameters has led to the identification of novel biomarkers that help predict key clinical outcomes. A promising area of research is the use of morphokinetic parameters to noninvasively predict embryo ploidy, as studies have shown that aneuploid embryos exhibit altered morphokinetics [56, 57]. The latest integration of artificial intelligence with morphokinetic models represents the latest advancement in this field, allowing for efficient processing of the extensive data generated by TLS [56, 57]. Although still an emerging area, this approach is anticipated to become a pivotal development in embryo assessment.

The future of TLSs in IVF is promising; as the technology continues to evolve, these systems are likely to improve embryo selection and IVF outcomes.

13.11.1 IMSI

Intracitoplasmatic morphologic sperm injection (IMSI) exploits a sperm selection method termed "motile sperm organelle morphology examination" (MSOME). This method involves the observation and selection of sperm based on the absence of vacuoles in the sperm head at high magnification (>6000x) [58].

However, current evidence including meta-analysis of randomized-control trials finds no benefit of IMSI on reproductive outcomes when compared to conventional ICSI [59].

References

1. Trounson A, Mohr L. Human pregnancy following cryopreservation, thawing and transfer of an eight-cell embryo. Nature. 1983;305(5936):707–9.
2. Dashti S, Eftekhar M. Luteal-phase support in assisted reproductive technology: an ongoing challenge. Int J Reprod Biomed IJRM. 2021;10:761–72.
3. Nosarka S, Kruger T, Siebert I, Grové D. Luteal phase support in in vitro fertilization: meta-analysis of randomized trials. Gynecol Obstet Investig. 2005;60(2):67–74.
4. van der Linden M, Buckingham K, Farquhar C, Kremer JAM, Metwally M. Luteal phase support for assisted reproduction cycles. Cochrane Database Syst Rev. 2015;2015(7):CD009154.
5. Nho EJ, Hong YH, Park JH, Kim SK, Lee JR, Jee BC, et al. Efficacy of dual progesterone administration (intramuscular and vaginal) for luteal support in fresh day 3 or day 4 embryo transfer cycles. Clin Exp Reprod Med. 2020;47(3):227–32.
6. Gari S, Al-Jaroudi D. Adding weekly intramuscular progesterone to a twice daily vaginal progesterone capsule for luteal phase support in IVF/ICSI cycles results in similar live birth rates. JBRA Assist Reprod. 2022;26(1):33–7.
7. Kol S. A rationale for timing of luteal support post gonadotropin-releasing hormone agonist trigger. Gynecol Obstet Investig. 2019;84(1):1–5.
8. Connell MT, Szatkowski JM, Terry N, DeCherney AH, Propst AM, Hill MJ. Timing luteal support in assisted reproductive technology: a systematic review. Fertil Steril. 2015;103(4):939–946.e3.
9. Schmidt KL, Ziebe S, Popovic B, Lindhard A, Loft A, Andersen AN. Progesterone supplementation during early gestation after in vitro fertilization has no effect on the delivery rate. Fertil Steril. 2001;75(2):337–41.
10. Aboulghar MA, Amin YM, Al-Inany HG, Aboulghar MM, Mourad LM, Serour GI, et al. Prospective randomized study comparing luteal phase support for ICSI patients up to the first ultrasound compared with an additional three weeks. Hum Reprod Oxf Engl. 2008;23(4):857–62.
11. Van Steirteghem AC, Smitz J, Camus M, Van Waesberghe L, Deschacht J, Khan I, et al. The luteal phase after in-vitro fertilization and related procedures. Hum Reprod Oxf Engl. 1988;3(2):161–4.

12. Ludwig M, Diedrich K. Evaluation of an optimal luteal phase support protocol in IVF. Acta Obstet Gynecol Scand. 2001;80(5):452–66.
13. Liu XR, Mu HQ, Shi Q, Xiao XQ, Qi HB. The optimal duration of progesterone supplementation in pregnant women after IVF/ICSI: a meta-analysis. Reprod Biol Endocrinol RBE. 2012;10:107.
14. European IVF Monitoring Consortium (EIM) for the European Society of Human Reproduction and Embryology (ESHRE), Smeenk J, Wyns C, De Geyter C, Kupka M, Bergh C, et al. ART in Europe, 2019: results generated from European registries by ESHRE†. Hum Reprod Oxf Engl. 2023;38(12):2321–2338.
15. Zaat T, Zagers M, Mol F, Goddijn M, van Wely M, Mastenbroek S. Fresh versus frozen embryo transfers in assisted reproduction. Cochrane Database Syst Rev. 2021;2(2):CD011184.
16. Ghobara T, Gelbaya TA, Ayeleke RO. Cycle regimens for frozen-thawed embryo transfer. Cochrane Gynaecology and Fertility Group, editor. Cochrane Database Syst Rev [Internet]. 2017 Jul 5 [cited 2022 Sep 18];2017(7). Available from: http://doi.wiley.com/10.1002/14651858.CD003414.pub3
17. Direito A, Bailly S, Mariani A, Ecochard R. Relationships between the luteinizing hormone surge and other characteristics of the menstrual cycle in normally ovulating women. Fertil Steril. 2013;99(1):279–285.e3.
18. Alonso-Mayo C, Kohls G, Santos-Ribeiro S, Soares SR, Garcia-Velasco JA. Modified natural cycle allows a window of 7 days for frozen embryo transfer planning. Reprod Biomed Online. 2024;49(1):103774.
19. Practice Committees of the American Society for Reproductive Medicine and the Society for Reproductive Endocrinology and Infertility. Diagnosis and treatment of luteal phase deficiency: a committee opinion. Fertil Steril. 2021;115(6):1416–23.
20. Olive DL. The prevalence and epidemiology of luteal-phase deficiency in normal and infertile women. Clin Obstet Gynecol. 1991;34(1):157–66.
21. Balasch J, Vanrell JA. Luteal phase deficiency: an inadequate endometrial response to normal hormone stimulation. Int J Fertil. 1986;31(5):368–71.
22. Rosenberg SM, Luciano AA, Riddick DH. The luteal phase defect: the relative frequency of, and encouraging response to, treatment with vaginal progesterone. Fertil Steril. 1980;34(1):17–20.
23. Shapiro DB, Pappadakis JA, Ellsworth NM, Hait HI, Nagy ZP. Progesterone replacement with vaginal gel versus i.m. injection: cycle and pregnancy outcomes in IVF patients receiving vitrified blastocysts. Hum Reprod Oxf Engl. 2014;29(8):1706–11.
24. Alsbjerg B, Labarta E, Humaidan P. Serum progesterone levels on day of embryo transfer in frozen embryo transfer cycles-the truth lies in the detail. J Assist Reprod Genet. 2020;37(8):2045–6.
25. Cédrin-Durnerin I, Isnard T, Mahdjoub S, Sonigo C, Seroka A, Comtet M, et al. Serum progesterone concentration and live birth rate in frozen-thawed embryo transfers with hormonally prepared endometrium. Reprod Biomed Online. 2019;38(3):472–80.
26. Labarta E, Sebastian-Leon P, Devesa-Peiro A, Celada P, Vidal C, Giles J, et al. Analysis of serum and endometrial progesterone in determining endometrial receptivity. Hum Reprod Oxf Engl. 2021;36(11):2861–70.
27. Roelens C, Santos-Ribeiro S, Becu L, Mackens S, Van Landuyt L, Racca A, et al. Frozen-warmed blastocyst transfer after 6 or 7 days of progesterone administration: impact on live birth rate in hormone replacement therapy cycles. Fertil Steril. 2020;114(1):125–32.
28. Xu M, Yan Y, Shen X, Sun H, Yan G, Kong N, et al. Prolonging the time of progesterone supplementation to improve the pregnancy outcomes of single day 6 blastocyst transfer in frozen-thawed cycles: study protocol for a randomized controlled trial. Trials. 2022;23(1):1024.
29. Zaat TR, Kostova EB, Korsen P, Showell MG, Mol F, Van Wely M. Obstetric and neonatal outcomes after natural versus artificial cycle frozen embryo transfer and the role of luteal phase support: a systematic review and meta-analysis. Hum Reprod Update. 2023;29(5):634–54.
30. Wilcox AJ, Baird DD, Weinberg CR. Time of implantation of the conceptus and loss of pregnancy. N Engl J Med. 1999;340(23):1796–9.

31. Garrido-Gómez T, Ruiz-Alonso M, Blesa D, Diaz-Gimeno P, Vilella F, Simón C. Profiling the gene signature of endometrial receptivity: clinical results. Fertil Steril. 2013;99(4):1078–85.
32. Díaz-Gimeno P, Ruiz-Alonso M, Blesa D, Bosch N, Martínez-Conejero JA, Alamá P, et al. The accuracy and reproducibility of the endometrial receptivity array is superior to histology as a diagnostic method for endometrial receptivity. Fertil Steril. 2013;99(2):508–17.
33. Ruiz-Alonso M, Blesa D, Díaz-Gimeno P, Gómez E, Fernández-Sánchez M, Carranza F, et al. The endometrial receptivity array for diagnosis and personalized embryo transfer as a treatment for patients with repeated implantation failure. Fertil Steril. 2013;100(3):818–24.
34. Tan J, Kan A, Hitkari J, Taylor B, Tallon N, Warraich G, et al. The role of the endometrial receptivity array (ERA) in patients who have failed euploid embryo transfers. J Assist Reprod Genet. 2018;35(4):683–92.
35. Amin J, Patel R, JayeshAmin G, Gomedhikam J, Surakala S, Kota M. Personalized embryo transfer outcomes in recurrent implantation failure patients following endometrial receptivity Array with pre-implantation genetic testing. Cureus. 2022;14(6):e26248.
36. Eisman LE, Pisarska MD, Wertheimer S, Chan JL, Akopians AL, Surrey MW, et al. Clinical utility of the endometrial receptivity analysis in women with prior failed transfers. J Assist Reprod Genet. 2021;38(3):645–50.
37. Cozzolino M, Diaz-Gimeno P, Pellicer A, Garrido N. Evaluation of the endometrial receptivity assay and the preimplantation genetic test for aneuploidy in overcoming recurrent implantation failure. J Assist Reprod Genet. 2020;37(12):2989–97.
38. Cohen AM, Ye XY, Colgan TJ, Greenblatt EM, Chan C. Comparing endometrial receptivity array to histologic dating of the endometrium in women with a history of implantation failure. Syst Biol Reprod Med. 2020;66(6):347–54.
39. Doyle N, Combs JC, Jahandideh S, Wilkinson V, Devine K, O'Brien JE. Live birth after transfer of a single euploid vitrified-warmed blastocyst according to standard timing vs. timing as recommended by endometrial receptivity analysis. Fertil Steril. 2022;118(2):314–21.
40. Cozzolino M, Diáz-Gimeno P, Pellicer A, Garrido N. Use of the endometrial receptivity array to guide personalized embryo transfer after a failed transfer attempt was associated with a lower cumulative and per transfer live birth rate during donor and autologous cycles. Fertil Steril. 2022;118(4):724–36.
41. Juárez-Barber E, Cozzolino M, Corachán A, Alecsandru D, Pellicer N, Pellicer A, et al. Adjustment of progesterone administration after endometrial transcriptomic analysis does not improve reproductive outcomes in women with adenomyosis. Reprod Biomed Online. 2023;46(1):99–106.
42. Gnainsky Y, Granot I, Aldo P, Barash A, Or Y, Mor G, et al. Biopsy-induced inflammatory conditions improve endometrial receptivity: the mechanism of action. Reprod Camb Engl. 2015;149(1):75–85.
43. Wong TY, Lensen S, Wilkinson J, Glanville EJ, Acharya S, Clarke F, et al. Effect of endometrial scratching on unassisted conception for unexplained infertility: a randomized controlled trial. Fertil Steril. 2022;117(3):612–9.
44. Bui BN, Lensen SF, Gibreel A, Martins WP, Torrance H, Broekmans FJ. Endometrial injury for pregnancy following sexual intercourse or intrauterine insemination. Cochrane Database Syst Rev. 2022;10(10):CD011424.
45. Izquierdo Rodriguez A, De La Fuente Bitaine L, Spies K, Lora D, Galindo A. Endometrial scratching effect on clinical pregnancy rates in patients undergoing egg donor in vitro fertilization cycles: the ENDOSCRATCH randomized clinical trial (NCT03108157). Reprod Sci. 2020;27(10):1863–72.
46. Lu X, Liu Y, Cao X, Liu SY, Dong X. Laser-assisted hatching and clinical outcomes in frozen-thawed cleavage-embryo transfers of patients with previous repeated failure. Lasers Med Sci. 2019;34(6):1137–45.
47. Li D, Yang DL, An J, Jiao J, Zhou YM, Wu QJ, et al. Effect of assisted hatching on pregnancy outcomes: a systematic review and meta-analysis of randomized controlled trials. Sci Rep. 2016;6:31228.

48. Busnelli A, Somigliana E, Cirillo F, Baggiani A, Levi-Setti PE. Efficacy of therapies and interventions for repeated embryo implantation failure: a systematic review and meta-analysis. Sci Rep. 2021;11(1):1747.
49. Lacey L, Hassan S, Franik S, Seif MW, Akhtar MA. Assisted hatching on assisted conception (in vitro fertilisation (IVF) and intracytoplasmic sperm injection (ICSI)). Cochrane Database Syst Rev. 2021;3(3):CD001894.
50. Salamonsen L, Shuster S, Stern R. Distribution of hyaluronan in human endometrium across the menstrual cycle. Cell Tissue Res. 2001;306(2):335–40.
51. Heymann D, Vidal L, Or Y, Shoham Z. Hyaluronic acid in embryo transfer media for assisted reproductive technologies. Cochrane Gynaecology and Fertility Group, editor Cochrane Database Syst Rev [Internet] 2020 Sep 2 [cited 2024 Aug 29];2020(9). Available from: http://doi.wiley.com/10.1002/14651858.CD007421.pub4
52. Yung SSF, Lai SF, Lam MT, Lui EMW, Ko JKY, Li HWR, et al. Hyaluronic acid–enriched transfer medium for frozen embryo transfer: a randomized, double-blind, controlled trial. Fertil Steril. 2021;116(4):1001–9.
53. Armstrong S, Bhide P, Jordan V, Pacey A, Farquhar C. Time-lapse systems for embryo incubation and assessment in assisted reproduction. Cochrane Database Syst Rev. 2018;5(5):CD011320.
54. Valera MÁ, Garg A, Bori L, Meseguer F, De Los Santos JM, Meseguer M. Undisturbed culture: a clinical examination of this culture strategy on embryo in vitro development and clinical outcomes. Fertil Steril. 2024;122(6):1037–47.
55. Jiang Y, Wang L, Wang S, Shen H, Wang B, Zheng J, et al. The effect of embryo selection using time-lapse monitoring on IVF/ICSI outcomes: a systematic review and meta-analysis. J Obstet Gynaecol Res. 2023;49(12):2792–803.
56. Giménez C, Conversa L, Murria L, Meseguer M. Time-lapse imaging: Morphokinetic analysis of in vitro fertilization outcomes. Fertil Steril. 2023;120(2):218–27.
57. Bamford T, Barrie A, Montgomery S, Dhillon-Smith R, Campbell A, Easter C, et al. Morphological and morphokinetic associations with aneuploidy: a systematic review and meta-analysis. Hum Reprod Update. 2022;28(5):656–86.
58. Bartoov B, Berkovitz A, Eltes F. Selection of spermatozoa with normal nuclei to improve the pregnancy rate with intracytoplasmic sperm injection. N Engl J Med. 2001;345(14):1067–8.
59. Teixeira DM, Hadyme Miyague A, Barbosa MA, Navarro PA, Raine-Fenning N, Nastri CO, et al. Regular (ICSI) versus ultra-high magnification (IMSI) sperm selection for assisted reproduction. Cochrane Database Syst Rev. 2020;2(2):CD010167.

14 Preimplantation Genetic Testing in IVF

Nathan R. Treff and Talia Metzgar

14.1 Introduction

As IVF (in vitro fertilization) technology continues to advance, one of the most significant innovations in recent years has been the development of preimplantation genetic testing (PGT) [20]. This testing, available in several forms, allows clinicians and patients to assess the genetic health of embryos before implantation, potentially improving outcomes by selecting embryos with the best chance of resulting in a healthy pregnancy). As IVF nurses, your role in supporting patients undergoing PGT is vital, as it involves not only specialized knowledge and expertise but also compassionate care and clear communication [23].

This chapter will provide an overview of the different types of PGT, the clinical applications of these tests, and the role of IVF nurses in the PGT process. Understanding PGT is crucial for nurses who work with IVF patients to ensure that they are informed, supported, and able to provide the highest quality care during this complex and sometimes emotional phase of treatment [11].

N. R. Treff (✉)
Nucleus Genomics Inc, New York, NY, USA

Department of Obstetrics, Gynecology, and Reproductive Sciences, Rutgers University, New Brunswick, NJ, USA
e-mail: nathan@mynucleus.com

T. Metzgar
Institute for Reproductive Medicine and Science, Livingston, NJ, USA
e-mail: talia.metzgar@yahoo.com

M. Das, M. H. Dahan (eds.), *A Comprehensive Guide to Reproductive Health and Infertility Medicine for Nurses*, https://doi.org/10.1007/978-3-032-24372-0_14

14.2 What Is Preimplantation Genetic Testing (PGT)?

PGT is a process used to examine embryos created through IVF for genetic abnormalities. By testing embryos before they are implanted into the uterus, PGT aims to reduce the risk of miscarriage, increase the chances of a successful pregnancy, and decrease the likelihood of passing on inherited genetic disorders [17].

PGT can help identify:

- Chromosomal abnormalities such as those associated with Down syndrome, Turner syndrome, or other aneuploidies (monosomy and trisomy).
- Single-gene disorders or monogenic diseases such as cystic fibrosis, sickle cell anemia, or Huntington's disease.
- Structural chromosome rearrangements that may affect fertility or lead to pregnancy loss.
- Polygenic disease risk, such as diabetes, cancer, and heart disease.

14.3 Types of Preimplantation Genetic Testing

There are four primary types of PGT, each serving a different purpose depending on the patient's needs [22]. They are as follows.

14.4 PGT-A (Preimplantation Genetic Testing for Aneuploidy)

PGT-A screens embryos for chromosomal abnormalities, specifically looking for aneuploidy, where there are extra or missing chromosomes, both whole chromosomes and partial or segmental chromosomes. This type of testing is often used by patients of advanced maternal age, those who have had multiple pregnancy losses, or individuals with known genetic conditions that predispose to aneuploidy.

Several methods of PGT-A are available for utilization including SNP array–based testing and next-generation sequencing (NGS)-based testing.

NGS-based PGT is the most commonly used laboratory method because of the ease of obtaining supplies for testing and its low cost of utilization [31]. As with most PGT methods, it involves whole genome amplification (WGA) in order to obtain enough DNA from a trophectoderm biopsy to perform analysis [10]. Common methods of WGA for NGS use random fragmentation of the genome and ligation of an adapter sequence that can then serve as a primer site for polymerase chain reaction (PCR). After amplification, ligation of additional adapters and DNA barcodes allow for multiple biopsies to be processed on the same sequencing run to reduce costs and increase throughput. Because each embryo biopsy will have added a unique sequence to its DNA, after sequencing is complete, the sequence derived from individual embryos can be separated computationally. Sequencing data is then analyzed to evaluate the number of reads per chromosome and compared to known normal samples in order to count each chromosome from each embryo biopsy [20].

Chromosomally normal embryos possess two of each autosome (chromosomes 1–22), and either one of each sex chromosome (XY), or two X chromosomes (XX) indicating a normal male or normal female embryo, respectively.

One controversial method of data analysis involves predicting mosaicism from intermediate copy numbers [28]. This is based on the concept that a trophectoderm biopsy typically contains multiple cells, and if some cells are euploid and some are aneuploid, the net result is an intermediate copy number. That is, when the result of counting a chromosome indicates a value in-between a whole number like 1, 2, or 3, then some labs have elected to interpret the results as evidence of mosaicism. Some labs use different thresholds, such as 20%, 30%, or 50%. For example, if an individual chromosome count results in observing a copy number of 2.3 instead of 2, some labs may interpret the results as being consistent with low-level mosaic trisomy since the result is 30% of a full trisomy. 100% trisomy would have given a copy number result of 3, and 70% would have resulted in a copy number of 2.7. Unfortunately, this method can potentially lead to a significant level of false positive abnormal diagnoses leading to embryo wastage [17]. Most of the embryos with intermediate copy number chromosomes are actually euploid due to the impact of technical artifact and noise from the method of testing (NGS).

Another method of PGT-A involves the use of SNP array technology [29, 30]. One advantage of SNP array-based testing is the availability of genotyping information that can be useful to avoid false positives from using copy number data alone. SNP arrays also require WGA to obtain enough DNA from the biopsy to perform testing. SNPs are positions in the genome in which individuals (or embryos) may possess different genotypes or alleles. For example, at a particular SNP position, some people may be homozygous for a T nucleotide (T:T), others maybe heterozygous for a T and a C (T:C), and some may be homozygous for the C nucleotide (C:C). This provides an opportunity to use allele ratios to better interpret results from embryo biopsies. For example, if a chromosome has the normal number of copies, 2, then the ratio of a heterozygous SNP's alleles would be 1:1 or 50:50—one T allele and one C allele. In contrast, a trisomy chromosome would possess two of one allele and one of the other, resulting in a 2:1 ratio (i.e., T:T:C). A monosomy chromosome only has one allele and would therefore have a 1:0 ratio (i.e., T only). Each of these situations can be distinguished by evaluating several thousand SNPs across each chromosome. It also allows for distinguishing between haploidy and triploidy where the entire genome has complete loss of heterozygosity (haploid) or a 2:1 ratio (triploidy) [14].

SNP arrays also provide an opportunity to determine whether aneuploidy originated from a meiotic error or a mitotic error [24]. Meiotic errors originate from the sperm or the oocyte and lead to uniform aneuploidy, while mitotic errors occur after fertilization leading to non-uniform aneuploidy in the embryo (mosaicism). This works by being able to determine, for example, whether the extra trisomy chromosome is a different homolog from one parent (meiotic origin) or an exact copy of the same homolog (mitotic error). This distinction is significantly more accurate at predicting true mosaicism than the use of intermediate copy number analysis because it is less prone to error from methodological noise, where the data is difficult to accurately interpret.

Key Benefits:

- Improves implantation rates by selecting euploid embryos (those with the correct number of chromosomes).
- Reduces the risk of miscarriage caused by chromosomal abnormalities.
- Can be particularly beneficial in women 35+ years of age, who are at a higher risk for aneuploidy.

14.5 PGT-M (Preimplantation Genetic Testing for Monogenic/Single Gene Disorders)

PGT-M is used to test for specific single-gene disorders, like cystic fibrosis, Tay-Sachs disease, or muscular dystrophy. This type of testing is typically recommended for couples who are carriers of a known genetic condition. Patients often determine their risk through expanded carrier screening, where a couple is found to be carriers of a disease-causing mutation in the same gene [15]. In a recessive disease, heterozygous carriers are unaffected by the disease. However, if both parents are carriers, then there is a 25% risk of having a child affected with the disease (homozygous for the mutation) [16]. In an autosomal dominant disease, one parent may already be affected by the disease and there is a 50% chance of having an affected child with the same mutation [11].

Several advances have been made to improve the accuracy of PGT-M. Because there are very few cells tested from the embryo, there is a risk of allele dropout of the mutation leading to misdiagnosis [10]. That is, if the embryo is heterozygous for an autosomal dominant disease (affected), on occasion the actual genotyping of the mutation may lead to failure to detect both the normal and mutant allele [5]. In this case, the embryo may be diagnosed as normal because the mutation was undetected. To avoid this, most laboratories incorporate testing the DNA sequence surrounding the mutation and can use Mendelian inheritance rules to indirectly determine what the embryo inherited. For example, if the carrier parent is heterozygous for an SNP near the mutation and the non-carrier parent is homozygous, genotyping that SNP in the embryo can be done to determine whether the embryo has the mutation or not [29]. This is done by using a trio. For example, an existing affected child can be genotyped at the nearby SNP to determine which of the two alleles it inherited from the carrier parent [18]. Then that allele can be used as a marker to determine whether sibling embryos also have the mutation or not. This method helps prevent misdiagnosis from direct mutation testing allele dropout.

Key Benefits:

- Enables the selection of embryos for transfer that do not carry the genetic mutations of concern.
- Reduces the risk of transmission of inherited diseases to offspring.

14.6 PGT-SR (Preimplantation Genetic Testing for Structural Rearrangements)

PGT-SR is utilized when one or both parents carry a structural chromosomal rearrangement, such as a translocation or inversion, that might not affect the individual but could impact the embryos [20]. This testing helps to identify embryos that may be balanced or normal and viable, thus improving the chances of a successful pregnancy [26].

Patients undergoing IVF for infertility are more likely to be carriers of a balanced translocation compared to the general population. This increased prevalence is due to the fact that carriers are more likely to experience miscarriage due to inheritance of unbalanced chromosomes. Although they possess the correct amount of DNA (2 copies), a portion of one chromosome maybe swapped with and connected to another chromosome (a reciprocal translocation) [9]. In this case, there is a risk that offspring may inherit an unbalanced karyotype, with extra material from one chromosome and missing material from the other. These abnormalities increase the risk of miscarriage and of having a child with significant abnormalities [19]. Often patients learn they are carriers only after experiencing a miscarriage and evaluating the karyotype of the loss.

Most methods of PGT-SR are unable to distinguish between an embryo that is normal from one that carries the same balanced translocation as their carrier parent. However, SNP array methods can tell the difference by evaluating genotypes near the breakpoints of the translocation and referencing either an unbalanced embryo or an existing child or parent of the carrier who has a known karyotype [29]. For example, if an embryo that appears to have normal copy number (balanced or normal) has similar genotypes to an embryo that is known to be unbalanced (carries one of the two abnormal derivative chromosomes), then that embryo can be determined to be a carrier of the balanced translocation (carries both derivative chromosomes). This method provides PGT-SR patients with the option to prevent transmitting the translocation to their children so they may avoid the same increased risk of miscarriage and infertility in their own future.

Key Benefits:

- Increases the chances of a successful pregnancy by selecting embryos with normal chromosomes (SNP array) or balanced carrier/normal chromosomes (other methods of PGT-SR).
- Helps reduce the risk of miscarriage due to unbalanced chromosomal arrangements.

14.7 PGT-P (Preimplantation Genetic Testing for Polygenic Disease Risk)

PGT-P can be used when parents have a family history of polygenic disease such as diabetes, cancer, or heart disease. A polygenic risk score (PRS) is a quantitative measure that reflects an individual's genetic predisposition to a particular disease based on multiple genetic variants across the genome. These variants are typically single-nucleotide polymorphisms (SNPs), each contributing a small effect to the overall risk. Advances in genome-wide association studies (GWAS) have allowed researchers to identify thousands of SNPs associated with a wide range of conditions (Fig. 14.1). By aggregating these small genetic effects, researchers can predict the likelihood that a person will develop certain diseases or susceptibility to conditions like schizophrenia, cancer, or Alzheimer's disease [3].

For an embryo, PRS can be calculated based on the inherited genetic material from both parents. The predictive accuracy of PRS in embryos depends on the availability of large datasets (such as the UK Biobank, All of Us, or the Thousand Genomes Project), refined algorithms, and comprehensive understanding of genetic-environmental interactions. While still a developing field, PRS has already shown promise in predicting risks for common diseases in adults [8].

One key application involves patients already affected with diabetes. It is estimated that over 3% of IVF patients have diabetes, twice as many patients as all PGT-M indications combined. Instead of selecting embryos based on morphology, these patients may benefit from choosing an embryo with the lowest risk of diabetes. Several studies have demonstrated 30–70% reduction in the risk of type 1 diabetes with the use of PGT-P-based selection compared to random selection [27]. These studies were done in existing cohorts of adult human siblings. Given that over 50% of IVF already involves PGT, there is little to no risk to adding information on polygenic risk prior to embryo selection and significant potential to help reduce risk of disease in future generations [6].

Key Benefits:

- Prioritizes embryos for transfer which have the lowest risk of developing a polygenic condition.
- Helps reduce the risk of polygenic disease in future generations.

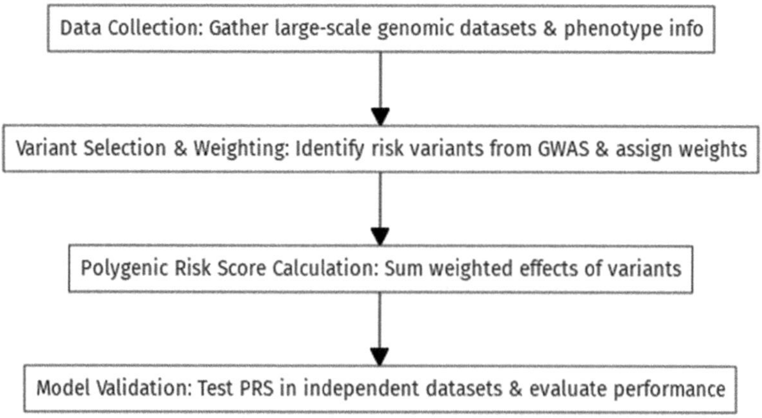

Fig. 14.1 Developing and validating polygenic risk scores (PRS) involves several key steps, from selecting genetic variants to evaluating the predictive power of the score. The process generally follows these stages

14.8 The PGT Process: Step by Step

The PGT process involves several key phases, from IVF embryo creation to testing and embryo transfer. Nurses play a critical role in supporting patients through each of these steps.

14.9 IVF and Embryo Culture

PGT begins with IVF (Fig. 14.2), where oocytes are retrieved from the ovaries, fertilized in the IVF laboratory, and cultured for several days. Typically, embryos are cultured to the blastocyst stage (day 5, 6, or 7) before biopsy. It is important to remember that not all embryos will survive the biopsy process, so careful embryo selection and culture are essential. It is also difficult to estimate the number of

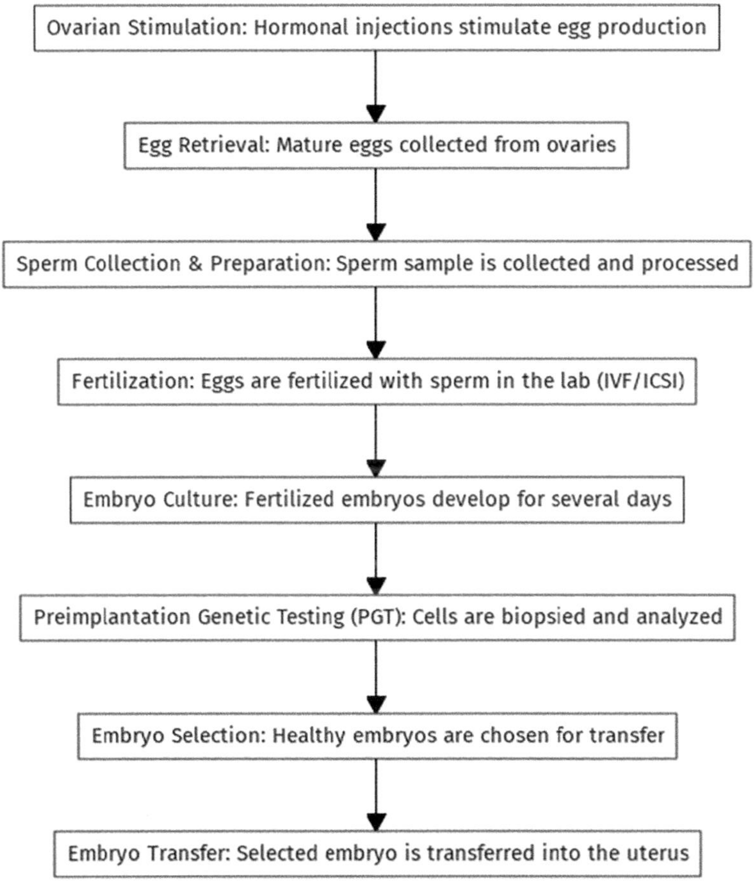

Fig. 14.2 Flowchart for the IVF and preimplantation genetic testing (PGT) process

usable blastocysts that will be available when counseling patients. The blastocyst rate is highly impacted by stimulation protocols, the quality of the embryology laboratory, and individual patient characteristics (i.e., maternal age and ovarian reserve). The Society for Assisted Reproduction and Technology (SART) does not currently track blastocyst formation rates by clinic, making it difficult to develop reasonable estimates for patients. Therefore, this data should be developed at each individual clinic in order to provide a resource for nurses to counsel patients on expectations [12].

Nurses' Role:

- Educate patients about the IVF process, including the stimulation, egg retrieval, and IVF laboratory procedures.
- Provide emotional support, as the IVF journey can be stressful and uncertain.

14.10 Embryo Biopsy for Genetic Testing

Once the embryos reach the blastocyst stage, a biopsy is performed (Fig. 14.3). This involves removing a small number of cells (usually from the trophectoderm, the outer layer of cells that will become the placenta). This process is typically done under the guidance of a skilled embryologist and requires precision to minimize any potential damage to the embryo [1].

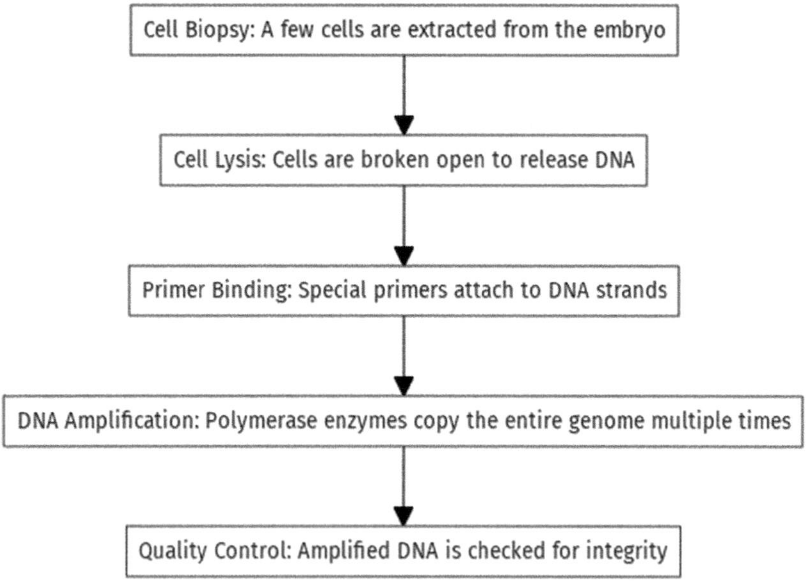

Fig. 14.3 Whole genome amplification (WGA) is a critical step in preimplantation genetic testing (PGT), allowing the analysis of a small number of embryonic cells by amplifying their DNA. The process generally follows these steps

There are several iterations of the blastocyst biopsy in use today. Some embryology labs perform laser-assisted hatching to aid in the release of trophectoderm cells from the zona pellucida. Some perform biopsy using several laser pulses to separate cells from the trophectoderm tissue layer followed by pipette suctioning to obtain cells for testing. Others may use a flicking method to avoid the use of a laser. In all cases, the biopsy is moved through loading buffer to wash excess material and obtain only intact cells for PGT.

The number of intact cells obtained from biopsy can be critical to optimal performance of PGT. Most PGT laboratories recommend 4–7 cells to obtain accurate results. It can be difficult to accurately determine the number of cells obtained as the trophectoderm is often compacted and difficult to visualize.

Finally, it is important for each embryology laboratory to perform test runs on biopsies of discarded embryos prior to clinical use of specific PGT laboratory providers. This test can help address any limitations that may exist with PGT laboratory specific biopsy loading procedures and downstream analysis methods. For example, mosaicism rates have been shown to be highly dependent on the clinic of origin, indicating the technical artifacts may result from methodological variations in embryo biopsy procedures [25, 32].

Nurses' Role:

- Ensure that patients are fully informed about the biopsy process, potential risks, and benefits.
- Help manage patient anxiety about the procedure and explain the importance of the biopsy in the broader context of genetic testing and embryo selection.

14.11 Genetic Testing

The biopsied cells are sent to a genetic testing laboratory, where DNA analysis is performed. This may involve techniques like whole genome amplification, next-generation sequencing, or SNP array–based analysis [31]. Procedures for handling biopsy specimens require care and PGT laboratories should have obtained CLIA and CAP accreditation in order to establish high-quality services [25]. Typically, each case includes a negative control to evaluate whether there is contamination in the biopsy or loading media. Contamination from sources including sperm, cumulus cells, or the laboratory technician can result in misdiagnosis. PGT laboratories operate under strict conditions and involve the use of DNA-free filtered pipette tips, personal protective equipment, and a laboratory space free from amplified DNA [7]. Reagents used to initiate whole genome amplification are also added in a manner to prevent loss of DNA from the biopsy, such as pipetting reagents onto the side of the PCR tube, instead of directly in the fluid containing the biopsy.

There are several quality control steps typically used by PGT labs to avoid sample mix-ups. These include the use of genotyping data on cohorts of biopsies to demonstrate sibling relationships within one case and unrelated status across different cases. In situations where discordance is observed, the PGT lab can investigate the root cause prior to issuing a report to avoid misdiagnosis and the use of embryos that may have been inaccurately prepared within the embryology lab.

Another set of quality control parameters involve the use of positive controls within each batch of testing. This allows the PGT laboratory to demonstrate obtaining the expected result from samples with previously known karyotypes or genotypes. Examples include the use of aneuploid cell lines previously testing with conventional karyotyping or rebiopsies of embryos previously found to possess a meiotic origin aneuploidy.

Additional quality control involves the ability to distinguish between true signal and artifactual noise. Sometimes biopsy samples do not perform as well as others. This can originate from issues related to the embryo quality, the number of cells obtained from the biopsy, the biopsy and loading procedures, sample shipping, and variation in the PGT laboratory sample processing. Some labs may inappropriately interpret unclear data as evidence of mosaicism or chaotic aneuploidy, while others may use metrics such as genotyping call rates, or median absolute pairwise difference (MAPD) to distinguish signal from unclear data. MAPD evaluates the concordance of copy number assignments at nearby positions in the genome. For example, if a chromosome is truly a trisomy, then all regions of analysis within that chromosome should indicate there are three copies. However, when sample data quality results are poor, these values may be found to have an unusually high level of discordance in assigned copy number values.

Nurses' Role:

- Explain the timeline of testing results (usually 5–10 days).
- Provide reassurance while waiting for the results and offer counseling support in case of any anxiety or difficult emotions related to genetic testing.

14.12 Embryo Selection and Transfer

Once the genetic testing results are available, the embryo(s) identified as chromosomally normal or free of specific genetic mutations are selected for transfer. Depending on the patient's history or underlying health concerns and IVF protocol, a single embryo or multiple embryos may be transferred. The frozen embryo transfer is the thawing and transfer of the embryo(s) that requires preparation of the endometrium (uterine lining) by using a patient's natural menstrual cycle versus synthetic preparation using synthetic hormones. The process can take several weeks.

It is important to set realistic expectations for patients utilizing PGT. There is no PGT method that results in 100% accuracy. The technical challenges of working with very few cells inevitably result in some errors in predicting the embryos genetic status. Embryo mosaicism, while not truly frequent, can result in sampling error that can led to misdiagnosis. Embryos can acquire chromosomal abnormalities after the blastocyst stage of development. While steps necessary to avoid error involving witnessing, duplicate review of results, quality controls, competency assessments, and proficiency testing are critical, errors still occur, and patients should be counseled on the potential for error as defined by each individual PGT laboratory [4, 21].

When specifically discussing the predictive value of PGT-A, several considerations are critical. Several randomized clinical trials have demonstrated that PGT-A improves outcomes for IVF patients. However, success rates vary by clinic and by the PGT laboratory used. Each individual clinic should routinely evaluate success rates by PGT provider in order to have accurate estimates for individual patients. Of course, success rates are highly dependent on maternal age and ovarian reserve. However, aneuploidy rates are highly dependent on the PGT methods used and can significantly impact patient success rates. For example, NGS-based testing typically results in 10% more aneuploidy than SNP array technology. This results in fewer embryos available for transfer and lower success rates when evaluated by cycle start (as opposed to success rates per transfer) [31].

Not all euploid embryos implant and result in a healthy pregnancy. Several factors beyond aneuploidy may impact success, including the embryo transfer procedure, health of the endometrium, unknown genetic factors, and individual patient characteristics [2].

Nurses' Role:

- Support patients in understanding their options based on the genetic testing results.
- Prepare patients for the embryo transfer procedure, providing them with information about the process and what to expect.
- Set realistic expectations for patients regarding accuracy and predictive value of PGT.

14.13 Pregnancy Test and Follow-Up

After the embryo transfer, patients will typically undergo a blood test (beta-hCG) about 10–14 days later to confirm pregnancy. If pregnancy is achieved, further monitoring is essential to assess the progression of the pregnancy.

Nurses' Role:

- Provide ongoing support during the two-week wait, which can be a stressful time for patients.
- Assist with follow-up appointments and monitor early pregnancy progression.

14.14 Counseling and Communication

The role of an IVF nurse is not limited to the technical aspects of the PGT process. Effective communication and counseling are critical components of patient care, especially when dealing with genetic testing results. The outcome of PGT can sometimes bring difficult news, such as the absence of viable embryos, the presence of genetic disorders, or results indicating aneuploidy in all embryos tested. Nurses must be prepared to offer empathetic support and to work closely with the fertility team to ensure that patients fully understand their options moving forward [13].

Key Points for Nurses:

- Use clear, non-judgmental language to explain genetic test results.
- Offer emotional support and direct patients to counseling services or support groups if needed.
- Encourage an open dialogue between patients and their reproductive endocrinologists to ensure informed decision-making.

14.15 Ethical Considerations

Preimplantation genetic testing raises several ethical questions, particularly when it comes to deciding which embryos should be transferred. Nurses may find themselves addressing patient concerns related to the potential for "designer babies," the moral implications of embryo selection, or the emotional impact of genetic information [17].

Considerations for Nurses:

- Be aware of personal biases and always provide care that respects patients' individual values and decisions.
- Encourage patients to ask questions and express their concerns, ensuring they feel supported regardless of the outcome of their testing.

14.16 Conclusion

Preimplantation genetic testing has revolutionized IVF by providing a means of screening embryos for genetic conditions before implantation, thus increasing the chances of a healthy pregnancy and reducing the risk of passing on inherited diseases. As IVF nurses, your role extends beyond technical assistance—you are essential to providing emotional support, clear communication, and compassionate care throughout the entire PGT process.

By understanding the different types of PGT, the procedural steps involved, and the potential emotional and ethical challenges that patients may face, you can help ensure that IVF patients are well informed and supported as they navigate the complexities of preimplantation genetic testing [4, 17].

References

1. Alikani M, Willadsen SM. Techniques in embryo micromanipulation. Semin Reprod Med. 2002;20(1):95–103. https://doi.org/10.1055/s-2002-23510.
2. Bacca D, et al. Factors influencing IVF success rates: the role of the embryo transfer procedure and endometrial receptivity. Fertil Steril. 2019;111(5):1003–12. https://doi.org/10.1016/j.fertnstert.2018.12.038.
3. Chatterjee A, et al. Polygenic risk scores: current progress and future potential in precision medicine. Genet Med. 2022;24(1):35–42. https://doi.org/10.1038/s41436-021-01151-2.
4. Chavez A, et al. Mosaicism and its implications for embryo selection: review of preimplantation genetic testing. Hum Reprod. 2021;36(2):345–52. https://doi.org/10.1093/humrep/deaa323.
5. De Rycke M, et al. Preimplantation genetic diagnosis for monogenic disorders: a systematic review on factors influencing pregnancy outcome. Hum Reprod Update. 2005;21(3):399–408.
6. Doria C, et al. Reducing polygenic disease risk in IVF embryos: opportunities and challenges. J Assist Reprod Genet. 2022;39(6):1449–57. https://doi.org/10.1007/s10815-022-02243-5.
7. Dreesen JT, et al. Quality control in preimplantation genetic testing: approaches for detecting contamination, allele dropout, and sample misidentification. Mol Hum Reprod. 2014;20(2):122–30. https://doi.org/10.1093/molehr/gat083.
8. Elliott P, et al. Challenges in implementing polygenic risk scores for disease prediction. Nat Rev Genet. 2021;22(1):27–39. https://doi.org/10.1038/s41576-020-00247-7.
9. Gardner RJM, Sutherland GR, Shaffer LG. Chromosome abnormalities and genetic counseling. 5th ed. Oxford University Press; 2018.
10. Handyside AH, et al. Avoiding misdiagnosis in preimplantation genetic diagnosis for single gene disorders: a close look at allele dropout and linked markers. Fertil Steril. 2010;94(1):41–8.
11. Harper JC, et al. The evolution of preimplantation genetic diagnosis as a reproductive technology. Reproduction. 2010;140(3):325–32.
12. Harris B, et al. Blastocyst development and viability in IVF: factors influencing success rates. Fertil Steril. 2020;113(6):1178–85. https://doi.org/10.1016/j.fertnstert.2020.02.026.
13. Harris M, et al. Counseling and communication in IVF: managing difficult genetic testing results. J Assist Reprod Genet. 2021;38(5):1091–9. https://doi.org/10.1007/s10815-021-02185-6.
14. Kratka C, Vadapalli PS, Mendola R, Garrisi J, Xu J, Treff NR, Marin D. Accurate detection and frequency of abnormal ploidy in the human blastocyst. F S Sci. 2023;4(2S):27–35. https://doi.org/10.1016/j.xfss.2023.02.003. Epub 2023 Mar 1. PMID: 36863445
15. Lazarin GA, et al. Carrier screening for severe genetic conditions in individuals of reproductive age: a clinical experience with expanded carrier screening. Genet Med. 2013;15(3):178–86.
16. Lebo RV, et al. Mendelian disorders and reproductive genetic screening. Am J Med Genet. 2019;179(2):179–91.
17. Miller E, et al. Ethical considerations in preimplantation genetic testing: a comprehensive review. Reprod Biomed Online. 2020;41(2):245–57. https://doi.org/10.1016/j.rbmo.2020.05.002.
18. Moutou C, et al. Preimplantation genetic diagnosis for single gene disorders: guidelines from the ESHRE PGD consortium. Hum Reprod. 2007;22(6):1280–6.
19. Munné S. Preimplantation genetic diagnosis for aneuploidy and translocations using array technology. Reprod Biomed Online. 2005;10(5):668–75.
20. Munné S, et al. Preimplantation genetic diagnosis significantly reduces pregnancy loss in infertile couples: a multicenter study. Fertil Steril. 2000;73(6):1184–8.
21. Munné S, Wells D. Preimplantation genetic testing: a review of clinical applications and future directions. Reprod Biomed Online. 2020;41(3):455–65. https://doi.org/10.1016/j.rbmo.2020.06.016.
22. Practice Committee of the American Society for Reproductive Medicine. Preimplantation genetic testing: a committee opinion. Fertil Steril. 2020;113(2):305–16. https://doi.org/10.1016/j.fertnstert.2019.11.025.

23. Quinn GP, et al. Knowledge and educational needs about pre-implantation genetic diagnosis (PGD) among oncology nurses. J Clin Med. 2014;3(2):632–45. https://doi.org/10.3390/jcm3020632.
24. Rana B, et al. Identifying parental and cell-division origins of aneuploidy in the human blastocyst. Am J Hum Genet. 2023;110(4):565–74. https://doi.org/10.1016/j.ajhg.2023.03.003. Epub 2023 Mar 27. PMID: 36977411; PMCID: PMC10119141
25. Scott R, et al. Quality control measures in preimplantation genetic testing: a review. Hum Reprod. 2021;36(4):877–89. https://doi.org/10.1093/humrep/deaa378.
26. Scriven PN, et al. Robertsonian translocations—reproductive risks and indications for preimplantation genetic diagnosis. Hum Reprod. 1998;13(8):2105–13.
27. Treff NR, et al. Preimplantation Genetic Testing for Polygenic Disease Relative Risk Reduction: Evaluation of Genomic Index Performance in 11,883 Adult Sibling Pairs. Genes (Basel). 2020;11(6):648. https://doi.org/10.3390/genes11060648. PMID: 32545548; PMCID: PMC7349610
28. Treff NR, Marin D. Marin D. The "mosaic" embryo: misconceptions and misinterpretations in preimplantation genetic testing for aneuploidy. Fertil Steril. 2021;116(5):1205–11. https://doi.org/10.1016/j.fertnstert.2021.06.027. Epub 2021 Jul 23. PMID: 34304887.
29. Treff NR, et al. Validation of concurrent preimplantation genetic testing for polygenic and monogenic disorders, structural rearrangements, and whole and segmental chromosome aneuploidy with a single universal platform. Eur J Med Genet. 2019;62(8):103647. https://doi.org/10.1016/j.ejmg.2019.04.004. Epub 2019 Apr 23. PMID: 31026593
30. Treff NR, et al. Accurate single cell 24 chromosome aneuploidy screening using whole genome amplification and single nucleotide polymorphism microarrays. Fertil Steril. 2010;94(6):2017–21. https://doi.org/10.1016/j.fertnstert.2010.01.052. Epub 2010 Feb 26. PMID: 20188357
31. Wells D, et al. Comparison of PGT-A methods: NGS versus SNP array for improved IVF outcomes. Fertil Steril. 2020;113(4):817–24. https://doi.org/10.1016/j.fertnstert.2019.12.020.
32. Widdows J, et al. Sample handling and contamination control in preimplantation genetic testing. J Reprod Genetic. 2020;9(4):202–14. https://doi.org/10.1016/j.jrg.2020.08.011.

15 Ovarian Hyperstimulation Syndrome, Other Complications and Their Management

Yousef Alebrahim and Raj Mathur

15.1 Ovarian Hyperstimulation Syndrome

15.1.1 Introduction

Ovarian hyperstimulation syndrome (OHSS) is the most significant short-term complication of assisted conception treatment due to ovarian stimulation with gonadotropins. This is a post-ovulatory phenomenon, strongly associated with human chorionic gonadotropin (hCG). OHSS is often associated with an 'excessive' ovarian response; however, it can also occur in cycles where the response has not been thought to be excessive. OHSS is usually self-limiting, but there is a risk of morbidity, and complications can be life-threatening if diagnosis or management is delayed. This chapter will explore the pathophysiology of OHSS, identifying patients at higher risk, evidence-based preventative strategies, a guide for assessment and principles of management.

15.1.2 Epidemiology

The true incidence of OHSS is unknown. Due to absence of mandatory reporting internationally and a lack of consensus on the use of a standardised classification system for severity, the incidence is likely to be significantly underestimated.

The risk of OHSS is modulated by patient characteristics and choice of stimulation protocol. Earlier studies reporting the incidence of OHSS using a GnRH

Y. Alebrahim (✉) · R. Mathur
Department of Reproductive Medicine, St Mary's Hospital, Manchester University NHS Foundation Trust, Manchester, UK
e-mail: Yousef.Alebrahim@mft.nhs.uk; rmathur@nhs.net

M. Das, M. H. Dahan (eds.), *A Comprehensive Guide to Reproductive Health and Infertility Medicine for Nurses*, https://doi.org/10.1007/978-3-032-24372-0_15

agonist protocol found an incidence of 20–33% for mild, 3–6% for moderate and 0.1–2% for severe OHSS [1].

The introduction of the GnRH antagonist substantially reduced the incidence of any grade of OHSS. The relative likelihood of OHSS in antagonist cycles is 50% lower compared with agonist cycles [2]. A Cochrane systematic review in 2016 reported the overall risk of OHSS following use of a GnRH agonist to be 11% (7% for moderate or severe), while the risk following GnRH antagonist would be between 6% and 9% (3% for moderate or severe) [3]. A recent 2020 UK study reported moderate and severe OHSS in 1.6% of treatment cycles receiving antagonist protocol [4]. A further study reported no cases of severe OHSS with the addition of an agonist trigger and elective embryo cryopreservation ('freeze-all') in high responders [5].

In 2023–2024, the HFEA received reports of 53 cases of severe and critical OHSS, occurring in less than 0.1% of all treatment cycles in the UK [6].

15.1.3 Pathophysiology and Clinical Features

The main feature of OHSS is enlargement of the ovaries [7]. To explain the features observed in OHSS, an understanding of the anatomy and physiology of the ovarian follicle is required. An ovarian follicle consists of a single oocyte surrounded by granulosa and theca cells. Granulosa cells express receptors for follicle-stimulating hormone (FSH) and luteinising hormone (LH). As a result of FSH stimulation, granulosa cells produce oestradiol (E2) [8, 9]. During ovarian stimulation, E2 levels elevate significantly due to increased granulosa cell activity [10]. Activation of the LH receptor transforms granulosa cells into the progesterone-producing granulosa-lutein cells within the corpus luteum [8, 9]. hCG, which has a similar molecular structure to LH, is used to stimulate LH receptors to induce oocyte maturation following ovarian stimulation. Compared to LH, hCG is more biologically active due to its longer half-life and affinity to the LH receptor [10].

hCG increases the production of vascular endothelial growth factor (VEGF). This is a potent molecule which promotes the growth of new blood vessels (angiogenesis) and increases vascular permeability [11]. The blood vessels become 'leaky', leading to movement of fluid out of the circulation. This fluid can collect in the abdominal cavity causing ascites, or in the pleural cavity (around the lungs) causing a pleural effusion [12].

An increase in immune cell populations is observed in follicular fluid. Activated immune cells produce cytokines such as interleukin-6 (IL-6), which contributes to ovarian neovascularisation and increased vascular permeability. IL-6 is also a potent inhibitor of hepatic albumin production and increases synthesis of acute phase reactants. There is a reduced level of serum albumin, which reduces oncotic pressure and further drives third-space fluid accumulation [7, 10].

The reduction in plasma volume makes the blood more concentrated ('haemoconcentration'). This is shown by a rise in haematocrit, white blood cells and platelets [7, 12].

The loss of fluid from the intravascular space also leads to hypovolaemia and hypotension. A compensatory increase in heart rate may occur [7]. These circulatory changes lead to reduced blood flow to critical organs including the kidney and liver. Reduced glomerular filtration causes oliguria (low urine output). In the liver, the production of anticoagulant factors is affected. Along with haemoconcentration, this increases the risk of thrombosis [12].

The renin-angiotensin system has also been implicated in the course of OHSS. The ovaries can synthesize pro-renin and renin. Higher concentrations of angiotensin-converting enzyme and angiotensin II have been reported in severe OHSS. Hypovolaemia can also activate the renin-angiotensin system, leading to secondary hyperaldosteronism [10].

Ovarian enlargement and rapid fluid accumulation in the peritoneal cavity lead to an increase in intra-abdominal pressure, which causes abdominal pain and distension. This can cause compression of the inferior vena cava, decreasing venous return to the heart and resulting in the aforementioned changes in circulation. Intestinal symptoms include nausea, vomiting, decreased appetite and constipation. An increase in intra-abdominal pressure can further impair hepatic and renal function. This can also cause elevation of the diaphragm, restricting lung expansion and leading to shortness of breath (dyspnoea) [12].

In summary, the exact pathophysiology of OHSS is unknown, and several mechanisms have been considered (Fig. 15.1). OHSS is characterised by cystic ovarian enlargement and the release of vasoactive substances and inflammatory mediators that lead to third-space fluid accumulation and deranged haematological, hepatic and renal parameters [12].

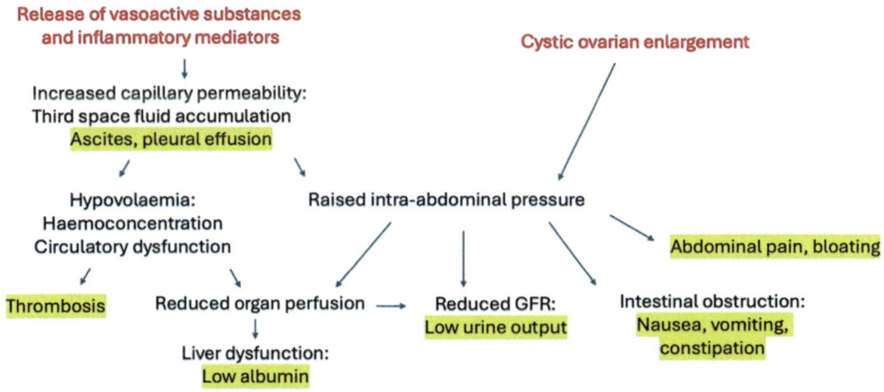

Fig. 15.1 Pathophysiology of OHSS

15.1.4 Diagnosis

15.1.4.1 Presentation

OHSS can be categorised into two distinct forms: 'early' and 'late'.

- Early OHSS is associated with the ovarian response during stimulation and is triggered by exogenous hCG (administration of hCG trigger). Symptoms of early OHSS present within 3–7 days of the ovulation trigger.
- Late OHSS exists almost exclusively in the context of pregnancy (endogenous hCG). Symptoms of late OHSS usually present 9–17 days post-trigger, after a fresh embryo transfer has taken place. Studies have shown that late OHSS is more likely to be severe. This can be explained by the increasing levels of hCG in early pregnancy causing greater and longer stimulation of the granulosa cells. Due to the higher levels of hCG, multiple pregnancy is associated with a higher risk of OHSS [13].

The earliest clinical features of OHSS are abdominal discomfort and distension (bloating). Progression of the condition causes nausea, vomiting, constipation, increasing discomfort and swelling of extremities. Patients with respiratory compromise may present with shortness of breath and chest pain or discomfort [14]. However, clinicians should be aware that these clinical features are not specific to OHSS, and alternative diagnoses should be considered such as haemorrhage, infection and ovarian torsion. These are discussed later in this chapter.

15.1.4.2 Assessment

The assessment of a patient with suspected OHSS should start with obtaining a relevant medical history. This includes confirmation of type of fertility treatment, symptom onset, type of trigger used, number of oocytes collected and whether embryo transfer has taken place and how many embryos were transferred. The number of follicles on the final ultrasound scan should be noted if this information was available. A diagnosis of polyendocrine metabolic ovarian syndrome (PMOS) identifies patients at risk of OHSS [15].

A general clinical examination may demonstrate signs of dehydration or presence of peripheral oedema. Abdominal examination may reveal large, palpable ovaries and presence of ascites. Lung auscultation for assessment of air entry and presence of added breath sounds may raise suspicion of pleural effusion, pulmonary oedema and/or pneumonia. This should be followed by obtaining baseline observations, including the heart rate, respiratory rate, blood pressure and peripheral oxygen saturation using pulse oximetry. Measurement of weight and abdominal circumference (girth) can be used for monitoring of disease progression [15].

Blood tests are used to determine severity of OHSS. A full blood count (FBC) may demonstrate haemoconcentration with elevation of the haematocrit, haemoglobin level, white cell count and platelet count. Renal profile may identify electrolyte imbalance such as hyponatraemia (low sodium) and/or hyperkalaemia (high potassium). Liver profile could demonstrate reduced albumin level and elevated liver enzymes (ALT, AST, ALP). A coagulation profile may be deranged. Serum osmolality may be reduced. Measurement of hCG levels is useful to determine pregnancy outcome, which is helpful to determine a diagnosis of late OHSS and raises caution regarding potential severity [15].

Ultrasound examination of the pelvis and abdomen should be performed for measurement of ovarian volumes, fluid in the pelvis and ascites [15].

In the presence of tachycardia and/or chest pain, an electrocardiogram (ECG) should be arranged. An echocardiogram could be considered if a pericardial effusion is suspected. If respiratory symptoms are reported, initial imaging with chest X-ray should be considered. Additional investigations such as arterial blood gas, D-dimer, CT pulmonary angiogram or ventilation/perfusion (VQ) scan should be considered if there is a clinical suspicion of pulmonary embolism [15].

15.1.4.3 Severity

Determining the severity of OHSS is helpful to guide decisions on place of care and management. Several classification systems are used internationally. A commonly used classification is proposed by the Royal College of Obstetricians and Gynaecologists (RCOG) [15].

- *Mild OHSS:* Patients usually present with abdominal distention and mild pain; ultrasound shows enlarged ovaries measuring less than 8 cm in maximum diameter.
- *Moderate OHSS:* Typically involves moderate abdominal pain with nausea and/or vomiting; ultrasound reveals ascites, with ovarian diameters between 8 and 12 cm.
- *Severe OHSS:* Characterised by the presence of clinical ascites, pleural effusion and/or reduced urine output, alongside haemoconcentration (haematocrit >0.45), electrolyte imbalance and/or hypoalbuminaemia (<35 g/L); ultrasound demonstrates ovaries exceeding 12 cm in diameter.
- *Critical OHSS:* Marked by tense ascites, large pleural effusions, minimal or absent urine output, thromboembolism and/or acute respiratory distress syndrome; blood tests show severe haemoconcentration (haematocrit >0.55) and/or leucocytosis (white cell count >25,000/mL) [15].

15.1.5 Risk Factors

Several patient-specific factors are associated with an increased risk of developing OHSS including young age, low body mass index (BMI), Black race, PMOS, high ovarian reserve markers such as antral follicle count (AFC) and anti-Mullerian hormone (AMH), excessive ovarian response in a previous treatment cycle and FSH receptor polymorphisms [16, 17].

Age: Younger women, under the age of 35, are reportedly more likely to develop OHSS [18]. Women with 'late' OHSS have been found to be significantly younger [13]. Meanwhile, women aged 40 and older with severe OHSS are at an increased risk of life-threatening complications [19].

BMI: Lower BMI has been associated with higher risk of OHSS [20]. However, there is no significant difference between risk of OHSS in normal-weight and overweight women [21].

Ethnicity: Black or African-American women are almost twice as likely to develop OHSS compared with white women, and their risk of severe OHSS is nearly threefold higher. Meanwhile, there is no statistically significant difference in risk of OHSS between other ethnicities [17].

Ovarian reserve markers: AFC is obtained using ultrasound examination of the ovaries, counting follicles between 2 and 10 mm in size. AMH is a hormone expressed by the granulosa cells of pre-antral and small antral follicles in the ovaries. Serum AMH levels and/or AFC are used as ovarian reserve markers and to predict the ovarian response in IVF treatment. The combination of these values is used to categorise patients into groups based on their predicted response—'low', 'normal' and 'high' responders. High responders are at a significantly increased risk of OHSS, and additional preventative measures are usually considered for this group [22, 23].

PMOS: Women with anovulatory PMOS typically have higher ovarian reserve and are at an increased risk of OHSS. Lower doses of gonadotropins are usually required as polycystic ovaries exhibit extreme sensitivity to stimulation [24].

Previous excessive response: Women with history of OHSS in a previous treatment cycle are generally recognised to be at risk for recurrence in future cycles [25].

FSH receptor polymorphisms: Mutations in the FSH receptor may influence ovarian response to stimulation with certain variants associated with higher incidence of OHSS [7].

15.1.6 Prevention Strategies

All patients undergoing ovarian stimulation should be counselled thoroughly about the risk of OHSS. Strategies to prevent OHSS factor in pre-treatment patient characteristics, stimulation protocols, in-treatment monitoring and choice of ovulation trigger. Several adjuvant therapies have been studied with variable benefit reported. Recent guidelines from the British Fertility Society (BFS) and American Society for Reproductive Medicine (ASRM) summarise current evidence [26, 27].

15.1.6.1 Pre-treatment

Prevention measures should be considered for predicted high responders [26]. Several thresholds for AFC and serum AMH level have been used to identify patients at high risk of OHSS. The risk of moderate or severe OHSS is almost fourfold higher in women with an AFC > = 24 [28]. A lower cut-off of 20 is associated with a sensitivity of 54.2% and specificity of 72.2% for moderate or severe OHSS. Meanwhile, an AMH level cut-off of 22.5 pmol/L has a sensitivity of 87.5% and specificity of 60.6% in predicting moderate or severe OHSS, while using a higher concentration of 35 pmol/L has a lower sensitivity of 54.2% but higher specificity of 99.1% [4].

15.1.6.2 Ovarian Stimulation

The use of GnRH antagonist protocols is associated with a significantly lower risk of OHSS in all patients undergoing ovarian stimulation. Antagonist protocols are particularly recommended to prevent OHSS in predicted high responders [26, 27].

Progestin-primed ovarian stimulation (PPOS) involves administration of progestins during the early follicular phase to prevent premature luteinisation by suppressing the LH surge. Fresh embryo transfer is not recommended due to the progestin-induced effects on the endometrium. Evidence does not show higher benefit of PPOS in reducing OHSS risk compared with use of GnRH antagonist protocols [29]. However, PPOS can be considered if fresh embryo transfer is not anticipated, thus eliminating the risk of late OHSS [26].

The use of ovarian reserve markers and patient characteristics to determine the starting gonadotropin dose can reduce risk of OHSS. Lower gonadotropin doses are recommended for predicted high responders in GnRH agonist cycles, meanwhile a conventional dose can be used in antagonist cycles. This is shown to decrease the risk of OHSS without affecting live birth rates [26, 27].

There is no difference in risk of OHSS with use of recombinant or urinary preparations of gonadotropins. Similarly, there is no difference in risk of OHSS with use of daily or long-acting recombinant gonadotropins for predicted normal responders [26].

Follitropin delta is a newer recombinant preparation of FSH. Dosing according to an algorithm using patient weight and AMH level has been shown to reduce risk of OHSS while improving the live birth rate [30].

15.1.6.3 'Excessive' Ovarian Response

It is well recognised that an 'excessive' ovarian response increases the risk of OHSS. Various thresholds are used to determine whether additional preventative measures should be taken. The perceived risk of OHSS is increased significantly if more than 17–19 follicles > = 11–12 mm in diameter are present on the final ultrasound scan prior to trigger. Clinicians should review choice of trigger in the event of 'excessive' response to reduce OHSS risk. Cycle cancellation reduces OHSS risk; however, this has significant psychological and financial implications and should only be considered in exceptional cases [26].

The incidence of OHSS is also proportional to the number of oocytes retrieved. The retrieval of 20 or more oocytes is associated with a sensitivity of 25% and specificity of 93% for moderate or severe OHSS in GnRH antagonist cycles. Embryo cryopreservation ('freeze-all') should be considered in this group of patients as this eliminates the risk of late OHSS [26].

Measurement of serum oestrogen (E2), progesterone or LH levels has not shown to reduce the risk of OHSS and should not be used for this purpose [26].

Coasting involves the discontinuation of gonadotropins in women who exhibit an 'excessive' response during ovarian stimulation. Coasting is effective in reducing risk of OHSS in GnRH agonist cycles, but this is not recommended as a primary prevention strategy in GnRH antagonist cycles due to lacking evidence and availability of alternate, more effective interventions such as use of an agonist trigger and embryo cryopreservation [26, 27].

15.1.6.4 Trigger

Final oocyte maturation in IVF cycles is achieved with administration of hCG, GnRH agonist or recombinant LH. The use of a hCG trigger plays a key role in the development of OHSS. Studies have shown that the use of a lower dose of hCG (below 5000 units) does not alter the incidence of OHSS. The use of a GnRH agonist trigger significantly reduces the risk of OHSS and is recommended for high responders and in women with an 'excessive' response and when fresh embryo transfer is not anticipated. Dual trigger, comprising of both hCG and GnRH agonist, does not increase the incidence of OHSS compared with use of hCG alone [26, 27, 31, 32].

15.1.6.5 Luteal Phase

Luteal phase support with progesterone is used to prepare the endometrium for pregnancy. The additional use of hCG for luteal phase support may increase pregnancy and live birth rates; however, this significantly increases the risk of OHSS and is not recommended for high responders. The addition of oestrogen or GnRH agonist for luteal phase support has not shown to affect the risk of OHSS [26, 33].

15.1.6.6 Adjuvant or Alternative Therapies

The use of a GnRH antagonist for a few days post-oocyte retrieval may reduce the incidence of OHSS by suppressing endogenous LH and inducing early luteolysis. This could be considered for prevention of moderate or severe OHSS if a fresh embryo transfer is not planned [26].

Metformin has been used during ovarian stimulation to reduce risk of OHSS in women with PMOS. Current evidence demonstrates benefit in GnRH agonist cycles only [34].

Dopamine agonists such as cabergoline, quinagolide and bromocriptine may selectively inhibit VEGF-induced vascular permeability, lowering risk of severe forms of OHSS. The evidence suggests benefit in both agonist and antagonist cycles. Dopamine agonists can be started following trigger or on the day of oocyte retrieval and continued for several days in patients who exhibit 'excessive' response [26, 27, 35, 36].

There is insufficient evidence for the use of other adjuvants such as aspirin, melatonin, inositol, albumin and/or calcium infusion during ovarian stimulation to reduce risk of OHSS. Current guidance recommends against their use for OHSS prevention [26].

In vitro maturation (IVM) treatment involves the retrieval of immature oocytes without supraphysiological ovarian stimulation. No cases of OHSS with IVM treatment have been reported in the literature. Where available, this could be considered to prevent OHSS in high responders [37].

15.1.7 Management

Place of Care: Mild and moderate OHSS can be managed conservatively with outpatient monitoring every 2–3 days. Monitoring may include repeat laboratory investigations or imaging; however, this should be individualised and guided by severity of OHSS. Women receiving outpatient management should be advised to seek urgent medical attention if they develop clinical features of worsening OHSS. Hospital admission with daily review is recommended for severe and critical OHSS. In some cases, outpatient management may also be appropriate for severe OHSS if patients are clinically stable and able to attend hospital appointments regularly for monitoring. Hospital admission can also be considered if patients are unable to control pain with over-the-counter analgesia or experience significant dehydration due to inability to maintain fluid intake. A diagnosis of critical OHSS should prompt urgent review for possible admission to critical care [15].

Analgesia: Simple analgesia is usually adequate for patients with mild or moderate OHSS. Opioids can be offered for management of severe pain, and this may require hospital admission for closer monitoring. Non-steroidal anti-inflammatory drugs (NSAIDs) should be avoided as they can be nephrotoxic, further decreasing urine output [15].

Fluid Replacement: Due to fluid shifts and resulting hypovolaemia, patients with OHSS are at risk of significant dehydration. Patients are encouraged to drink to thirst, which is usually adequate to correct intravascular dehydration. However, intravenous fluid therapy should be considered for patients with nausea and vomiting who are unable to maintain fluid intake. Anti-emetics should also be offered. Correction of electrolyte imbalances may be required. Strict fluid balance monitoring should be in place for all hospitalised patients with OHSS [15].

Albumin: Intravenous colloid therapy, such as human albumin infusion, can be used as a plasma volume expander. Albumin therapy increases oncotic pressure, shifting fluid back into the intravascular space. This can be administered in doses of 50–100 g over 4 hours and repeated 4–12-hourly [15].

Fluid Drainage: Ultrasound-guided drainage of ascites (therapeutic paracentesis) should be considered for patients with severe pain or abdominal distension, respiratory compromise or persistent oliguria despite fluid replacement. Drainage of pleural effusions (thoracocentesis) is less commonly indicated. Albumin infusion should be considered in patients undergoing paracentesis or thoracocentesis to prevent circulatory dysfunction. Diuretics should be avoided as they can worsen intravascular dehydration [15].

Venous Thromboembolism (VTE) Prophylaxis: All patients should be advised adequate hydration and mobilisation to reduce risk of VTE. Mechanical prophylaxis (stockings) can be offered. All women hospitalised with OHSS should receive low molecular weight heparin (LMWH) due to their increased risk of VTE. LMWH can be offered for women with moderate OHSS if other risk factors for VTE are present. In pregnant patients, local VTE prophylaxis guidelines should be followed, and LMWH may be extended until the end of the first trimester [15].

Other: The use of GnRH antagonists or dopamine agonists may reduce risk of OHSS; however, there is no evidence of benefit in established OHSS [15].

15.2 Other Complications

15.2.1 Haemorrhage

Peri-operative vaginal bleeding is often minor, occurring in up to 8.6% of cases. Haemostasis is usually achieved in under a minute spontaneously or with local compression. In severe cases, vaginal tamponade or application of a suture may be required [38].

Intra-abdominal bleeding is rare and has been reported in 0.02–0.3% of cases, and this can be life-threatening if severe [38]. This is mostly caused by trauma to the ovarian capsule, bleeding from the ruptured follicles or rarely from injury to adjacent large vessels or pelvic organs [38–40]. Stimulated ovaries are highly vascular, and operators should limit vaginal punctures with careful ultrasound visualisation of peripheral follicles to reduce risk of vascular or pelvic organ injury [39, 41]. Continuous movement of the retrieval needle should be avoided as this can cause lacerations within the ovaries [39]. The use of intra-operative colour Doppler sonography can be considered; however, this may not definitively exclude active bleeding from small vessels [40, 42].

Studies suggest that an average blood loss of 230 mL within 24 hours is expected post-oocyte retrieval [38, 42]. A decrease of up to 5% in haematocrit and/or 16 g/L in haemoglobin is considered acceptable [42].

Lean patients with PMOS are at an increased risk of bleeding, where typically higher numbers of oocytes are retrieved and ovarian tissue can be more fragile [39].

Women with known bleeding disorders are at risk of haemorrhagic complications. Severe cases of intra-abdominal haemorrhage have been reported in patients with Von Willebrand disease, essential thrombocytopaenia and factor XI deficiency. Although there are no specific guidelines for prophylaxis in this group of patients undergoing oocyte retrieval, it is good practice to consult with haematology to assess the peri-operative bleeding risk and create an individualised care plan that may involve administration of blood products [41].

Earliest signs of bleeding may present within an hour of oocyte retrieval. Most cases present in the first 24 hours post-operatively. However, approximately 7% may be asymptomatic at first and could present days later. Patients may present with severe abdominal pain, nausea, vomiting, dizziness, weakness and tachycardia [40]. Pelvic fluid and clots may be seen on ultrasound scan; however, this does not always indicate active bleeding [39].

Hospitalisation for close observation and serial measurement of haemoglobin should be considered if suspicion of significant bleeding. Fluid resuscitation and blood transfusion may be required. A conservative management approach is recommended to avoid handling fragile ovarian tissue; however, a diagnostic laparoscopy should be considered if there were signs of haemodynamic instability and/or decreasing haemoglobin levels [40]. Laparoscopy or laparotomy may be indicated for evacuation of haematoma, coagulation of bleeding sites, application of haemostatic agents and/or ovariectomy [38–40]. Embolisation of vaginal or uterine arteries can be considered for stable patients [40]. Despite the acute and life-threatening nature of this complication, recovery is often quick and unlikely to impact treatment outcome [39].

15.2.2 Infection

Symptomatic pelvic infection may occur following oocyte retrieval, although this is rare with an incidence of 0.25–0.6% [43]. Approximately half of pelvic infections post-oocyte retrieval are severe and can be life-threatening [44]. Most infections are likely caused by pelvic contamination with vaginal flora. Ovarian puncture may cause collection of blood in the aspirated follicles or accumulation of free fluid in the pelvis, both of which serve as a rich culture medium for bacterial proliferation [45–47]. Bowel injury and puncture of hydrosalpinges may also cause infection, though this is less likely [46, 47].

Risk factors for pelvic infection include endometriosis, pelvic adhesions, previous pelvic inflammatory disease, ovarian cysts, hydrosalpinges, multiple ovarian punctures and a prolonged procedure [43, 47]. Routine administration of prophylactic antibiotics pre-procedure is not proven to significantly reduce risk of infection [43]. However, the use of broad-spectrum antibiotics with anaerobic cover should be considered in patients with risk factors, especially in the presence of endometriomas or if suspected cyst puncture [46].

Patients usually present with abdominal pain and fever [44]. Symptoms may be masked by or mistaken for OHSS [43]. Leucocytosis and elevation of inflammatory markers such as ESR and CRP are common [45]. Onset of symptoms is usually within 3 days of oocyte retrieval; however, this can be as early as a few hours or up to 8 weeks later [44]. Infection may continue into pregnancy, carrying a risk of sepsis, miscarriage and preterm birth [45].

Prompt treatment of pelvic infections is necessary to prevent significant clinical deterioration and life-threatening complications of sepsis [43]. Medical treatment with antibiotic therapy is successful in 34–87.5% of cases [44]. Bacterial cultures should be considered in severe cases to confirm antibiotic choice [43]. Laparoscopy or laparotomy for drainage of abscesses and excision of infected tissue may be required if there was diagnostic uncertainty or failure of clinical improvement with antibiotics within 72 hours. Alternatively, colpotomy or ultrasound-guided drainage can be performed; however, the latter carries a 6.6% risk of recurrence due to residual infected material [44]. Infected endometriomas are associated with a high risk of oophorectomy [46].

15.2.3 Ovarian Torsion

Ovarian torsion is a rare complication of ovarian stimulation, occurring in 0.025–0.2% of treatment cycles [48]. This is a gynaecological emergency during which the ovary completely or intermittently rotates over its supporting ligaments and vascular supply. As a result, blood flow to the ovary is reduced or lost, leading to ischaemia and risk of necrosis if untreated. Significant ovarian enlargement during stimulation or after developing OHSS can predispose the ovaries to torsion [49]. This can occur at any stage during an IVF cycle, with cases reported prior to and after oocyte retrieval, after embryo transfer and during pregnancy [48–50]. Other risk factors for ovarian torsion include endometriosis, past abdominal surgery, ovarian cysts and previous ovarian torsion [48].

Diagnosis of ovarian torsion can be difficult due to the non-specific clinical features, and this can be mistaken for OHSS, appendicitis or pyelonephritis [50, 51]. Patients may present with acute onset abdominal and/or pelvic pain, nausea, vomiting and fever. Leucocytosis is often present. Pelvic examination may reveal a palpable mass. Ultrasound examination may aid diagnosis by using colour flow Doppler to evaluate ovarian blood flow, which may be absent or reduced. Torsion can also lead to oedema and increase in ovarian size with a risk of cyst rupture and intraperitoneal haemorrhage [50].

Management of ovarian torsion involves emergency surgery to detort or rotate the ovary back into its normal position. A laparoscopic approach is usually preferred for enhanced recovery and lower risk of complications if the patient is pregnant. For optimal outcomes, surgical intervention should be performed within 24 hours of symptom onset. Delays may lead to ovarian tissue necrosis, necessitating an oophorectomy, and risk of pregnancy loss [49]. Torsion occurring prior to egg collection may impact oocyte potential and IVF treatment outcome [48].

References

1. Delvigne A, Rozenberg S. Epidemiology and prevention of ovarian hyperstimulation syndrome (OHSS): a review. Hum Reprod Update. 2002;8(6):559–77.
2. Al-Inany HG, Youssef MAFM, Aboulghar M, Broekmans F, Sterrenburg M, Smit J, et al. GnRH antagonists are safer than agonists: an update of a Cochrane review. Hum Reprod Update. 2011;17(4):435.
3. Al-Inany HG, Youssef MA, Ayeleke RO, Brown J, Lam WS, Broekmans FJ. Gonadotrophin-releasing hormone antagonists for assisted reproductive technology. Cochrane Database Syst Rev. 2016;4
4. Sood A, Goel A, Boda S, Mathur R. Prediction of significant OHSS by ovarian reserve and ovarian response—implications for elective freeze-all strategy. Hum Fertil. 2022;25(2):390–6.
5. Fernández-Sánchez M, Fatemi H, García-Velasco JA, Heiser PW, Daftary GS, Mannaerts B. Incidence and severity of ovarian hyperstimulation syndrome (OHSS) in high responders after gonadotropin-releasing hormone (GnRH) agonist trigger in "freeze-all" approach. Gynecol Endocrinol. 2023;39(1):2205952.
6. Human Fertilisation and Embryology Authority. State of the fertility sector 2023/24 2024. Available from: https://www.hfea.gov.uk/about-us/publications/research-and-data/state-of-the-fertility-sector-2023-2024/.
7. Rizk B. Genetics of ovarian hyperstimulation syndrome. Reprod Biomed Online. 2009;19(1):14–27.
8. Kishi H, Kitahara Y, Imai F, Nakao K, Suwa H. Expression of the gonadotropin receptors during follicular development. Reprod Med Biol. 2018;17(1):11–9.

9. Disler ER, Ng NW, Nguyen TG, Anchan CJ, Waldman IN, Anchan RM. Chapter 6—Induced pluripotent stem cell derived from ovarian tissue. In: Birbrair A, editor. Cell sources for iPSCs, vol. 7. Academic Press; 2021. p. 107–35.
10. Nastri CO, Ferriani RA, Rocha IA, Martins WP. Ovarian hyperstimulation syndrome: pathophysiology and prevention. J Assist Reprod Genet. 2010;27(2–3):121–8.
11. Ferrara N, Gerber H-P, LeCouter J. The biology of VEGF and its receptors. Nat Med. 2003;9(6):669–76.
12. Grossman LC, Michalakis KG, Browne H, Payson MD, Segars JH. The pathophysiology of ovarian hyperstimulation syndrome: an unrecognized compartment syndrome. Fertil Steril. 2010;94(4):1392–8.
13. Mathur RS, Akande AV, Keay SD, Hunt LP, Jenkins JM. Distinction between early and late ovarian hyperstimulation syndrome. Fertil Steril. 2000;73(5):901–7.
14. Borase H, Mathur R. Ovarian hyperstimulation syndrome: clinical features, prevention and management. Obstetr Gynaecol Reprod Med. 2012;22(7):186–90.
15. Royal College of Obstetricians and Gynaecologists. The Management of Ovarian Hyperstimulation Syndrome: Green-top Guideline No. 5 2016. Available from: https://www.rcog.org.uk/guidance/browse-all-guidance/green-top-guidelines/the-management-of-ovarian-hyperstimulation-syndrome-green-top-guideline-no-5/.
16. Drakopoulos P, Khalaf Y, Esteves SC, Polyzos NP, Sunkara SK, Shapiro D, et al. Treatment algorithms for high responders: What we can learn from randomized controlled trials, real-world data and models. Best Pract Res Clin Obstet Gynaecol. 2023;86:102301.
17. Luke B, Brown MB, Morbeck DE, Hudson SB, Coddington CC 3rd, Stern JE. Factors associated with ovarian hyperstimulation syndrome (OHSS) and its effect on assisted reproductive technology (ART) treatment and outcome. Fertil Steril. 2010;94(4):1399–404.
18. Abbara A, Patel B, Parekh I, Garg A, Jayasena CN, Comninos AN, et al. Ovarian Hyperstimulation Syndrome (OHSS) requiring Intensive Care Unit (ICU) admission between 1996–2020 in England, Wales, and Northern Ireland. Front Endocrinol. 2022;13
19. Selter J, Wen T, Palmerola KL, Friedman AM, Williams Z, Forman EJ. Life-threatening complications among women with severe ovarian hyperstimulation syndrome. Am J Obstet Gynecol. 2019;220(6):575.e1–e11.
20. Schirmer DA 3rd, Kulkarni AD, Zhang Y, Kawwass JF, Boulet SL, Kissin DM. Ovarian hyperstimulation syndrome after assisted reproductive technologies: trends, predictors, and pregnancy outcomes. Fertil Steril. 2020;114(3):567–78.
21. Koning AM, Mutsaerts MA, Kuchenbecker WK, Broekmans FJ, Land JA, Mol BW, et al. Complications and outcome of assisted reproduction technologies in overweight and obese women. Hum Reprod. 2012;27(2):457–67.
22. Zegers-Hochschild F, Adamson GD, Dyer S, Racowsky C, de Mouzon J, Sokol R, et al. The International Glossary on Infertility and Fertility Care, 2017. Fertil Steril. 2017;108(3):393–406.
23. Ulrich ND, Marsh EE. Ovarian reserve testing: a review of the options, their applications, and their limitations. Clin Obstet Gynecol. 2019;62(2):228–37.
24. Homburg R, Howles CM. Low-dose FSH therapy for anovulatory infertility associated with polycystic ovary syndrome: rationale, results, reflections and refinements. Hum Reprod Update. 1999;5(5):493–9.
25. Whelan JG, Vlahos NF. The ovarian hyperstimulation syndrome. Fertil Steril. 2000;73(5):883–96.
26. Tsampras N, Palinska-Rudzka K, Alebrahim Y, Craciunas L, Mathur R. Prevention of ovarian hyperstimulation syndrome (OHSS): British Fertility Society policy and practice guideline. Hum Fertil (Camb). 2025;28(1):2441827.

27. Practice Committee of the American Society for Reproductive Medicine. Prevention of moderate and severe ovarian hyperstimulation syndrome: a guideline. Fertil Steril. 2024;121(2):230–45.
28. Jayaprakasan K, Chan Y, Islam R, Haoula Z, Hopkisson J, Coomarasamy A, et al. Prediction of in vitro fertilization outcome at different antral follicle count thresholds in a prospective cohort of 1,012 women. Fertil Steril 2012;98(3):657–663.
29. Guan S, Feng Y, Huang Y, Huang J. Progestin-primed ovarian stimulation protocol for patients in assisted reproductive technology: a meta-analysis of randomized controlled trials. Front Endocrinol (Lausanne). 2021;12:702558.
30. Nelson SM, Shaw M, Alrashid K, Anderson RA. Individualized dosing of follitropin delta affects live birth and safety in in vitro fertilization treatment: an individual participant data meta-analysis of randomized controlled trials. Fertil Steril. 2024;122(3):445–54.
31. Youssef M, Van der Veen F, Al-Inany HG, Mochtar MH, Griesinger G, Nagi Mohesen M, et al. Gonadotropin-releasing hormone agonist versus HCG for oocyte triggering in antagonist-assisted reproductive technology. Cochrane Database Syst Rev. 2014;10
32. Hu K-L, Wang S, Ye X, Zhang D, Hunt S. GnRH agonist and hCG (dual trigger) versus hCG trigger for follicular maturation: a systematic review and meta-analysis of randomized trials. Reprod Biol Endocrinol. 2021;19(1):78.
33. van der Linden M, Buckingham K, Farquhar C, Kremer JAM, Metwally M. Luteal phase support for assisted reproduction cycles. Cochrane Database Syst Rev. 2015;7
34. Tso LO, Costello MF, Albuquerque LET, Andriolo RB, Macedo CR. Metformin treatment before and during IVF or ICSI in women with polycystic ovary syndrome. Cochrane Database Syst Rev. 2020;12(12):Cd006105.
35. Soares SR. Etiology of OHSS and use of dopamine agonists. Fertil Steril. 2012;97(3):517–22.
36. Tang H, Mourad SM, Wang A, Zhai SD, Hart RJ. Dopamine agonists for preventing ovarian hyperstimulation syndrome. Cochrane Database Syst Rev. 2021;4(4):CD008605.
37. Siristatidis CS, Maheshwari A, Vaidakis D, Bhattacharya S. In vitro maturation in subfertile women with polycystic ovarian syndrome undergoing assisted reproduction. Cochrane Database Syst Rev. 2018;11(11):CD006606.
38. Bodri D, Guillén JJ, Polo A, Trullenque M, Esteve C, Coll O. Complications related to ovarian stimulation and oocyte retrieval in 4052 oocyte donor cycles. Reprod Biomed Online. 2008;17(2):237–43.
39. Liberty G, Hyman JH, Eldar-Geva T, Latinsky B, Gal M, Margalioth EJ. Ovarian hemorrhage after transvaginal ultrasonographically guided oocyte aspiration: a potentially catastrophic and not so rare complication among lean patients with polycystic ovary syndrome. Fertil Steril. 2010;93(3):874–9.
40. Nouri K, Walch K, Promberger R, Kurz C, Tempfer CB, Ott J. Severe haematoperitoneum caused by ovarian bleeding after transvaginal oocyte retrieval: a retrospective analysis and systematic literature review. Reprod Biomed Online. 2014;29(6):699–707.
41. Peavey M, Steward R, Paulyson-Nunez K, James A. Successful prophylactic regimens for transvaginal oocyte retrieval in women with bleeding diatheses. Haemophilia. 2013;19(3):e189–91.
42. Vloeberghs V, Peeraer K, Pexsters A, D'Hooghe T. Ovarian hyperstimulation syndrome and complications of ART. Best Pract Res Clin Obstet Gynaecol. 2009;23(5):691–709.
43. El-Toukhy T, Hanna L. Pelvic infection after oocyte retrieval: a preventable complication or an inevitable risk? J Obstet Gynaecol. 2006;26(7):701–3.
44. Kelada E, Ghani R. Bilateral ovarian abscesses following transvaginal oocyte retrieval for IVF: a case report and review of literature. J Assist Reprod Genet. 2007;24(4):143–5.
45. Sharpe K, Karovitch AJ, Claman P, Suh KN. Transvaginal oocyte retrieval for in vitro fertilization complicated by ovarian abscess during pregnancy. Fertil Steril. 2006;86(1):219.e11–3.
46. Yaron Y, Peyser MR, Samuel D, Amit A, Lessing JB. Infected endometriotic cysts secondary to oocyte aspiration for in-vitro fertilization. Hum Reprod. 1994;9(9):1759–60.
47. Howe RS, Wheeler C, Mastroianni L Jr, Blasco L, Tureck R. Pelvic infection after transvaginal ultrasound-guided ovum retrieval. Fertil Steril. 1988;49(4):726–8.

48. Smith LP, Oskowitz SP, Barrett B, Bayer SR. IVF and embryo development subsequent to ovarian torsion occurring during the resumption of meiosis. Reprod Biomed Online. 2010;21(3):418–21.
49. Tsai H-C, Kuo T-N, Chung M-T, Lin MYS, Kang C-Y, Tsai Y-C. Acute abdomen in early pregnancy due to ovarian torsion following successful in vitro fertilization treatment. Taiwan J Obstetr Gynecol. 2015;54(4):438–41.
50. Pinto AB, Ratts VS, Williams DB, Keller SL, Odem RR. Reduction of ovarian torsion 1 week after embryo transfer in a patient with bilateral hyperstimulated ovaries. Fertil Steril. 2001;76(2):403–6.
51. Zhu L, Zhang D, Yang Y. A case of excision of ovarian torsion necrosis due to luteoma in a female who conceived a twin pregnancy through in vitro fertilization misdiagnosed with acute appendicitis. Gynecol Endocrinol. 2022;38(10):885–8.

16 Third-Party Reproduction

Francesca Steyn

16.1 Introduction

Third-party reproduction provides pathways to parenthood for individuals and couples facing complex fertility challenges [1]. Whilst there is a physical medical process that takes place, these routes involve additional emotional, legal, and ethical dimensions. Nurses are central to supporting patients on these journeys, ensuring informed consent, appropriate counselling, coordination with specialists, and ongoing emotional support and well-being [2].

16.2 Understanding Third-Party Reproduction

Type of Third-Party Reproduction	Description
Donor sperm	A donor provides sperm to achieve pregnancy in another individual
Donor egg	A donor provides eggs for use by another person or couple
Donor embryo	Both sperm and egg are donated (often anonymously or from surplus embryos)
Surrogacy	A surrogate carries a pregnancy for intended parent(s)
Reciprocal IVF	One partner provides eggs, the other carries the pregnancy (typically in same-sex female couples)

F. Steyn (✉)
Department of Obstetrics and Gynecology, Wales Fertility Institute, Port Talbot, UK
e-mail: Francesca.steyn@wales.nhs.uk

M. Das, M. H. Dahan (eds.), *A Comprehensive Guide to Reproductive Health and Infertility Medicine for Nurses*, https://doi.org/10.1007/978-3-032-24372-0_16

In Britain, third-party reproduction is governed by the Human Fertilisation and Embryology Act (1990, amended 2008), which sets out conditions for consent, parenthood, donation, and surrogacy [3]. These guidelines are similar in many countries which permit third-party reproduction with slight variations expected.

16.3 The Nurse's Role

Nurses provide individualised care, continuity, coordination, and compassionate care throughout all treatment types. According to the *RCN Fertility Nursing Framework* (2023) [2], competencies specific to third-party reproduction include:

Core Nursing Responsibilities in Third-Party Reproduction

- Facilitating informed consent discussions
- Coordinating screening and counselling appointments
- Supporting access to donor gamete selection and surrogacy organisations
- Providing legal and ethical guidance
- Liaising with multidisciplinary teams (MDTs)
- Ensuring compliance with HFEA Code of Practice
- Provision of information and education on treatments and timelines

16.4 Donor Conception

16.4.1 Clinical and Ethical Considerations

Donor conception may be indicated in cases of:

- Severe male factor infertility
- Premature ovarian insufficiency
- Genetic conditions
- Same-sex couples or single parents by choice

In the UK, the current legal and clinical guidelines set by the Human Fertilisation and Embryology Authority (HFEA) state that sperm donors must be between 18 and 45 years old, while egg donors must be between 18 and 35 years old [3]. Although the upper age limit for egg donors is not explicitly outlined in legislation, most clinics adhere to the British Fertility Society (BFS) recommendation to limit donation to those under 36 years due to declining egg quality with age. All donors are required to undergo thorough screening for infectious and genetic conditions and must provide valid, informed consent for the use and storage of their gametes. Since 2005, UK law also requires all new donors to agree to be identifiable to donor-conceived individuals once they reach the age of 18 [4]. Although these specific-age cut-offs may not apply in other countries, the concepts behind them remain valid that pregnancy rates will decline with increasing donor age and that donors not of the age of maturity are at risks of exploitation by their elders. Other issues to consider are the donor and recipient related and could the recipient exert untold pressure on the donor preventing true informed consent.

Screening required for donors	Examples
Virology	HIV, hepatitis B/C, syphilis, gonorrhoea, chlamydia
Genetics	Karyotype, CF screen, ethnicity-linked disorders
Lifestyle and medical history review	Smoking, alcohol, family history, medications, illicit drug use
Counselling and legal consent	Identity release rules, storage, withdrawal

16.4.2 Emotional Support

Implications counselling is a vital component of third-party reproduction, providing individuals and couples with the opportunity to explore the emotional, social, legal, and ethical aspects of using donor gametes, embryos, or a surrogate. This type of counselling helps patients consider the potential impact on their future family, including issues of disclosure, identity, and the long-term well-being of donor-conceived children. It also supports decision-making by ensuring that all parties understand the consequences of treatment before proceeding. The British Infertility Counselling Association (BICA) strongly advocates for the integration of implications counselling into fertility care, highlighting its importance in promoting informed consent and emotional preparedness [4]. BICA's professional guidelines emphasise that counselling should be delivered by qualified fertility counsellors and be accessible at all key stages of the treatment journey. This is the case in most countries with fertility counselling requiring additional expertise and training.

Patients may experience complex emotions around donor conception. BFS and HFEA guidance recommend mandatory implications counselling to explore:

- Feelings around lack of genetic link or non-biological parent status
- Disclosure to future children
- Family and cultural dynamics
- Coping with identity or loss

Nurses can play a key role in assessing readiness and providing reassurance while ensuring referral to specialist counselling services.

16.5 Surrogacy

Surrogacy provides a valuable route to parenthood for individuals and couples unable to carry a pregnancy themselves. There are two primary types: traditional surrogacy, where the surrogate uses her own egg and is therefore genetically related to the child, and gestational surrogacy, where the surrogate carries an embryo created from the intended parents' or donors' gametes, with no genetic link to the surrogate. In the UK, surrogacy is governed by the Human Fertilisation and Embryology Act 1990 (as amended), which stipulates that the surrogate is the legal mother at birth, regardless of genetic connection [5]. Legal parenthood is transferred to the intended parents through a parental order post-birth. Fertility nurses play a crucial role in supporting all parties through the clinical process, coordinating care, ensuring legal compliance, and providing emotional support throughout the surrogacy journey.

16.5.1 Types of Surrogacies

Surrogacy Type	Description
Gestational	Embryo created via IVF using intended parents' or donor gametes; surrogate has no genetic link
Traditional	Surrogate uses her own egg and donor/involved sperm; carries and delivers the baby

The surrogacy coordinator plays a pivotal role within fertility clinics, acting as the primary liaison between intended parents, surrogates, and the multidisciplinary team. Their responsibilities include guiding patients through the complex surrogacy process, ensuring that all legal, ethical, and clinical requirements are met in accordance with regulations and national guidance. This includes verifying that all parties have received appropriate counselling, that informed consent is accurately documented, and that legal advice has been sought where necessary. The coordinator also supports the emotional wellbeing of both the surrogate and intended parents, facilitates communication, and helps manage expectations throughout treatment and into the postnatal period. Fertility nurses are particularly well placed to take on this role, given their established skills in patient coordination, counselling support, and regulatory compliance. By maintaining clear oversight of timelines, documentation, and interprofessional collaboration, the surrogacy coordinator ensures a structured, safe, and compassionate experience for everyone involved [6, 7].

16.5.2 Legal and Policy Considerations

- It should be noted that in some countries, surrogacy agreements are *not legally enforceable.*
- The *birth mother is the legal mother at birth.*
- A *Parental Order* must be obtained post-birth to transfer legal parenthood.

- Reasonable expenses may be paid, but commercial surrogacy is illegal in many countries such as the UK and Canada, while it is legal in other countries such as the USA.
- In other countries, the *commissioning couples are* automatically recognized as *the birth parents* with their names placed on the birth certificate.

Nurses must advise patients to seek independent legal advice to support timely parental order applications.

Nurse's Checklist for Best Practice in Surrogacy Cases Should Include

- Life insurance for all parties
- Wills for all parties
- Informed consent
- Screening in line with donation guidance as intended parents providing eggs and sperm will need to be screened and registered as donors in some countries
- Quarantine timeframes for stored gametes
- Legal parenthood and parental responsibility
- Legal advice and support
- Implications counselling
- Welfare of the child assessment

16.5.3 Emotional Impact and Counselling

Surrogacy can involve complex feelings of attachment, anxiety, and loss for surrogates and intended parents. Counselling sessions will cover:

- Roles, expectations, and communication
- Managing birth and handover
- Involvement of partners and family
- Postnatal emotional support

Fertility nurses play a key liaison role, particularly as births may occur outside the treatment centre.

16.6 Reciprocal IVF

Reciprocal IVF—sometimes called "shared motherhood"—allows one partner in a same-sex female couple to provide the egg, while the other carries the pregnancy. It offers a meaningful shared parenting experience, but adds complexity to consent, medical care, and expectations.

Step	Nurse consideration
Stimulation of partner A	Support egg provider with medication and monitoring
Embryo transfer to partner B	Ensure understanding of legal and clinical steps
Legal parenthood	Consent to parenthood forms must be correctly completed
Counselling	Explore feelings around roles, expectations, outcomes

In general, *both partners should consent* to parenthood and understand the implications. Nurses are critical in coordinating consent and supporting clear communication between partners.

16.7 Informed Consent and Documentation

Third-party reproduction involves multiple layers of consent. Nurses must ensure compliance with the local Code of Practice whilst also adhering to their governing body and their professional code of conduct.

In fertility clinics, nurses play a vital role in the consent process by providing patients with clear, comprehensive information about treatments, risks, benefits, and alternatives, ensuring that patients fully understand their options. They support patients emotionally and assess their understanding to facilitate truly informed and voluntary consent. Nurses assist in completing and documenting consent forms in accordance with legal and regulatory frameworks. They act as key communicators within the multidisciplinary team, ensuring that patient wishes are respected throughout treatment. Importantly, nurses should recognise that consent is an ongoing process, revisiting discussions as treatment plans evolve. Nurses emphasize patient autonomy and safeguard informed decision-making in a sensitive and complex clinical environment.

16.8 Multidisciplinary Collaboration Team (MDT)

Third-party treatments require coordination across a wide MDT, including:

- Clinicians
- Embryologists and lab teams
- Fertility nurses
- Specialist counsellors
- Surrogacy organisations
- Family lawyers—to support with legal parenthood matters

16.9 Ethical and Cultural Considerations

Nurses must approach third-party reproduction with sensitivity to religious, cultural, and personal values. Scenarios may include:

- Religious opposition to gamete donation or surrogacy
- Cultural stigma around infertility or non-biological parenting
- Language barriers to informed consent

Ethical Practice Principles
- Respect autonomy and diversity
- Avoid assumptions; ask open questions
- Ensure equal access to information and support
- Refer to ethics committees if needed

Reflective practice is a fundamental part of nursing, encouraging nurses to critically evaluate their actions, decisions, and experiences to improve their professional skills and patient care. In the context of third-party reproduction, such as egg or sperm donation and surrogacy, reflective practice allows nurses to explore the complex ethical considerations involved, including issues of consent, confidentiality, and respect for all parties' rights and well-being. By regularly reflecting on challenging cases and ethical dilemmas, nurses can develop greater awareness of their own values and biases, enhance empathy, and ensure they uphold professional standards and legal frameworks. This ongoing self-evaluation supports nurses in providing sensitive, individualised patient care that balances the needs of intended parents, donors, and surrogates within a respectful and ethically sound framework.

16.10 Conclusion

Third-party reproduction expands access to parenthood but presents unique clinical, emotional, and legal challenges. Fertility nurses play a central role in supporting patients, coordinating care, and safeguarding ethical standards. Through adherence to HFEA regulations, professional guidelines, and professional standards, nurses can empower diverse families to make informed, supported choices in building their families.

References

1. National Institute for Health and Care Excellence (NICE). Fertility problems: assessment and treatment. NICE guideline [CG156]; 2017.
2. Royal College of Nursing (RCN). Career and competence framework for fertility nursing. London: RCN Publishing; 2023.

3. British Fertility Society. New guidelines for screening of sperm, egg and embryo donors in the UK. 2008. Retrieved from https://www.britishfertilitysociety.org.uk/press-release/new-guidelines-for-screening-of-sperm-egg-and-embryo-donors-in-the-uk/.
4. British Infertility Counselling Association. Guidelines for good practice in fertility counselling. 4th ed. BICA; 2019. Retrieved from https://www.bica.net/item/1/BICA/Guidelines-for-Good-Practice-in-Infertility-Counselling.html.
5. Department of Health and Social Care. Care in surrogacy: guidance for the care of surrogates and intended parents in surrogate births in England and Wales. 2024. Retrieved from https://www.gov.uk/government/publications/having-a-child-through-surrogacy/care-in-surrogacy-guidance-for-the-care-of-surrogates-and-intended-parents-in-surrogate-births-in-england-and-wales
6. Human Fertilisation and Embryology Authority (HFEA). Code of Practice [Internet]. HFEA: London; [cited 2025 May 21]. Available from: https://www.hfea.gov.uk.
7. Human Fertilisation and Embryology Act 1990, as amended by the Human Fertilisation and Embryology Act 2008.

17 The First Trimester of Pregnancy

Richard Brown

17.1 Introduction

The first trimester, spanning from conception to the end of the 12th week, represents the foundation of pregnancy, encompassing not only the key periods of embryologic and fundamental fetal development but also the establishment of placental development and function and a time of significant maternal adaptation to pregnancy. It is therefore a period of rapid development and profound physiological change.

For women who have not planned a pregnancy, more than a third of this period can pass prior to the presence of a pregnancy even being recognized. For women planning a pregnancy, preparation prior to conception permits preparations and groundwork that can positively influence the many processes that will occur in these crucial weeks.

Understanding the many changes occurring during this period will provide caregivers with the knowledge to be able to provide comprehensive care and support to pregnant patients.

Following successful fertilization that typically happens in the fallopian tube within 24 h of ovulation, the zygote undergoes rapid mitotic divisions (cleavage) as it travels toward the uterus, forming a morula and then a blastocyst by day 5. The blastocyst consists of an inner cell mass, which will become the embryo, and an outer layer of trophoblast cells, which will form the placenta—the normal development of both being essential for a healthy pregnancy. Implantation generally occurs at around days 6–10 post-fertilization when the blastocyst attaches to the endometrial lining of the uterus. These initial stages follow an altered physiologic course

R. Brown (✉)
Division of Maternal Fetal Medicine, Department of Obstetrics and Gynaecology, McGill University Health Centre & McGill University, Montreal, QC, Canada
e-mail: richard.brown@mcgill.ca

M. Das, M. H. Dahan (eds.), *A Comprehensive Guide to Reproductive Health and Infertility Medicine for Nurses*, https://doi.org/10.1007/978-3-032-24372-0_17

when in vitro fertilization replaces the natural passage of the fertilized egg into the uterus with direct injection of the embryo or blastocyst into the uterine cavity.

17.1.1 Physiologic Changes and Maternal Adaptation

The trophoblast cells secrete enzymes that facilitate implantation and transformation into the placenta. Following implantation, the trophoblast also secretes human chorionic gonadotropin (hCG) which maintains and supports the corpus luteum (CL) in its production of progesterone, which is essential for sustaining the endometrial lining, inhibiting uterine contractions, and supporting early pregnancy development. As the placenta develops, this organ will assume the role of progesterone production; the placenta and CL both also produce estrogen which promotes uterine growth and increases blood flow to the uterine vessels (and therefore to the placenta itself). Estrogen also initiates the stimulation of breast tissue development for later lactation.

As can be seen, progesterone is crucial for the development of an early pregnancy. That is why in cases where there is no corpus luteum (CL), as may arise in certain types of IVF frozen embryo transfer cycles or when the CL is injured by a needle during egg collection, progesterone replacement is essential to maintain the pregnancy.

Human placental lactogen (hPL) is also generated by the placenta and modulates maternal metabolism to support fetal growth and development.

The combination of hormonal influences contributes to the maternal physiological adaptations that commence within the first trimester and continue throughout pregnancy. These include an increase in the maternal blood volume by approximately 30–50% across pregnancy with a concurrent increase in the maternal cardiac output that is jointly contributed to by an elevated heart rate and an increased cardiac stroke volume.

Vasodilatation and decreased systemic vascular resistance contribute to slight decreases in blood pressure toward the end of the first trimester. Both decreased vascular resistance and increased cardiac output contribute to the 50–80% increase in renal blood flow with a glomerular filtration rate (GFR) that rises by 40–50%, supporting increased waste elimination. Meanwhile respiratory rate and pulmonary tidal volume also increase, resulting in higher minute ventilation and enhancing oxygen delivery.

The benefits of the hormonal changes in some systems, although not fully understood, also contribute to several of the symptoms associated with pregnancy. For example, progesterone not only relaxes the uterine muscle to reduce contractions but also relaxes smooth muscle in general, which within the gastrointestinal system contributes to slower gastric emptying and reduced gastrointestinal motility that in turn contributes to symptoms including nausea, vomiting, and constipation.

17.1.2 Embryologic Development

Rapid and dramatic growth and structural changes in the fetus occur across the first trimester. The zygote having undergone rapid mitotic division forms a cluster of cells called the blastomere, which by 3–4 days post-fertilization becomes a solid ball-like cluster of cells termed the "morula". Over the next 24–48 h, this develops into a blastocyst, consisting of an outer trophoblast layer and an inner cell mass (ICM) with a fluid-filled cavity (blastocoele). By day 6–7, this implants into the uterine wall—erroneous implantation potentially resulting in extra-uterine gestations including ectopic (tubal, ovarian, cornual, etc.), scar, and cervical pregnancies.

The inner cell mass forms two layers (a bilaminar disc) comprising the epiblast (which will give rise to the embryo) and the hypoblast (which contributes to the yolk sac). Meanwhile the trophoblast differentiates into two layers: the cytotrophoblast (inner layer) and syncytiotrophoblast (outer layer), which invades the uterine lining to establish the placenta.

In the third week after fertilization, a structure called the primitive streak appears on the surface of the epiblast, marking the beginning of gastrulation, a process in which cells migrate through the primitive streak, forming the three primary germ layers—ectoderm, mesoderm, and endoderm—that are fundamental to the development of tissues and organs.

These layers undergo distinct differentiation. The ectoderm develops into the nervous system, skin, and hair. The mesoderm will form the skeleton, muscles, cardiovascular system, and reproductive organs while the endoderm becomes the gastrointestinal tract, liver, pancreas, and lungs.

The rudimentary cardiac tube also develops with cardiac activity evident from around days 22–23 post-fertilization; over the coming weeks, this undergoes a complex folding process to form the heart.

Over the next 2 weeks (weeks 4–5), the ectoderm thickens to form the neural plate which then folds to form the neural tube, which will develop into the brain and spinal cord.

Cells at the edges of the neural tube migrate to form neural crest cells, which contribute to the development of the peripheral nervous system, facial cartilage, and other structures. In parallel with the above, the mesodermal cells become organized into segmental areas or somites, which will form the vertebrae, ribs, and skeletal muscles.

At the periphery of the structure, limb buds begin the development of the arms and legs.

During weeks 6–8, the heart has continued its folding process and undergoes further development, with the formation of the four chambers and major blood vessels. In parallel, the brain divides into five distinct regions, and the neural tube closes completely. The primitive gut forms and begins to differentiate into the stomach, intestines, liver, and pancreas. The early formation of the lungs begins as outpouchings from the foregut.

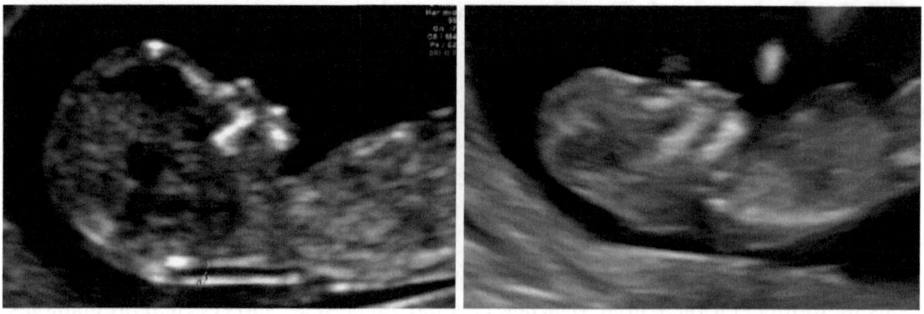

Fig. 17.1 The fetus on the left demonstrates a normal cranial vault and skull contour. The fetus on the right demonstrates acrania and early damage to the brain resulting from the lack of skull protection that leads to the acrania–exencephaly–anencephaly sequence

Limb buds elongate and differentiate into the future arms and legs, with the formation of digits (fingers and toes). Early facial features begin to form, including the eyes, ears, and nasal structures.

Weeks 5–8 represent the most active period of organogenesis and therefore a critical period during which teratogenic exposures (be those drugs, infections, substances, poorly controlled medical conditions) can interfere with these processes and result in congenital malformations. Errors of neural tube folding give rise to the neural tube defect spectrum of disorders that includes acrania/anencephaly (Fig. 17.1) and spina bifida, while the heart with its complex folding is also particularly prone to maldevelopment.

In the next few weeks (9–12), the embryo transitions into its appearance as a fetus with both rapid growth and further refinement of organs and body systems.

The brain continues to develop and grow, with increased complexity and function.

Bones begin to ossify, and muscles strengthen, allowing for early movements.

The kidneys start producing urine, and the external genitalia begin to differentiate.

The appearances of the fetus as it evolves over these weeks are depicted in Fig. 17.2.

Alongside fetal development there is a parallel process of development and maturation of the placenta with it becoming a fully functional organ charged with providing nutrients and oxygen to the growing fetus while simultaneously removing waste products. The umbilical cord connects the placenta to the fetus which occupies a fluid-filled sac surrounded by a thin membrane, the amnion. Surrounding the amniotic sac, there is a second space contained by another membrane, the chorion. Typically, by 15 weeks, the chorion and amnion fuse so that only a single fluid-filled amniotic sac is seen.

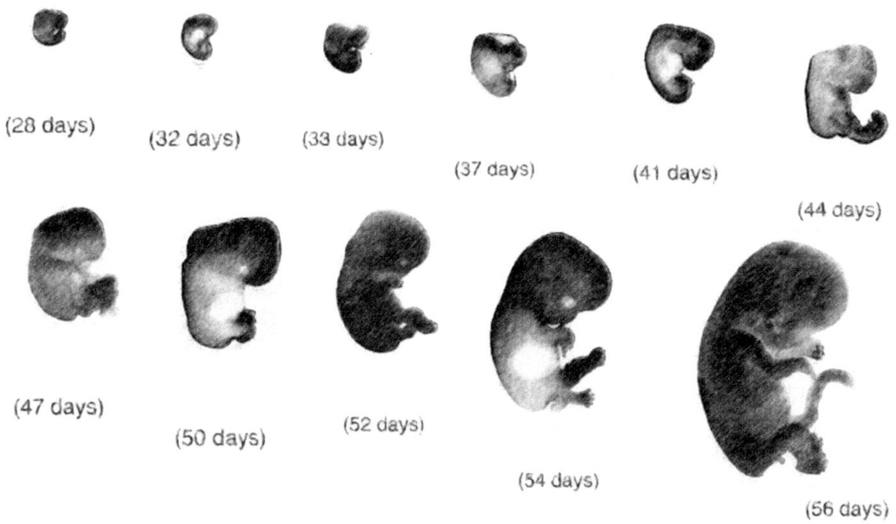

Fig. 17.2 Depictions of the developmental stages of a human embryo (from 28 to 56 days post-ovulation)

17.2 Complications of the First Trimester of Pregnancy

As this is a critical period marked by rapid fetal and placental development as well as maternal adaptation and physiological changes to the pregnant state, it is also a time when each of these processes may be vulnerable to complications.

The role of nurses in the early recognition of complications, providing prompt intervention and compassionate care, is vital in ensuring the best possible outcomes for both the mother and the developing fetus. Understanding the risk factors, clinical presentations, diagnostic approaches, and management strategies for these complications enables the patient to be supported and appropriately guided through this crucial and often stressful phase of pregnancy.

17.2.1 Miscarriage/Early Pregnancy Loss/Spontaneous Abortion

The spontaneous loss of a pregnancy most commonly occurs within the first trimester and represents the most frequent complication of early pregnancy. Many phrases have been used to describe pregnancy failure with the currently preferred term being "early pregnancy loss" (EPL). This is categorized by the presence of a nonviable, intrauterine pregnancy comprising either an empty gestational sac or a gestational sac containing an embryo or fetus without fetal heart activity within the first trimester. This occurs in 10–20% of recognized pregnancies but affects up to 30% of conceived pregnancies overall, as a significant proportion (~20%) will be lost before clinical recognition of a pregnancy, with these cases only being identified using biochemical evaluation of hCG [1, 2].

The contributing risk factors for pregnancy loss are broad and diverse, although over half of pregnancy losses arise due to a fetal aneuploidy [3]. As aneuploidy rates increase with maternal age, the overall loss rate observed also increases with maternal age. For younger women (<30), a rate between 9% and 17% has been reported, rising to 40% by age 40 and 80% by age 45 [4].

In addition to advanced maternal age (>35) being a risk factor, a history of prior EPL, chronic and particularly poorly controlled medical conditions such as diabetes, thyroid or autoimmune disorders, are significant risks. Lifestyle factors particularly smoking, alcohol use, or illicit drug use can also adversely impact the developing pregnancy resulting in early loss. Maternal infections such as rubella are less frequent with high overall vaccination rates, particularly in the developed world, but must be considered especially given trends toward vaccine hesitancy in some populations. Cytomegalovirus, influenza, zika, malaria, bacterial vaginosis, and syphilis as well as other infections may contribute to up to 15% of EPLs [5].

Genetic abnormalities, for example, balanced or unbalanced translocations, may result in the passage of severe or lethal genetic defects to the embryo and therefore also contribute to the toll of pregnancy losses.

The signs and symptoms include vaginal bleeding, which may range from minimal to heavy, sometimes with the passage of tissue or clots from the vagina, abdominal cramping or pain, and a decrease or loss in pregnancy symptoms. Bleeding itself however is also common in ongoing pregnancies, as is non-specific pelvic pain or discomfort. The diagnosis may in some cases be clinical, when for example products of conception are seen being expulsed through the cervix, but most often relies upon either ultrasound findings or the serial measurement of serum hCG values.

Management of a confirmed EPL may be expectant (i.e., allowing the process to proceed along its natural course without medical intervention), medical, or surgical. Medical approaches rely on the administration of drugs such as misoprostol that accelerate expulsion of residual pregnancy tissue, while surgical management involves performing a dilation and curettage (D&C) to remove the fetal tissue from the uterine cavity. Whichever method is used, there should always be consideration for offering emotional support and counseling.

17.2.2 Subchorionic Hemorrhage

A subchorionic hemorrhage arises from bleeding between the chorion and the uterine wall. It is one of the commonest abnormal findings in early pregnancy being identified by ultrasound in up to 20% of pregnancies (Fig. 17.3). The use of anticoagulant medications or the presence of a bleeding disorder will increase the risk, as may the presence of uterine malformations.

Frequently this may be an incidental finding on ultrasound in an asymptomatic case, but it also may be associated with vaginal bleeding that may range from light

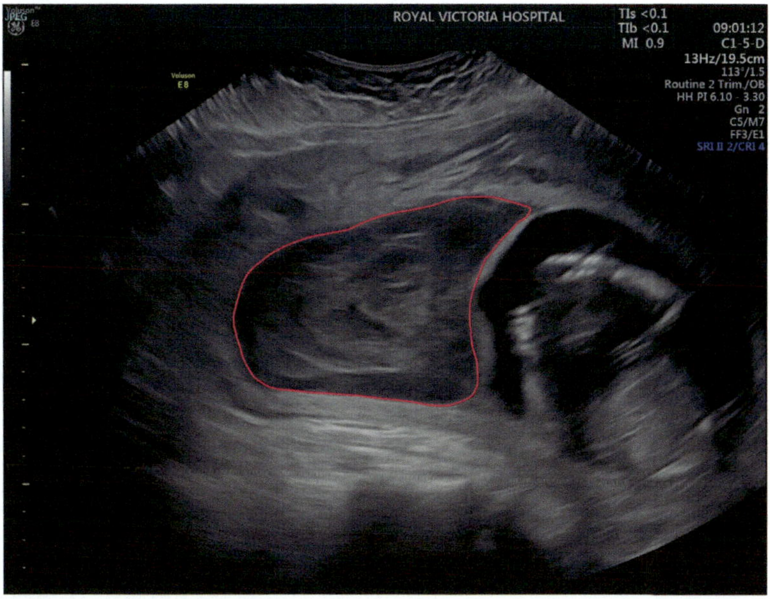

Fig. 17.3 An image from a first trimester pregnancy demonstrating a large subchorionic hematoma (contained within the red border)

spotting to heavy bleeding and consist of either fresh or old blood, which may or may not be accompanied by abdominal cramping. Management is expectant with observation and follow-up ultrasound imaging. Temporary modification or reduction of physical activity may be appropriate, as may temporary cessation of anticoagulant medication, if this is deemed otherwise safe for the woman.

17.3 Pregnancy of Unknown Location and Ectopic Gestations

17.3.1 Pregnancy of Unknown Location

Pregnancy of unknown location (PUL) is a term used when a pregnancy test is positive, but the location of the pregnancy cannot be determined through transvaginal ultrasound (TVS). An intrauterine pregnancy can be identified at its earliest by the presence of a gestational sac within the endometrial cavity by TVS as of 5 weeks of gestation. Prior to this, a pregnancy cannot be identified by ultrasound. Sometimes even after an expected gestation of at least 5 weeks, TVS may fail to identify an intrauterine gestation. This scenario presents a diagnostic challenge as it can represent a normal early intrauterine pregnancy, a miscarriage, or an ectopic pregnancy. Proper management and follow-up are critical to ensure patient safety and optimal outcomes.

There are four possible outcomes of PUL. An intrauterine pregnancy (IUP) may eventually be identified. This may be because of the presence of a normal early pregnancy that was too small to be detected by ultrasound at the initial time of evaluation, most typically because of a variation or error in the dating of the pregnancy. The pregnancy may be identified as ectopic, discussed further below. Failure to identify the pregnancy may be indicative of a failed intrauterine pregnancy that may have already been expelled or that had never reached the size that would have been identified by ultrasound. The most challenging scenario may be when the location of the pregnancy remains unknown even after initial evaluation and follow-up and further assessments are required.

Given the diverse possible outcomes for PUL, the risk factors include those that predispose to either ectopic gestation or early pregnancy failure. These include previous ectopic pregnancy or history of tubal damage for example due to pelvic inflammatory disease (PID) or tubal surgery, pregnancies resulting from assisted reproductive technologies (ART); the presence of an intrauterine device (IUD), a history of recurrent pregnancy loss, of advanced maternal age, or of harmful habits such as smoking.

As in these cases ultrasound is non-diagnostic, other investigations are used. Serial serum hCG measurements are critical. In a normal intrauterine pregnancy, hCG levels typically double approximately every 48 h in early pregnancy. Abnormal rise patterns may suggest an ectopic pregnancy as may static values; the latter or falling values may often be indicative of an EPL. It must be borne in mind though that even with ectopic gestations, the rate of rise of hCG may be comparable to that of a healthy intrauterine gestation.

Expectant management is appropriate for patients with stable vital signs and no significant pain and consists of close symptom monitoring combined with serial hCG measurements and repeat ultrasounds until the pregnancy location is determined or hCG levels return to the non-pregnant range. Although the initial TVS may not be revealing, this must be done by an operator able to thoroughly examine the pelvis to rule out an intrauterine or extrauterine pregnancy, and repeat ultrasounds after a suitable time interval should be performed to reevaluate if the pregnancy can now be located.

Some centers advocate the evaluation of progesterone levels, as low values are associated with non-viable pregnancies, while higher levels suggest a potentially viable pregnancy. PUL with significant maternal symptoms or cardiovascular instability may justify diagnostic laparoscopy.

In asymptomatic women with plateauing or sub-optimally rising hCG levels indicative of a non-normally advancing pregnancy, medical management, as for an ectopic gestation, can be considered. This is typically with methotrexate therapy, which inhibits cell division resulting in resolution of the pregnancy, whatever its location. Additional doses of methotrexate or surgical intervention may be necessary if hCG levels do not decline as expected.

Patient compliance is paramount in the safe, especially conservative, management of PUL and therefore the importance of follow-up, and the rationale for serial hCG measurements and ultrasounds must be carefully explained and understood by the patient. Vital signs and pain must be assessed at each evaluation, and clear instructions regarding signs and symptoms that require immediate medical attention, such as severe abdominal pain, heavy vaginal bleeding, or syncope, must be offered. Although when compliance is questionable early laparoscopy is sometimes considered, it must be appreciated that early ectopics may not be identified by laparoscopy in the same way ultrasound failed to identify them.

17.3.2 Ectopic Pregnancies

An ectopic pregnancy occurs in up to 1–2% of conceptions, when the fertilized egg implants outside of the uterine cavity, most commonly in the fallopian tube but also on the ovary, on peritoneal surfaces, or within the cervix [6]. It is a potentially life-threatening condition if rupture of the structure supporting or containing the gestational sac results in significant internal bleeding.

A previous ectopic pregnancy increases the risk of recurrence, with the incidence also being elevated in women who have suffered prior tubal damage, for example, due to PID or prior tubal surgery. Although IUDs effectively prevent intrauterine implantation, they do not prevent ectopic implantation and, therefore, among IUD users, the rates of ectopic gestation are greater, although the incidence itself is not increased overall. Although ART, particularly in vitro fertilization (IVF) as opposed to intrauterine insemination (IUI), has been associated with increased ectopic gestation rates, more recent data following the introduction of controls to the number of embryos transferred demonstrates that rates following ART have improved with time [7].

Ectopic pregnancies located in the cervix account for only around 0.1% of ectopic gestations but present a significant risk for maternal morbidity and mortality, given the risk of the ectopic eroding into the cervical vessels and resulting in massive hemorrhage [8]. The appropriate management (conservative or surgical) remains to be established.

Cervico-isthmic pregnancies are perhaps even more rare given that the incidence remains undetermined. This can pose more of a dilemma in diagnosis and management with cases progressing well beyond the first trimester and even with term livebirths of such cases having been reported, even in the case of a twin gestation [9, 10]. Nonetheless, these are very high-risk situations with a risk of hemorrhage at any gestation or with potential need for surgical interventions given that placenta accreta spectrum is almost always found in such cases.

Implantation of a pregnancy into the scar site of a prior caesarean birth has become an increasingly appreciated entity over the last two decades, and although the true incidence remains undetermined, it is estimated to arise in around 1 in every 2000 pregnancies in women who have had a prior caesarean birth. The mechanism of implantation at the scar site remains unclear and the role of several risk factors may predispose a woman to persistent uterine scar defect after CD. The impact of the type of closure of the uterine incision at caesarean remains controversial, although caesarean delivery in the second stage and infective complications do appear to be risk factors [11].

Approximately 1:10000 live births or less results from an abdominal pregnancy, an ectopic that implants within the peritoneal cavity (outside of tubal, ovarian, or broad ligament locations). Although full-term abdominal pregnancies are reported and known to occur, the risks of maternal morbidity and mortality are significantly increased and largely impacted by the site or organ upon which the placenta implants with vascularized structures posing the greatest risks [12, 13].

Ectopic gestations may be diagnosed by ultrasound in asymptomatic women or may be identified following presentations most typically with abdominal or pelvic pain, vaginal bleeding, referred shoulder pain (in cases with intraperitoneal bleeding), or maternal syncope and shock. Ultrasound and the rate of rise of hCG are key elements in the diagnosis with surgical evaluation (laparoscopy) being indicated in those cases where the diagnosis is uncertain, and observation is inappropriate. Medical management such as methotrexate to cause cell death in the developing pregnancy and stop its growth and development is appropriate for early, unruptured ectopic pregnancies. In larger ectopic gestations or where rupture is suspected, laparoscopy with salpingectomy or salpingostomy is indicated. Conservative management may be appropriate in those cases where spontaneous resolution is suspected. For those sites where ectopic gestations are rarely encountered (e.g., cervical), case experience is limited such that there is no consensus on the best management approach.

17.4 Hyperemesis Gravidarum

Hyperemesis gravidarum (HG) impacts 0.5–2% of pregnant women and is an extreme presentation of the nausea and vomiting that physiologically arises in most pregnancies. At its most severe, this can lead to significant maternal dehydration, electrolyte imbalance, and weight loss. Although more frequent in multiple gestations or other situations where hCG levels are abnormally elevated (including molar pregnancies), this can arise in uncomplicated singleton gestations. Certain ethnicities (Asian and Middle Eastern) seem to be more prone to HG. Although infrequently overt hyperthyroidism can contribute to the development of HG, in many cases of HG, a transient hyperthyroidism will be noted which is likely due to presence of a less sialylated form of hCG, which stimulates the TSH receptor [14]. A prior history or family history of HG is also a risk factor for its occurrence or recurrence and may in some cases be due to hypersensitivity to hCG caused by a TSH receptor mutation.

Evaluation includes a clinical assessment of the severity of symptoms; laboratory analysis including electrolyte levels, liver function tests, and thyroid function tests; as well as ultrasound to rule out multiple gestations and molar pregnancy, both of which increase the risks of hyperemesis gravidarum.

Management is focused on the use of antiemetic medications (for example metoclopramide of ondansetron) or dietary modifications—small, frequent meals with a bland diet, hydration and electrolyte replacement which may require intravenous replacement if not achieved orally. In severe cases, hospitalization for both intravenous fluids and nutritional support (parenteral nutrition) may become indicated, which includes the administration of thiamine, as in severe cases of HG, thiamine deficiency can lead to the development of Wenicke's encephalopathy, an acute neurological disorder characterized by visual signs including nystagmus and diplopia, ataxia, and even altered mental status [16].

17.5 Gestational Trophoblastic Disease (GTD)

Gestational trophoblastic disease (GTD) encompasses a spectrum of conditions, including hydatidiform mole (molar pregnancy), invasive mole, and choriocarcinoma. GTD is characterized by abnormal growth of trophoblastic tissue. Molar pregnancies occur in about 1 in 1000 pregnancies with this being found more frequently in women of advanced maternal age (over 40 years), those with a history of previous molar pregnancy, and in those with some nutritional deficiencies (e.g., low carotene, folic acid) [17].

As noted above, molar pregnancy can cause HG and may also present with bleeding, which is more often dark in nature or may contain vesicle or grape-like structures. The uterine size may be disproportionately larger than expected for gestational age, and serum hCG levels will be much higher than expected. hCG levels may raise suspicion of the diagnosis as may ultrasound findings (Fig. 17.4). Hydropic trophoblast degeneration in a spontaneous abortion may often mimic the ultrasound appearances but will not be associated with the high hCG values. The

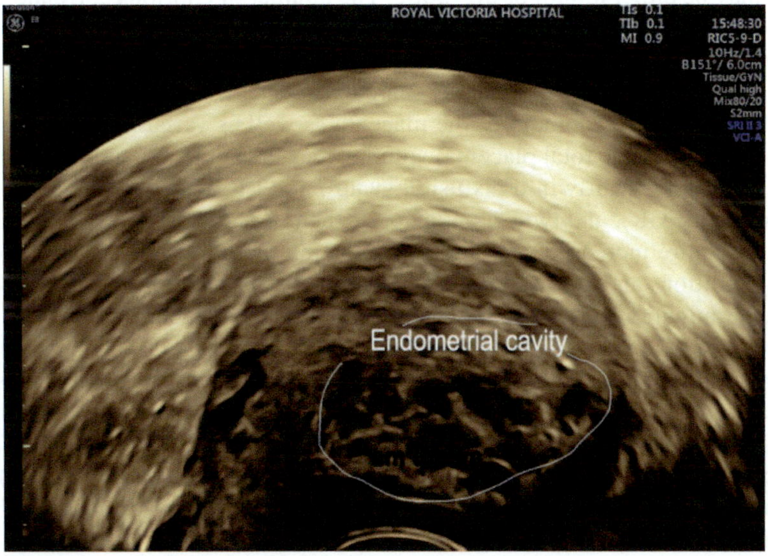

Fig. 17.4 The uterus is seen to contain multiple cystic spaces (highlighted) and no evident gestation. Histology later confirmed the vesicular appearances of the placenta to be a complete hydatidiform mole

supraphysiologic hCG levels may result in ovarian hyperstimulation, and the presence of multiple theca lutein cysts, together with the snowstorm or vesicular appearances of the uterine contents on ultrasound supports the diagnosis. Ultimately, however, histopathological examination of evacuated tissue obtained at suction curettage will be diagnostic.

Post curettage, complete removal of tissue as well as detection of possible malignancy (choriocarcinoma) relies on serial hCG monitoring. A minimum weekly evaluation for at least three consecutive weeks after hCG values have become undetectable is required, while for a complete mole, subsequent monthly monitoring should continue for 6 months [18]. The difference in follow-up duration is because invasive mole or persistent GTD arises in around 15% of women who have had complete molar pregnancy compared to 1% or less after a partial molar pregnancy.

Chemotherapy is indicated in malignant GTD and, after successful treatment, monitoring for at least 6–12 months is advised with adequate contraception to ensure that there is no confounding pregnancy to mask possible recurrence.

17.6 Multiple Pregnancy

Globally, twins account for 1–3% of all pregnancies with rates having doubled since the 1980s mostly due to the use of ART and advancing maternal age (a risk factor for multiple gestation). Around 65% of twin pregnancies are dizygotic and 35% are monozygotic. All monochorionic twins are monozygotic. Dichorionic twins may be either mono- or dizygotic. The number of chorions correlates to the number of placentas. Monochorionic gestations, although less prevalent, account for the larger proportion of complications associated with twinning. Due to their placental arrangement of a single shared placenta with vascular connections between each twin's domain of the placenta as well as variation in the distribution or sharing of the total placental volume, they are subject to unique complications, including twin-twin transfusion syndrome (TTTS), selective fetal growth restriction (SFGR), and twin anemia polycythemia sequence (TAPS). Such pregnancies require increased surveillance following the first trimester to screen for these conditions and allow appropriate and timely intervention where applicable. The determination of chorionicity is therefore key to determining the future course of a twin gestation. Determination of chorionicity is most reliably achieved at the end of the first trimester between the 10th and 13th weeks. The evaluation of the junction of the amnion and chorion at the placenta surface, characterized as the lambda sign "λ" in dichorionic gestations and the "T" sign in monochorionic gestations, has an accuracy of close to 100% (Fig. 17.5) [19]. This is more reliable than evaluation of the number of yolk sacs or other characteristics at earlier gestations.

Mostly resulting from ART and mostly from IUI, especially in those domains where IVF is regulated limiting the number of embryos that are transferred, pregnancies with 3–8 viable fetuses may infrequently arise (Fig. 17.6).

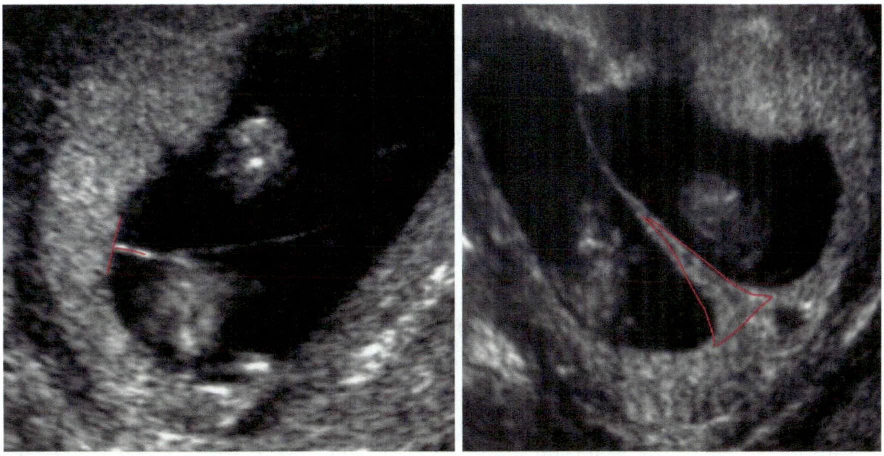

Fig. 17.5 In the image on the left, the inter-twin membrane is thin, and where it meets the placental surface, the junction resembles a T (marked in red)—this is a monochorionic twin gestation. In the image on the right, the membrane is thicker and at its placental junction also has placental tissue in-between the membranes in a "λ" shape (highlighted)—this is a dichorionic twin gestation

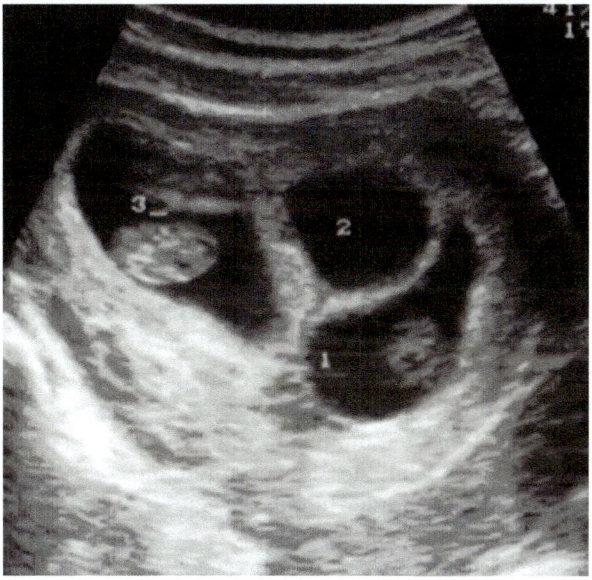

Fig. 17.6 Figure depicting a trichorionic triamniotic triplet gestation

17.7 Screening in the First Trimester

The first trimester presents the earliest opportunity for screening for pregnancy complications and abnormalities that will impact the future health of the fetus and course of the pregnancy.

Evaluation of fetal health comprises screening for the presence of major chromosome abnormalities and structural malformations. Evaluations of maternal adaptation to pregnancy can help predict uteroplacental pathologies that may result in conditions such as fetal growth restriction and pre-eclampsia. The advantages of early screening include early recourse to further investigation, ability to consider termination at earlier gestations when justified, to permit early parental preparation for potential problems and providing an opportunity to initiate treatments that may influence the development of complications.

17.8 Screening for Fetal Aneuploidy

Aneuploidy (a reduction or increase from the normal number of chromosomes) screening has advanced over the last 40 years from an initial selection for invasive testing based solely on maternal age, to a first trimester–focused approach. Early screening and diagnosis allow for earlier termination of affected pregnancies where permitted and desired, as well as ensuring earlier parental reassurance when screening is low risk or more time for preparation and adjustment to the possibility of having a child who may have special needs when the risk is high or aneuploidy is confirmed. The most frequently encountered and clinically significant aneuploidies are Down syndrome (trisomy 21), Edwards syndrome (trisomy 18), Patau syndrome (trisomy 13), and Turner syndrome (monosomy X). First trimester screening for fetal aneuploidy may involve a combination of maternal blood tests and ultrasound imaging to assess the likelihood of these conditions.

Recent advances in next-generation sequencing (NGS) have revolutionized prenatal screening by enabling highly accurate and comprehensive analysis of fetal DNA from a maternal blood sample. In noninvasive prenatal screening (NIPS), NGS is used to sequence cell-free fetal DNA (cffDNA) circulating in the mother's bloodstream, allowing for the detection of chromosomal abnormalities including trisomies 13,18, and 21. NGS can offer a high sensitivity (>99%) and specificity compared to traditional screening methods, significantly reducing false positives and negatives. It can also be performed from 10 weeks of gestation. Its ability to screen for a broader range of genetic conditions, including microdeletions and duplications, has made it a powerful tool in early pregnancy care. These techniques however remain costly and have only been routinely embraced in a limited number of public healthcare settings remaining a paid option in most countries [20, 21].

First trimester screening for aneuploidy is performed between the 11th and 14th weeks of pregnancy and combines serum and ultrasound screening techniques.

Although various serum markers have been employed, the two most robust first trimester markers are pregnancy-associated plasma protein-A (PAPP-A) and β-hCG. PAPP-A is produced by the placenta with abnormally low levels being associated with chromosomal abnormalities, while with free β-hCG, also produced by the placenta, abnormally high levels are associated with an increased risk of aneuploidy, especially Down syndrome.

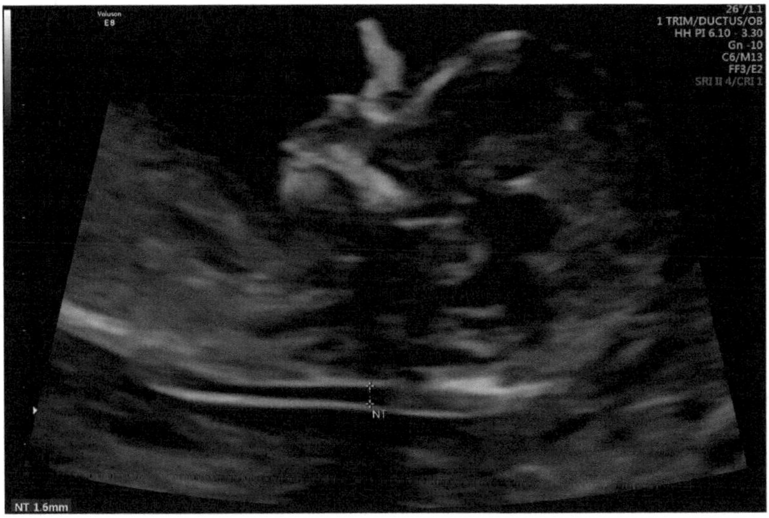

Fig. 17.7 Ultrasound imaging in a Mid-sagittal plane of the fetal heard and thorax demonstrating assessment of the nuchal translucency (NT, identified between the yellow + marks)

The key to ultrasound screening for aneuploidy is evaluation of the Nuchal Translucency (NT) (Fig. 17.7). The NT measurement represents the thickness of the fluid-filled space at the back of the fetus' neck. Chromosomal abnormalities, particularly Down syndrome, various genetic conditions, and cardiac anomalies often have an increased nuchal translucency. An NT measurement of 3.0 mm or higher may be considered abnormal, prompting further testing, but with appropriate software (Fetal Medicine Foundation), each measurement can be used to individually modify a woman's age-related background risk for an aneuploidy. Additional ultrasound markers may be combined with the NT to improve the ultrasound screening detection rate. These include assessment of the nasal bone—the absence or underdevelopment of the nasal bone can act as a marker for Down syndrome but is also impacted by patient ethnicity—and evaluation of the Ductus Venosus—the pattern of blood flow in this vessel can act as a marker for both fetal aneuploidy and congenital heart disease [22].

The results from the serum screening and NT ultrasound are combined with other factors that define the baseline risk (predominantly maternal or oocyte age). These factors are used to calculate a risk score for each chromosomal abnormality that is expressed as a probability, representing the likelihood of the fetus having each chromosomal condition. Detection rates may be in the range of 75–95% depending on the combination of serum and ultrasound markers being used.

In twin gestations, serum screening (PAPP-A and β-hCG) performs poorly and therefore ultrasound screening or NIPS is used.

If the screening indicates an increased risk (typically defined as greater than 1:150–300, depending on local practice), then either further screening using NIPS or diagnostic testing may be recommended. Diagnostic tests include chorionic villus sampling (CVS) or amniocentesis, which provide a definitive diagnosis by directly analyzing the fetal chromosomes, in the case of CVS from a placental biopsy and in the case of amniocentesis from an amniotic fluid sample.

It is essential to understand that first trimester screening cannot diagnose chromosomal abnormalities but can only assess the risk; this is currently considered true even with high sensitivity NIPS. Any screening test may also produce false-positive or false-negative results. A false-positive result indicates a high risk when the fetus does not have an abnormality, while a false-negative result indicates a low risk when there is a chromosomal abnormality. These possibilities underscore the importance of follow-up diagnostic testing for definitive evaluation especially when the risk is considered high. It is also important that parents realize that this screening is targeted for the aneuploidies noted and is not screening for genetic conditions in general. Although diagnostic tests allow for more extensive genetic evaluation, in the context of confirmation of a positive aneuploidy screen, testing may still be limited to these few chromosomes with more extensive testing only being performed if indicated by the presence of genetic conditions within the family history or in the context of fetal structural or functional abnormalities.

17.9 Screening for Structural Fetal Anomalies

With present ultrasound techniques, including the use of high-frequency endovaginal probes, careful fetal evaluation allows the detection of many fetal abnormalities even in the late first trimester. Later evaluation remains essential as due to ongoing fetal structural development since not all structures can be assessed or evaluated in the first trimester—for example, the corpus callosum only forms by 16 weeks of gestation. Nonetheless, particularly in higher risk pregnancies, many anomalies can be identified early [23, 25]. These will be reviewed briefly by anatomical region.

Cranial, facial and spine: Acrania/anencephaly (Fig. 17.1) can be detected in all cases by the late first trimester. Encephaloceles can be identified and together with renal anomalies and polydactyly may suggest a genetic condition, Mekel-Gruber. Alobar and lobar holoprosencephaly (failures in the development of two hemispheres) can be detected at 11–13 weeks and may be associated with aneuploidies (Fig. 17.8).

Evaluation of the intracranial translucency (Fig. 17.9) may be an earlier marker for neural tube defects. Major facial defects including larger facial clefts can also be identified.

Limb abnormalities: Conditions like amelia (absence of limbs) or talipes (clubfoot) may be detected in early ultrasounds, though detailed anatomy scans later in pregnancy are more informative and can better evaluate skeletal malformations and dysplasias.

Thorax and heart: 50% of diaphragmatic hernias may be identified within the first trimester. A proportion of congenital cardiac defects can be detected (Fig. 17.10) although the rates of detection increase appreciably if the period of examination

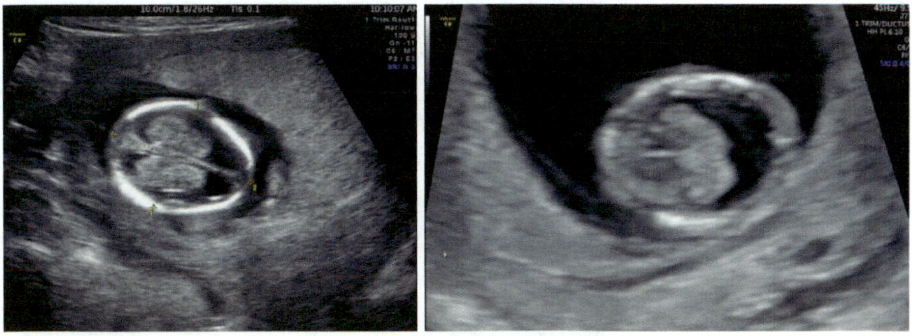

Fig. 17.8 The fetus on the left demonstrates the normal midline division of the brain, the gray areas inside the skull being the choroid plexuses. The fetus on the right demonstrates alobar holoprosencephaly with a single large anterior ventricle that crosses the midline with failure of division of the forebrain into its two hemispheres

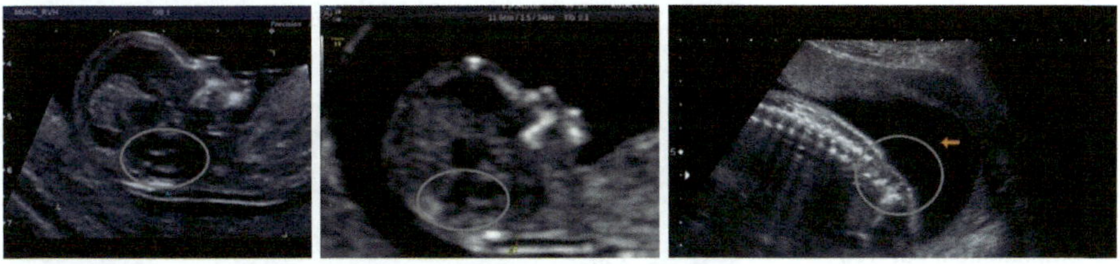

Fig. 17.9 The fetus in the left image demonstrates a normal intracranial translucency (highlighted), the center image demonstrates a fetus with obliteration of the cisterna magna (the lowest horizontal black space in the highlighted area of the left image), an early marker of NTD with an open spina bifida seen in the right image which demonstrates a defect exposing neural tissue at the base of the spine (highlighted)

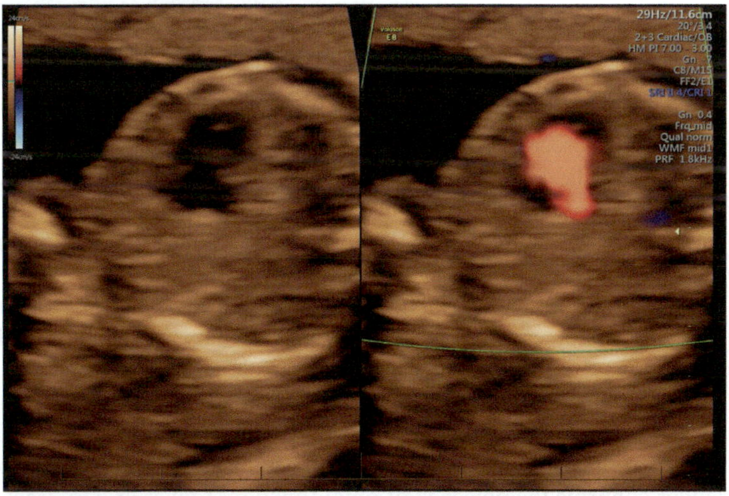

Fig. 17.10 Figure of the heart showing a single ventricle in place of two distinct ventricles being seen in a case of hypoplastic left heart, the right hand image applies colour Doppler to demonstrated blood flow and highlights the presence of only a single ventricle

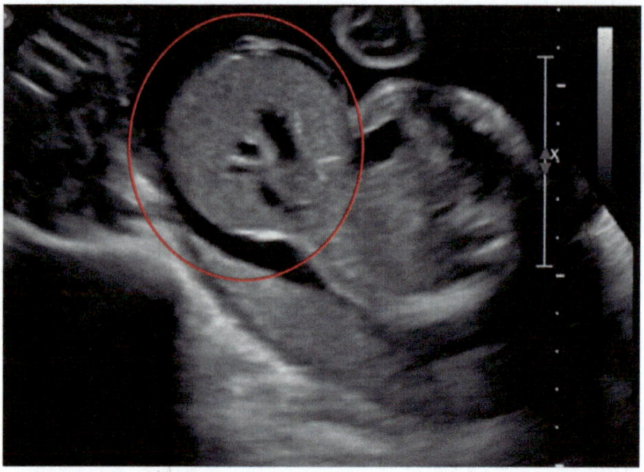

Fig. 17.11 Fetus with an omphalocele. The highlighted area identifies an omphalocele extruding beyond the adjacent abdomen and containing solid organs structures including the liver

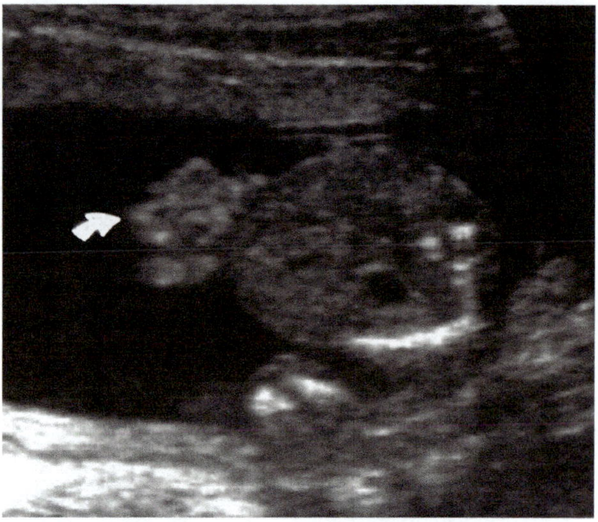

Fig. 17.12 Figure showing a gastroschisis. In this fetus with an abdominal wall defect, free loops of bowel are indicated by the arrow, These are not contained within a membrane as in an omphalocele but free floating in the amniotic fluid

extends into the early second trimester (<15 weeks) [28]. Combined cardio-thoracic malformations like the pentalogy of Cantrell, where the heart sits outside of the chest wall (ectopia cordis) are readily evident by 13 weeks.

Abdomen: Although all fetuses have a physiologic bowel herniation (due to the rate of growth of the bowel exceeding that of the abdomen), this is typically present from 8 + 3 to 10 + 4 weeks at which time the hernia reduces. The presence of an abdominal wall defect can be confirmed with certainty beyond the end of the 11th week and may represent either an omphalocele (Fig. 17.11) (which may be related with fetal aneuploidy) or gastroschisis (Fig. 17.12).

Kidneys and bladder: The kidneys can be seen by the end of the first trimester, but their absence although suspected may not be confirmed until later. The presence of the bladder confirms the presence of renal function. Lower urinary tract outflow obstruction may present with massive dilatation of the bladder—megacystis (Fig. 17.13).

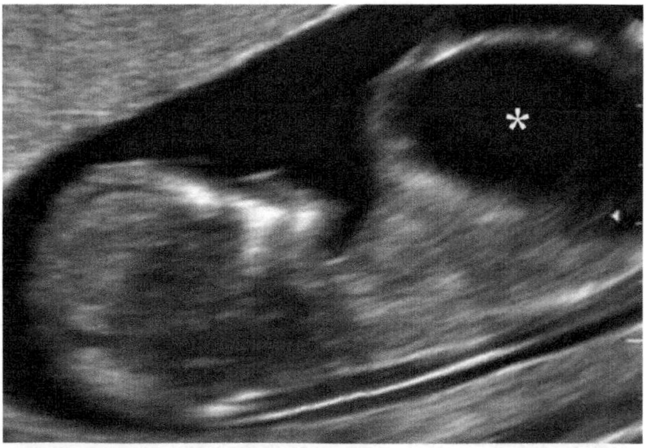

Fig. 17.13 Megacystis. In this 12-week fetus, a lower urinary tract obstruction (LUTO) has resulted in massive distension of the bladder (indicated by the star)

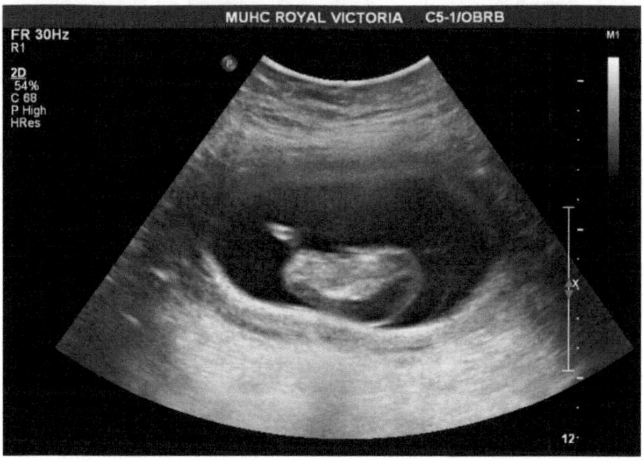

Fig. 17.14 The demised "acardiac" twin in a case of twin-reverse arterial perfusion sequence demonstrates no normal cephalic structures and an increased nuchal translucency extending into generalized skin edema (the black space seen beneath the body)

Anomalies of twinning: Cases of twin reverse arterial perfusion sequence, a rare complication of monochorionic twins, can be identified often by the end of the first trimester. In this condition, one twin's heart either never forms properly or stops; however, because of the anastomoses that exist between the twin's circulations in the shared placenta, the surviving twin continues to perfuse itself and its' demised sibling. This demised fetus may continue to grow, but with incomplete perfusion of the limbs and extremities, including the head, which may atrophy resulting in an amorphous torso; which gave rise to the prior name of this condition describing the demised twin as an "acardic monster" (Fig. 17.14).

17.10 Screening for Pre-eclampsia and Fetal Growth Restriction

Uterine artery Doppler (Fig. 17.15) is a valuable screening tool used in early pregnancy to assess the risk of preeclampsia, a serious hypertensive disorder that can complicate pregnancy and early onset fetal growth restriction (FGR). Increased

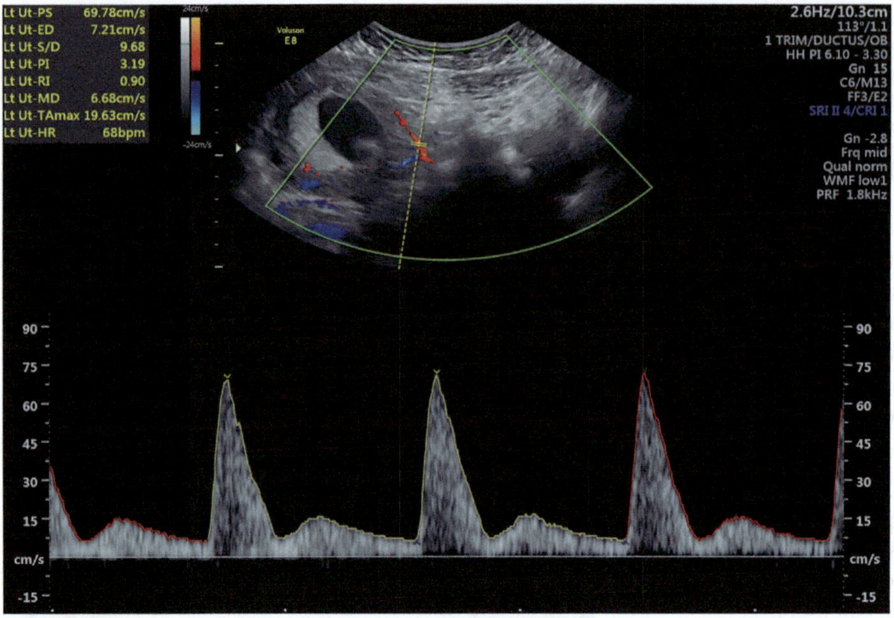

Fig. 17.15 Example of assessment of the uterine artery Doppler, used together with maternal risk factors and biochemical markers in the screening for preeclampsia

resistance in the uterine arteries, reflected by high pulsatility indices on Doppler evaluation, may indicate impaired blood flow to the placenta and a higher risk for these conditions. Between 11 and 14 weeks of gestation, uterine artery Doppler screening may be combined with other risk factors, such as maternal history and biochemical markers, including placental-like growth factor (PLGF), to improve predictive accuracy. Early identification of women at high risk allows for potential interventions, such as low-dose aspirin (150–175 mg), that has been shown to reduce the likelihood of early-onset preeclampsia and its associated complications and of early-onset FGR.

References

1. Wilcox AJ, et al. Incidence of early loss of pregnancy. N Engl J Med. 1988;319(4):189–94.
2. Zinaman MJ, et al. Estimates of human fertility and pregnancy loss. Fertil Steril. 1996;65(3):503–9.
3. Stephenson MD, Awartani KA, Robinson WP. Cytogenetic analysis of miscarriages from couples with recurrent miscarriage: a case-control study. Hum Reprod. 2002;17(2):446–51.
4. Practice Committee of the American Society for reproductive. Evaluation and treatment of recurrent pregnancy loss: a committee opinion. Fertil Steril. 2012;98(5):1103–11.
5. Giakoumelou S, et al. The role of infection in miscarriage. Hum Reprod Update. 2016;22(1):116–33.
6. Panelli DM, Phillips CH, Brady PC. Incidence, diagnosis and management of tubal and non-tubal ectopic pregnancies: a review. Fertil Res Pract. 2015;1:15.

7. Santos-Ribeiro S, Tournaye H, Polyzos NP. Trends in ectopic pregnancy rates following assisted reproductive technologies in the UK: a 12-year nationwide analysis including 160 000 pregnancies. Hum Reprod. 2016;31(2):393–402.
8. Singh S. Diagnosis and management of cervical ectopic pregnancy. J Hum Reprod Sci. 2013;6(4):273–6.
9. Iloabachie GC, Igwegbe AO, Izuora KL. Cervico-isthmic twin pregnancy carried to 37 weeks. Int J Gynaecol Obstet. 1993;40(1):59–61.
10. Kayem G, et al. Conservative management of a near-term cervico-isthmic pregnancy, followed by a successful subsequent pregnancy: a case report. Fertil Steril. 2008;89(6):1826 e13–5.
11. Lin R, DiCenzo N, Rosen T. Cesarean scar ectopic pregnancy: nuances in diagnosis and treatment. Fertil Steril. 2023;120(3 Pt 2):563–72.
12. Atrash HK, Friede A, Hogue CJ. Abdominal pregnancy in the United States: frequency and maternal mortality. Obstet Gynecol. 1987;69(3 Pt 1):333–7.
13. Hymel JA, et al. Late abdominal pregnancies (>/=20 weeks gestation): a review from 1965 to 2012. Gynecol Obstet Investig. 2015;80(4):253–8.
14. Brent GA, Hershman JM. In: Martini L, editor. Thyroid disease and pregnancy, in Encyclopedia of endocrine diseases. Academic Press; 2004. p. 395-400.
15. Oudman E, et al. Wernicke's encephalopathy in hyperemesis gravidarum: a systematic review. Eur J Obstet Gynecol Reprod Biol. 2019;236:84–93.
16. Ngan HYS, et al. Update on the diagnosis and management of gestational trophoblastic disease. Int J Gynaecol Obstet. 2018;143(Suppl 2):79–85.
17. Eiriksson L, et al. Guideline no. 408: management of gestational trophoblastic diseases. J Obstet Gynaecol Can. 2021;43(1):91–105.
18. Sepulveda W, Sebire NJ, Nicolaides KH. The lambda sign in twin pregnancies. Ultrasound Obstet Gynecol. 1996;8(6):429.
19. Gadsboll K, et al. Current use of noninvasive prenatal testing in Europe, Australia and the USA: a graphical presentation. Acta Obstet Gynecol Scand. 2020;99(6):722–30.
20. Van Den Bogaert K, et al. Outcome of publicly funded nationwide first-tier noninvasive prenatal screening. Genet Med. 2021;23(6):1137–42.
21. Papatheodorou SI, et al. First-trimester ductus venosus screening for cardiac defects: a meta-analysis. BJOG. 2011;118(12):1438–45.
22. Rossi AC, Prefumo F. Accuracy of ultrasonography at 11-14 weeks of gestation for detection of fetal structural anomalies: a systematic review. Obstet Gynecol. 2013;122(6):1160-7.
23. Simula N, et al. Committee opinion no. 418: the complete 11-14 week prenatal sonographic examination. J Obstet Gynaecol Can. 2021;43(8):1013-21.
24. Carvalho JS. Fetal heart scanning in the first trimester. Prenat Diagn. 2004;24(13):1060-7.

The Role of the Mental Health Professional in the ART Clinic

18

Alice D. Domar, Michele Martens, and Margaux Eller

Key PointsSymptoms of anxiety and depression are common in the infertility patient population; REI nurses are frequently burdened with the need to support and counsel patients without adequate training or time; mental health professionals specially trained in this field can help relieve this burden.

18.1 Introduction

Infertility is increasingly becoming an obstacle for individuals and couples trying to get pregnant both in the United States and across the world. The World Health Organization defines infertility as "a disease of the male or female reproductive system defined by the failure to achieve pregnancy after 12 months or more of regular unprotected sexual intercourse" [9]. The causes of infertility can be diverse, ranging from tubal disorders in both men and women, uterine or ovary disorders, endocrine/hormonal disorders, and obstructions of the reproductive tract [9]. Additionally, lifestyle factors, including smoking, alcohol consumption, obesity, and exposure to pollutants, can also play a role in one's fertility [9]. Regardless of the root cause of

A. D. Domar (✉)
Inception Research Institute, Harvard Medical School, Houston, TX, USA
e-mail: adomar@inceptionllc.com

M. Martens
Department of Nursing, Vanderbilt University School of Nursing, Nashville, TN, USA
e-mail: michele.martens@vanderbilt.edu

M. Eller
Inception Research Institute, Inception Fertility, Middlebury College,
Houston, TX: Middlebury, VT, USA

M. Das, M. H. Dahan (eds.), *A Comprehensive Guide to Reproductive Health and Infertility Medicine for Nurses*, https://doi.org/10.1007/978-3-032-24372-0_18

infertility, its impacts can vary extensively, affecting intimacy and the psychosocial and financial aspects of a relationship. Further, the psychological effects can manifest emotionally, mentally, or physiologically. Not only can the impacts of infertility be pervasive in one's daily life, but the impact of fertility treatment can be quite burdensome. Fertility treatment options can vary; however, most require extensive appointments and doctor's visits resulting in emotional and financial stress. Furthermore, many people pursue fertility treatments without success, resulting in additional stress and turmoil leading to a variety of health and psychological effects.

Infertility can be a long journey for many people. Due to the high stress associated with it, healthcare workers can play an important role in managing some of the impacts of infertility. In particular, nurses are vital to supporting patients during fertility treatment and offer other parallel support. This can include educational material on fertility treatment, emotional support, as well as physical support throughout the treatment process [24]. Because of the support needed, this often creates close relationships between nurses and their infertility patients which can increase the emotional burden associated with the field. Nurses across all healthcare fields are experiencing burnout, but nurses working in assisted reproductive services showed significantly higher levels of burnout including emotional exhaustion, depersonalization, and low personal accomplishment [21]. Again, this could be for many reasons, but may be due to the highly emotional and delicate nature of the field. This, in turn, can lead to nurses experiencing burnout and mental exhaustion from supporting their patients.

Further exploration of the impact of infertility, treatment, and pregnancy loss can provide a deeper understanding of this common issue faced by many. Currently, there is a lack of nursing textbooks on fertility care and assisted conception. Therefore, increasing knowledge about the psychological effects of these issues can better prepare healthcare workers, primarily nurses, who frequently interact with fertility patients. This will enhance their ability to provide comprehensive care by equipping them with background information on infertility and its wide-ranging impacts on overall well-being.

18.2 Impact of Infertility

Infertility can have wide-ranging effects on an individual's life, including physiological, financial, social, and psychological. These effects can be significant for both men and women and may involve emotional and mental health challenges in addition to physical concerns.

The physical effects of infertility in women can include hormonal imbalances, stress-related symptoms, and treatment-related side effects. Hormones and inflammatory markers play a crucial role in reproductive functioning, making it essential to understand these mechanisms when addressing infertility as a broader issue. Ovulatory disorders account for up to half of infertility cases among couples and individuals trying to get pregnant [20], so discussing these disorders and their physical effects on women is vital for a comprehensive understanding of infertility. Polyendocrine metabolic ovarian syndrome (PMOS) is one of the most common reproductive disorders, affecting 4–29% of women of reproductive age [22]. PMOS not only increases the risk of health complications, such as obesity and insulin resistance, but also negatively impacts fertility and pregnancy outcomes. In addition to PMOS, other endocrine disorders—including congenital adrenal hyperplasia, prolactinomas or pituitary tumors, and hypothalamic dysfunction—can impair reproductive health [20]. These conditions affect hormone levels, which can influence mood, energy levels, and metabolism, further exacerbating fertility issues. Hormonal imbalances may lead to weight fluctuations and digestive problems. When these physical challenges are combined with the emotional stress of infertility, they can further complicate the well-being of those affected.

Infertility not only affects one physically but also has significant psychological impacts. Receiving an infertility diagnosis can be overwhelming and distressing for those trying to get pregnant, leading to feelings of anger, guilt, sadness, depression, and anxiety [18]. Psychosocially, people may experience low self-esteem, reduced quality of life, and social isolation [18]. Research has shown that approximately 40% of couples seeking infertility treatment meet the criteria for a preexisting psychiatric disorder [13]. Among these conditions, generalized anxiety disorder is the most common, followed by major depressive disorder and dysthymia. Infertility patients also report significantly higher rates of depression and anxiety—ranging from 25% to 60% higher—compared to their fertile counterparts [13]. Additionally, there is a six times higher prevalence of eating disorders in infertile patients undergoing fertility treatment compared to pregnant individuals with no history of infertility [11]. The psychological burden of infertility is significant. Despite clear evidence of distress, accurately assessing the emotional suffering in women with infertility remains challenging, partly due to the limitations of self-report measures. Some researchers suggest that women may "fake good" in order to appear healthier than they actually are [16]. Many women choose to conceal their emotional struggles as a coping mechanism or to maintain an outward appearance of optimism during infertility treatment. However, numerous studies have shown that both women and men dealing with infertility report higher levels of depression and anxiety compared to their fertile counterparts. For example, a longitudinal study conducted in California revealed that 56.5% of women and 32.1% of men scored in the clinical range for depressive symptoms, while 75.9% of women and 60.6% of men fell in the clinical range for anxiety [15]. These findings highlight the widespread psychological distress experienced by individuals coping with infertility.

18.3 The Impact of Fertility Treatment

For many individuals pursuing pregnancy, fertility treatment represents the hope of having a biological child. However, it is essential to recognize that the process of fertility treatment is rarely straightforward. Not only is treatment a significant financial commitment, but it also involves numerous doctor's appointments and various medical procedures. While infertility is not uncommon and fertility treatments are increasingly utilized to assist many in conceiving, the journey can be burdensome. Continuous treatment can profoundly affect an individual's overall well-being. Numerous studies have explored the psychological impacts of fertility treatments, particularly those involving assisted reproductive technology (ART), revealing that these treatments can have varied and complex effects on women undergoing treatment [18]. The psychological effects of infertility and infertility treatment can be profound and life-altering. To contextualize this, one study compared the psychological symptoms of infertile women with those of patients suffering from other chronic medical conditions, including chronic pain, cardiac rehabilitation needs, cancer, hypertension, and those who are HIV-positive. The participants completed a symptoms checklist, and the results showed that infertile women had overall symptom scores equivalent to those of patients with cancer, those requiring cardiac rehabilitation, and those with hypertension. However, their scores were lower than those of patients experiencing chronic pain and those who are HIV-positive [5]. These findings reveal that the psychological symptoms faced by infertile individuals are equivalent to those associated with other serious medical conditions. Therefore, appropriate medical and psychological interventions, which are typically implemented for chronic conditions, should similarly be implemented for those undergoing infertility treatment. A recent stressor that has impacted many individuals' lives is/was the COVID-19 pandemic. It has had a significant psychological effect on individuals, influencing various aspects of life, including economic, political, and social dimensions. A study surveying non-pregnant women found that the stress of infertility has become a significant concern comparable to the stress of the pandemic itself [23].

For pregnant women undergoing assisted reproductive technology (ART), one study revealed that during the early stages of the pandemic, COVID-19 was a stressor; however, those still facing infertility ranked it as a greater source of stress than the pandemic [4]. Additionally, patients who became pregnant after ART reported heightened stress levels related to the pandemic [4]. Receiving fertility treatment and reproductive therapy is already a challenging, and the pandemic compounded these difficulties, disrupting the treatment process for many patients. Pregnant individuals also faced significant concerns about contracting the virus and its effects on pregnancy outcomes. Given the circumstances surrounding COVID-19 and the ongoing threat of airborne illnesses, medical personnel who work with infertility patients should incorporate stress reduction strategies into their treatment protocols. Moreover, more research is needed on stress management for pregnant women who have undergone ART. It is crucial for healthcare providers working in the fertility field to understand and recognize the various treatments that can impact their patients. Evidence indicates that a perceived lack of empathy from healthcare professionals can significantly increase the distress experienced by couples undergoing fertility treatment [13]. This emotional disconnect can adversely affect treatment outcomes and may lead some to discontinue treatment if they feel unsupported.

Practicing empathy and understanding with patients can help prevent psychological distress and alleviate some of the burdens associated with infertility. A study evaluated how training physicians in empathic skills affected patient satisfaction after their first consultation in a fertility clinic. Researchers used a self-rating questionnaire to assess various aspects of care, including information provided, the dynamics of the visit, the time dedicated, patient-physician interaction, and physician expertise. The results indicated that empathic training led to higher satisfaction scores from patients and a decreased likelihood of lower ratings across all evaluation criteria [8]. Thus, training physicians, nurses, and other medical personnel involved in the fertility treatment process can enhance patient satisfaction and begin to mitigate some of the psychological challenges such treatment often entails.

The burden of fertility treatment can be significant, and it becomes even more challenging when treatments are unsuccessful. Studies have shown that recurrent pregnancy loss following assisted reproduction can be a triggering factor for prolonged grief and mourning [3]. One study found that 30–40% of women undergoing fertility treatment experience varying levels of depressive or anxious symptoms [2]. Although the relationship between psychological stress and treatment success is not well understood, some studies suggest that the stress experienced during fertility treatments may negatively impact conception rates [14]. Therefore, it is essential to recognize the psychological toll that fertility treatment can impose, both for patient care and to enhance future treatment protocols. Fertility treatment presents significant emotional and psychological challenges, highlighting the need for psychosocial care and support for women before, during, and after treatment. This support is essential not only for short-term coping but also for long-term psychological recovery. Unfortunately, such support is often inadequate, and partners may unintentionally dismiss the emotional pain women experience throughout the treatment process [3]. Healthcare providers should be equipped to address these concerns and offer the emotional and psychological support necessary to help their patients navigate the complexities of infertility treatment.

Fertility treatments can have a range of physical side effects in addition to their psychological impacts. Common side effects include weight fluctuations, bloating, hot flashes, bruising from injections, and pelvic discomfort. The severity and types of side effects can vary among individuals. Many fertility treatments involve hormone therapy, which may lead to symptoms such as spotting, breast tenderness, nausea, and mood changes [1]. As the treatment continues, particularly if egg stimulation is required, women may experience headaches, nausea, bloating, hot flashes, and breast tenderness [1]. After egg retrieval, patients may also face additional symptoms, such as vomiting, constipation, and exacerbated bloating [1]. When fertility treatment is unsuccessful, the emotional impact can be significant, often resulting in grief and frustration for women and their partners.

As infertility treatments continue to evolve, it is essential for healthcare professionals to understand the various challenges their patients encounter. This awareness is necessary not only to improve treatment outcomes but also to provide comprehensive care that addresses the emotional, psychological, and physical needs of those undergoing these treatments. Future research continues to investigate the complex interactions between psychological, physiological, and systemic factors to create more supportive, patient-centered treatment models.

18.4 The Role of the Mental Health Professional in the ART Clinic

Several decades ago, it was common for infertility clinics to have an "embedded" mental health professional (MHP) who was an integral part of the health care team. They would be available to patients in crisis, such as when a prenatal scan did not show a heartbeat, or a patient woke up in the PACU and had fewer oocytes retrieved than anticipated. They were also available to employees, especially nurses, who needed immediate support, such as when a patient lost their temper at them or a favorite patient suffered yet another pregnancy loss. The MHP would also see individuals and couples for therapy, to discuss marital issues exacerbated by the infertility, coping skills for infertility and treatment, supporting them after a pregnancy loss, discussing the psychological ramifications of moving on to more intensive treatment, supporting them throughout that treatment, and helping them cope and make decisions when genetic parenthood was determined to be unlikely. Some clinics had/have a policy that all new patients had to meet with one of the MHPs to receive support and information even before treatment began. That way, if the patients(s) needed more support or faced a crisis, they already had their own MHP with whom to reconnect. However, as time went on, the role of the MHP slowly changed to primarily providing the psychological testing for patients moving on to third-party treatment.

Currently, there are only a few infertility clinics in the USA, which actually still employ an MHP, and these are primarily academic medical centers. Most private clinics maintain a list of recommended MHPs in the area and distressed patients are simply provided with this list. The main responsibility of MHPs in the USA is to do the third-party testing to meet ASRM guidelines.

The lack of inclusion of MHPs in the infertility clinic during current times is likely due to financial factors—some clinics provided their services for free to patients, paying the salary themselves, while other clinics billed insurance, which likely did not cover the cost of the MHP's salary. So many embedded MHPs were let go, primarily because of the cost burden.

However, this seems to be short-sighted. Patients drop out of treatment frequently; uninsured patients because of cost, but insured patients drop out because of the emotional burden of treatment. If an embedded MHP can support one patient per month to stay in treatment rather than dropping out, that would likely cover their salary. Furthermore, REI nursing turnover has increased significantly over the past few years (internal ASRM data), and some estimate that the cost of losing a nurse can reach $300,000 (RMA-Philadelphia presented data). If an embedded MHP can provide support and coping skills to just one nurse per year who decides to remain in her job, then that again would cover the MHP's salary for a couple of years.

An author of this chapter (ADD) is trying to reverse this trend by piloting a program in the Inception/Prelude network of clinics where she is employed. The model is to have a psychologist on site for 4 h/week (i.e., a half day) to see any patients or employees in crisis and then to be available via phone or remote for an additional hour/week. The cost to the clinic is minimal, and treatment termination rates and staff turnover are being tracked to determine the impact of the embedded MHP. If successful, the same model will be applied to the other clinics in the network.

18.5 Psychological Interventions

Infertility and its treatment can lead to a wide array of psychological, physical, and emotional challenges. Therefore, it is essential to implement interventions that address these issues, especially if there is no embedded MHP in the patient's clinic. Specifically, strategies aimed at reducing distress are essential for enhancing psychological well-being. Improving psychological health can lead to a better quality of life and may also potentially increase the chances of achieving a successful pregnancy. Previous research and literature reviews have shown mixed results regarding the efficacy of psychological interventions. A meta-analysis conducted in 2022 demonstrated that the number of randomized control trials testing the efficacy of psychological interventions for infertility outcomes and pregnancy rates has more than doubled over the past 10 years [6] This meta-analysis found that there were beneficial effects on psychological outcomes, but this varied by location internationally [6]. However, they found that in most regions of the world, psychological interventions were associated with reductions in distress and had modest effects on conception. In an earlier study, one meta-analysis from 2005 found that both individual/couple therapy and group interventions effectively reduced emotional distress and increased conception rates [19]. More recently, research has indicated that women who receive psychological intervention are approximately twice as likely to become pregnant compared to those who did not receive such support, with noticeable improvements in general psychological symptoms such as anxiety and depression [7]. Additionally, a meta-analysis of 39 studies revealed that psychosocial interventions, particularly cognitive behavioral therapy and mindfulness-based interventions, are highly beneficial in reducing distress and improving pregnancy outcomes in ART [7]. An additional meta-analysis of 15 randomized controlled trials assessed the impact of psychosocial intervention on pregnancy outcomes in women and couples undergoing ART treatment [10]. The findings suggest that psychosocial interventions are positively associated with significant increases in pregnancy rates in infertile women and couples undergoing ART treatment [10]. Decreasing the psychological stressors associated with infertility can significantly improve quality of life and may enhance one's ability to cope with stress, potentially increasing the likelihood of pregnancy. Therefore, medical providers should take these findings into account during fertility treatment. They should also strive to implement and enhance psychological and psychosocial interventions to optimize outcomes for their patients facing infertility challenges.

18.5.1 Impact of Pregnancy Loss

Infertility is a challenging struggle that many individuals and couples encounter while trying to conceive. Coping with pregnancy loss during this journey can be particularly traumatic and emotionally devastating. To comprehend the impact of pregnancy loss, it is essential to first define the various types of loss that individuals may experience. Pregnancy loss, which includes miscarriage and ectopic pregnancy, refers to any loss that occurs prior to 20 weeks of gestation. In contrast, stillbirth is defined as the death of a fetus after 20 weeks of pregnancy, while neonatal death refers to the death of a newborn within the first 28 days post-birth miscarriages. Additional forms of pregnancy loss include chemical pregnancies (a positive pregnancy test that then decreases to zero within a few days or a week) and early miscarriages. Research has shown that experiences such as abortion, fetal death, and reproductive failure can significantly impact the psychological well-being of infertile couples and individuals trying to get pregnant, often leading to profound emotional suffering [17].

The psychological effects of pregnancy loss can be profound and far-reaching. Common emotional responses include intense sadness, depression, irritability, anxiety, and worry. A study examining 316 women undergoing infertility treatment found that the most frequently reported negative emotional reactions to pregnancy loss include depression, despair, guilt, anger, anxiety, and frustration, particularly when treatment was unsuccessful [3]. Notably, reactions to pregnancy loss was the most common symptom reported among women coping with infertility and pregnancy loss. These emotional responses can be further intensified by the already significant emotional burden of infertility itself.

Experiencing pregnancy loss is extremely challenging and having a strong support system can be crucial in coping with associated grief. Unfortunately, some individuals undergoing fertility treatment may not have a robust support network, which can increase their emotional burden. For these individuals, receiving support from their healthcare providers is especially important, as they may be particularly susceptible to feelings of isolation and distress. Healthcare professionals, especially nurses, have a vital and unique role in providing care and emotional support to patients who have experienced pregnancy loss. Nurses are often heavily involved in fertility treatment and are positioned to offer empathy and compassionate care. Unless their clinic has an embedded MHP, or one readily available, it falls to the nursing staff to provide this care. It is crucial for medical staff to use language that reflects the sensitivity of the situation. For example, nurses can provide supportive phrases such as:

- I am truly sorry to share this information with you.
- I know this is not what you were hoping or expecting to hear.
- This news can be very difficult to process and you may find it surprising and shocking.
- You may have many questions after receiving this news. Please feel free to call me when you're ready to talk.
- Most people prefer not to be alone after receiving this type of information. Would you like to have your partner, a parent, or a close friend with you for support?

Pregnancy loss is a topic that is not widely discussed, and as a result, many experiencing it may often feel confused or lost. It is essential for healthcare providers to recognize that, according to the American College of Obstetricians and Gynecologists, early pregnancy loss occurs in approximately 10% of confirmed pregnancies [12].

Additionally, stillbirths—defined as the loss of a fetus after the 20th week—occur in about 1 in 160 deliveries [12]. Studies estimate that 15–20% of all pregnancies end in miscarriage, with 75% of these losses occurring within the first 12 weeks [12]. Furthermore, 75% of pregnancies in women over the age of 45 result in miscarriage. These statistics highlight the prevalence of pregnancy loss and emphasize the importance of providing psychological support to patients facing these challenges.

In addition to emotional support, healthcare providers can offer patients various coping strategies to help them navigate the challenging experience of pregnancy loss. These strategies include:

- Practicing self-compassion and being kind to oneself
- Leaning on social support systems, such as family and friends
- Establishing a relaxation routine that may include meditation, imagery, yoga, autogenic training, breath focus, or mindfulness
- Creating space for mourning and allowing time for emotional processing
- Encouraging emotional expression and communication

Infertility and pregnancy loss present complex challenges that require comprehensive, empathetic, and evidence-based psychological support. Because most clinics don't have an MHP on site or readily available, healthcare providers must recognize and integrate the profound psychological impact of reproductive health issues into fertility care protocols. Future research should continue to investigate the complex relationship between physiological reproductive issues and psychological well-being. Such research will help develop more sophisticated, holistic approaches to fertility treatment, ultimately providing patients a more supportive and comprehensive care experience. Ideally, the old model of having an embedded MHP in the infertility clinic will in fact "make a comeback,' providing patients with the emotional support and coping skills training they need, leaving the nursing staff to do the jobs they were trained to do, and lessening the burdens they experience.

References

1. Alicea B. In vitro fertilization (IVF) side effects at each stage. Illume Fertility; 2023. https://www.illumefertility.com/fertility-blog/in-vitro-fertilization-ivf-side-effects-at-each-stage.
2. Chen T-H, Chang S-P, Tsai C-F, Juang K-D. Prevalence of depressive and anxiety disorders in an assisted reproductive technique clinic. Hum Reprod. 2004;19(10):2313–8. https://doi.org/10.1093/humrep/deh414.
3. de Castro MHM, Mendonça CR, Noll M, de Abreu Tacon FS, do Amaral WN. Psychosocial aspects of gestational grief in women undergoing infertility treatment: a systematic review of qualitative and quantitative evidence. Int J Environ Res Public Health. 2021;18(24):13143. https://doi.org/10.3390/ijerph182413143.
4. Domar AD, Shah JS, Gompers AD, Meyers AJ, Hacker MR, Penzias AS, Sakkas D, Toth TL, Vaughan DA. The psychological impact of the COVID-19 pandemic on women pregnant following art: a longitudinal study. Fertil Steril. 2021;116(3):e364. https://doi.org/10.1016/j.fertnstert.2021.07.977.

5. Domar AD, Zuttermeister PC, Friedman R. The psychological impact of infertility: a comparison with patients with other medical conditions. J Psychosom Obstet Gynaecol. 1993;(14 Suppl):45–52.
6. Dube L, Bright K, Hayden KA, Gordon JL. Efficacy of psychological interventions for mental health and pregnancy rates among individuals with infertility: a systematic review and meta-analysis. Hum Reprod Update. 2023;29(1):71–94. https://doi.org/10.1093/humupd/dmac034.
7. Frederiksen Y, Farver-Vestergaard I, Skovgård NG, Ingerslev HJ, Zachariae R. Efficacy of psychosocial interventions for psychological and pregnancy outcomes in infertile women and men: a systematic review and meta-analysis. BMJ Open. 2015;5(1):e006592. https://doi.org/10.1136/bmjopen-2014-006592.
8. García D, Bautista O, Venereo L, Coll O, Vassena R, Vernaeve V. Training in empathic skills improves the patient-physician relationship during the first consultation in a fertility clinic. Fertil Steril. 2013;99(5):1413–8. https://doi.org/10.1016/j.fertnstert.2012.12.012.
9. Infertility. (2024). https://www.who.int/news-room/fact-sheets/detail/infertility.
10. Katyal N, Poulsen CM, Knudsen UB, Frederiksen Y. The association between psychosocial interventions and fertility treatment outcome: a systematic review and meta-analysis. Eur J Obstet Gynecol Reprod Biol. 2021;259:125–32. https://doi.org/10.1016/j.ejogrb.2021.02.012.
11. Le Floch M, Crohin A, Duverger P, Picard A, Legendre G, Riquin E. Prevalence and phenotype of eating disorders in assisted reproduction: a systematic review. Reprod Health. 2022;19:38. https://doi.org/10.1186/s12978-022-01341-w.
12. Management of Stillbirth. (n.d.). Retrieved 15 Dec 2024, from https://www.acog.org/clinical/clinical-guidance/obstetric-care-consensus/articles/2020/03/management-of-stillbirth.
13. Martens M, Schroer M, Williams T, Kennedy B. Identifying mental health issues associated with infertility. J Nurse Pract. 2023;19(2):104471. https://doi.org/10.1016/j.nurpra.2022.09.024.
14. Matthiesen SMS, Frederiksen Y, Ingerslev HJ, Zachariae R. Stress, distress and outcome of assisted reproductive technology (ART): a meta-analysis. Hum Reprod. 2011;26(10):2763–76. https://doi.org/10.1093/humrep/der246.
15. Pasch LA, Holley SR, Bleil ME, Shchab D, Katz PP, Adler NE. Addressing the needs of fertility treatment patients and their partners: are they informed of and do they receive mental health services? Fertil Steril. 2016;106(1):209–215.e2. https://doi.org/10.1016/j.fertnstert.2016.03.006.
16. Rooney KL, Domar AD. The relationship between stress and infertility. Dialogues Clin Neurosci. 2018;20(1):41–7. https://doi.org/10.31887/DCNS.2018.20.1/klrooney.
17. Schwerdtfeger KL, Shreffler KM. Trauma of pregnancy loss and infertility for mothers and involuntarily childless women in the contemporary United States. J Loss Trauma. 2009;14(3):211–27. https://doi.org/10.1080/15325020802537468.
18. Sharma A, Shrivastava D. Psychological problems related to infertility. Cureus. 2022;14(10):e30320. https://doi.org/10.7759/cureus.30320.
19. Strauss B, de Liz TM. Differential efficacy of group and individual/couple psychotherapy with infertile patients. Hum Reprod. 2005;20(5):1324–32. Oxford Academic. Retrieved January 27, 2025, from https://academic.oup.com/humrep/article-abstract/20/5/1324/2356650.
20. Unuane D, Tournaye H, Velkeniers B, Poppe K. Endocrine disorders & female infertility. Best Pract Res Clin Endocrinol Metab. 2011;25(6):861–73. https://doi.org/10.1016/j.beem.2011.08.001.
21. Urteaga R, & Díaz A. (2024). Burnout in assisted reproduction professionals: The influence of stressors in the workplace. Healthcare, 12(21), 2136. https://doi.org/10.3390/healthcare12212136.
22. Vannuccini S, Clifton VL, Fraser IS, Taylor HS, Critchley H, Giudice LC, Petraglia F. Infertility and reproductive disorders: impact of hormonal and inflammatory mechanisms on pregnancy outcome. Hum Reprod Update. 2016;22(1):104–15. https://doi.org/10.1093/humupd/dmv044.
23. Vaughan DA, Shah JS, Penzias AS, Domar AD, Toth TL. Infertility remains a top stressor despite the COVID-19 pandemic. Reprod Biomed Online. 2020;41(3):425–7. https://doi.org/10.1016/j.rbmo.2020.05.015.
24. Wang J, Li L, Zhou J, Pan X, Qi Q, Sun H, & Wang L. (2024). Patient satisfaction with nursing care in infertility patients: A questionnaire survey. Global Health & Medicine, 6(2), 141–148. https://doi.org/10.35772/ghm.2023.01044

Religious and Social Views, Ethics and Legislation

19

Rabbi Gideon Weitzman

In contrast to the rest of this volume, the current chapter does not deal with what can be done but, rather, with what should be done. Each society has restrictions and guidelines[1] when dealing with fertility testing and treatment. These constraints will impact the operation of fertility clinics and are dependent on the particular society. It is, therefore, imperative that the medical professionals are familiar with the particular precincts that are relevant to the lives of their patients.

We will discuss these in three areas: a. religious beliefs and practices, as they relate to fertility and reproductive technology, b. ethical considerations and principles to be considered when administering fertility treatment, and c. legal regulations in the practice of fertility medicine.

19.1 Religion[2]

Each religion holds a system of beliefs regarding the sanctity of life and preservation of such sanctity. Religions can be categorized based on their view of man's ability to interact with the divinely created world, and when the boundaries of

[1] 1 Be they formal or informal, they possess varying degrees of obligation and consequence if transgressed. These range from legal action, social shunning, and the fear of divine retribution and damnation.

[2] I have relied heavily on Eric Blyth and Ruth Landau's comprehensive book, Faith and Fertility, which is highly recommended for those seeking to expand their knowledge on this subject. I was honored to contribute a chapter to their volume, on Orthodox Judaism and fertility.

R. G. Weitzman (✉)
PUAH Institute, Jerusalem, Israel
e-mail: questions@puah.org.il

M. Das, M. H. Dahan (eds.), *A Comprehensive Guide to Reproductive Health and Infertility Medicine for Nurses*, https://doi.org/10.1007/978-3-032-24372-0_19

interfering with God's creation have been traversed. All religions and religious adherents have a relationship and an interaction with God and the Divine.

While each religion has its own expression, creed, and deed, there are common elements to each religion. Religions believe in a higher power that they consider holy and sacred. Religion is concerned with the correct way the adherents are to live and the sanctity of life.[3]

People's religiosity may affect their approach to fertility, although there may be a great range of adherence to religious injunction, even among those who consider themselves religious or members of a religious faith. Observance of religious practice may vary, and it cannot always be assumed that religion will, or will not, be a deciding factor in the eventual decision made by the couple.

Even when religion does not have a clear directive regarding fertility and fertility treatment, it has been shown that religion influences fertility and utilizing fertility treatment.[4] Since most religions promote and cherish procreation,[5] it has been claimed that women who are unable to conceive are devalued in religious societies.[6] This could well be part of the impetus for religious women to seek fertility treatment, especially for secondary infertility.

Despite religion's pronatalist stance, specific religions may place significant limitations on utilizing fertility treatment and even oppose some treatments, especially third-party treatments that can be viewed as compromising the sanctity of the exclusive marital bond between husband and wife. This has an impact on legal limitations in countries with a dominant religious population.[7]

In the following passages, we will briefly review some of the attitudes of the more prevalent religions regarding fertility treatment. It should be stressed that some of the information here is the official approach of the religion, and not every congregant will follow the exact injunctions of their religion. No patient should be made to feel inadequate or impious for acting in a way that does not follow entirely the official stance.

---

[3] Many religions believe in an afterlife where reward and punishment are realized, but for the purposes of this chapter we will concentrate on how religion dictates the mode of behavior in this world. For more on the afterlife see the academic work, Philip C Almond, *Afterlife: A History of Life after Death*, London and Ithaca NY: I.B. Tauris and Cornell University Press, 2015, or the more popularist Alan F. Segal, *Life After Death: A History of the Afterlife in Western Religion*, Doubleday, 2004.

[4] Lehrer, E.L. Religion as a determinant of marital fertility. *J Popul Econ* **9**, 173–196 (1996).

[5] See e.g. Adsera A., Religion and changes in family-size norms in developed countries. *Review of Religious Research* **47**, 3, 271–286 (2006).

[6] Inhorn, M.C., (1996) *Infertility and Patriarchy: The Cultural Politics of Gender and Family Life in Egypt*, p. 259, Philadelphia, PA, University of Pennsylvania Press, and Blyth, E., Landau, R., ed. (2009) *Faith and Fertility: Attitudes Towards Reproductive Practices in Different Religions from Ancient to Modern Times*, p. 21, London, Jessica Kingsley Publishers.

[7] See Blyth, E., Landau, R., eds. (2004) *Third Party Assisted Conception Across Cultures: Social, Legal and Ethical Perspectives*, London, Jessica Kingsley Publishers, especially the chapter by Luisa Baron on Argentina and Eleonora Bielawska-Baratowicz on Poland.

In addition, some religions give their spiritual leaders and clergy a degree of autonomy to make decisions that will be followed by their constituents that can depart somewhat from the party's norm. Thus, the medical professional may treat one patient according to the instructions that they received from their clergy and assume that this is what that religion adheres to. Whereas another patient, a co-religionist of the former patient, may have received distinctly different instructions. The medical professional cannot make assumptions regarding how each religious person will act and react. This stresses the need for an open and respectful conversation between the medical professional and the religious patient, and, when necessary, their cleric.

19.2 Catholicism

Catholicism is the religion with the most members worldwide and is family-centric, seeing "God Himself is the author of marriage"[8] and physical contact between man and wife is a divine act and the children produced are "the supreme gift of marriage."[9] Catholicism opposes homosexuality[10] and single women who conceive.[11] The Catholic Church sees the embryo as life and requires that it be cared for like any other human,[12] and does not approve of the storage of embryos. This is true even when the embryo was conceived through in vitro fertilization from the sperm and eggs from a married couple.[13] These limitations can have a serious impact on the normal workings of the fertility clinic. Catholicism does not permit third-party fertility treatment and sees it as immoral and denying the right of the child to know their father and mother, who are married to each other. (Third-party reproduction includes donor sperm, donor eggs, and surrogacy).

The American Catholic Conference of Bishops has presented a slightly more nuanced approach. They stated that "Unfortunately, most Catholics are not aware of the Church's teaching, do not know that IVF is immoral, and some have used it in attempting to have children. If a couple is unaware that the procedure is immoral, they are not subjectively guilty of sin. Children conceived through this procedure

[8] Second Vatican Council, 1998, p. 590.

[9] The Catechism in 2002, which also permitted adoption as a last resort when all other efforts to procreate have failed. It should be stated that the Pontifical Council for Justice and Peace in 2004 stated that marriage is not solely for procreation and marriage is valued and sanctified even of no children were born to the couple.

[10] Catechism, 2002.

[11] Trujillo, A.L., 2003, *The family and life in Europe*, Vatican City, Pontifical Council for the Family, "First, the expression "single-parent family" contains a contradiction in terms. A child *always* has two parents. To speak about a "single-parent family" is to deny the existence of the absent parent, usually the father, and to give credit to the growing matriarchal model." https://www.vatican.va/roman_curia/pontifical_councils/family/documents/rc_pc_family_doc_20030614_family-europe-trujillo_en.html

[12] Catechism 2002.

[13] Donum Vitae, 1987.

are children of God and are loved by their parents, as they should be. Like all children, regardless of the circumstances of their conception and birth, they should be loved, cherished and cared for."[14]

The Catholic Church is clearly opposed to the use of egg donation both on the part of the recipient and the donor[15] as well as the surrogacy and the use of donor sperm.

In conclusion, the Catholic Church is quite strict in its opposition to the use of almost all fertility treatment but does de facto accept and protect the rights of any child conceived in this manner. An exception would be ovarian stimulation and intercourse or insemination, which would not be an issue.

19.3 Protestantism

Protestantism is a reformed Christian religious movement that holds numerous denominations, including Methodist, Presbyterian, Lutheran, Baptist, and Pentecostal. Protestants do not have a pope but a series of ministers and clergy who diffuse the power structure of the church from one monolithic authority.

Martin Luther himself wrote that in the case of childless couple, the wife was permitted to have relations with the husband's brother or close relative in order to have a child.[16] While this could be viewed as a permission for all aspects of fertility treatment, in truth, Protestants vary in their beliefs on IVF, and unlike the Catholic Church, there is not one set of ethical guidelines for Protestant couples to follow regarding its use.[17] Those who support IVF limit its use to married couples. All the embryos must be replaced into the uterus, and selective reduction in the case of high-order pregnancy, which could place the life of the mother or fetuses at risks, is not allowed.[18]

Protestantism treats embryos with respect but does not forbid using preimplantation diagnosis that will lead to the destruction of embryos.[19]

Generally, Protestant denominations have become more accepting of in vitro fertilization and fertility treatments but are less agreeable to third-party treatments.[20]

---

[14] Haas, 1998, *Begotten not made: A Catholic view of reproductive technology,* https://www.usccb.org/issues-and-action/human-life-and-dignity/reproductive-technology/begotten-not-made-a-catholic-view-of-reproductive-technology, Accessed on 12/07/24.

[15] Pontifical Academy for Life, 2004, Tenth General Assembly.

[16] Martin Luther, 1552, *The Estate of Marriage.*

[17] It is indicative to note that one of the few comprehensive discussions of in vitro fertilization and surrogacy, the 1996 Report of the Commission on Theology and Church Relations of The Lutheran Church—Missouri Synod, entitled Christians Procreative Choices, is purposely vague and does not present a directive or a conclusion, rather a number of discussion points to ponder and contemplate.

[18] Sallam HN, Sallam NH. *Religious aspects of assisted reproduction. Facts Views Vis Obgyn.* 2016 Mar 28;8(1):33–48.

[19] Panicola, M., "Remaking ourselves? The ethics of stem-cell research," *Commonweal* 125 (December 4, 1998), 9–10.

[20] Waters, E., Protestant Denominations Need Stronger Leadership on Assisted Reproductive Technology, https://www.heritage.org/marriage-and-family/commentary/protestant-denominations-need-stronger-leadership-assisted, Accessed on 12.30.24.

19.4 Islam

Islam promotes an absolute and unconditional submission to God as revealed in the surah, verses, of the Qur'an.[21] In addition, the prophets' sayings, Hadith; the prophet's actions, Sunnah; and the jurist's decisions, Shariah, guide Islamic creed and deed.[22] Decisions by Islamic lawmakers may also rely on logic, public interest, local custom, and accepted consensus.[23] There is no single authority to determine specific binding laws, and this permits a debate as to how to interpret the Qur'an in any novel situation. Islam does not have a binary view of law as either forbidden or permitted but has five categories of human behavior: wajh, obligatory; haram, prohibited; sunna, recommended; makruh, discouraged; and mubah, permitted.

Different sects of Islam, such as Sunni and Shi'i, have differing opinions in many areas of life, including related to fertility and procreation, but all sects of Islan promote the importance and primacy of family and family connections. This explains the negative approach to third-party reproduction. In Islam it is the father who confers the religion on the child.

Islam promotes childbirth, "wealth and progeny are adornments for the life of this world"[24] and condones seeking a cause for infertility. But Islam does not promote the use of artificial reproductive technology without medical justification. Therefore, homosexual couples are not permitted to undergo fertility treatments, nor are single women able to use donor sperm to conceive.

Islam permits the use of in vitro feralization if (a) the couple are married, (b) the sperm comes from the husband and the egg from the wife, (c) surrogacy is not involved, (d) there is a competent team performing the procedure to eliminate the chances of failure or inadvertent mix-ups, and (e) only the appropriate number of fertilized eggs are transferred to the uterus.[25] Frozen embryos must be used by the couple if they are still married. No third-party fertility is permitted by Sunni scholars, but some Shia authorities have been more permissive,[26] with the use of egg donation permitted in Iran.

Cryopreservation is permitted by Islamic law, but frozen embryos are the exclusive property of the married couple and cannot be transferred to anyone else.[27] Sperm cannot be stored during a man's lifetime for the purpose of use posthumously.

---

[21] Edge, I., (1996), *Islamic Law and Legal Theory*, Aldershot, Dartmouth.

[22] Reinhart, A. K., (1983). Islamic Law as Islamic Ethics, *Journal of Religious Ethics* 11 (2):186–203.

[23] Iqbal, M., and Noble, R., 2009, *Islamic identity and the ethics of assisted reproduction*, in Blyth, E., and Landau, R., eds Faith and fertility, London, Jessica Kingsley Publications.

[24] Qur'an 18:46.

[25] Al-Bar MA, Chamsi-Pasha H. *Contemporary Bioethics: Islamic Perspective* Cham (CH): Springer; 2015. P. 175.

[26] Such a fatwa was issued by Ayatollah Khamenei himself, see Serour GI (2013) Ethical issues in human reproduction: Islamic perspectives. *Gynecol Endocrinol* 29(11):949–952. However, other Shia authorities concur with the Sunni view that all third-party reproduction is forbidden by Islam.

[27] Al-Bar and Chamsi-Pasha, op. cit. p. 179.

Fertilized eggs are not considered life[28] and those that will not be used can be destroyed, and this is not considered "killing" the embryos. Gender selection is a matter for God and is not permitted in Islam.[29]

19.5 Hinduism

In many ways Hinduism is not strictly a religion; it has no founding fathers, no church or clergy; rather, it is a way of life embracing several different philosophies, beliefs, and doctrines.[30] Hindu morality is based on Bhagavad Gita and other ancient scriptures. Hinduism believes in Cosmic Oneness, that the self is connected with the Cosmic Ultimate Reality, everyone has some divinity with them, and the Supreme Consciousness is inherent in everything. Hinduism believes in eternity and rebirth, life is eternal, humans have a special quality, Dharma, which is distinct for humans. Hinduism also believes in Karma, which guides the soul through its journey on earth to achieve merger with the Absolute. Hinduism believes in one human family and promotes universal well-being. Hindus are to be altruistic and be true to their inner voice, as well as maintain an open mind to accept new ideas.

Like other religions and religious philosophies, Hinduism sees the act of procreation, and even fertilization, as a sacred occurrence, "under the supervision of the Supreme Lord and according to the result of his work, the living entity, the soul, is made to enter into the womb of a woman through the particle of male semen to assume a particular type of body."[31] Accordingly, human life starts at conception, whereas another source suggests that life starts at the seventh month of embryonic development.[32] Reproduction is seen as a duty and a debt to previous generations. The "white seed," [semen] shukra, is a medium for the soul and joins with rajas, the "red seed" from the female, that forms the flesh. "Indian men are known for their obsession with virility,"[33] which refers to physical strength, mental agility, sexual energy, and the ability to father children. This can be significant when treating this population, as even performing a semen analysis can bring one's virility into question.

---

[28] As life begins 120 days after conception.

[29] Ibid. p. 183.

[30] Kishore, R.R., 2019, *Assisted Reproductive Technologies, challenges and values: Global milieu and a journey through the Hinduism,* Presented at Workshop on Protecting the Future Generations and the Ethics of Human Reproduction, organized by UNESCO, Casablanca, Morocco, 11–13 November, 2019, and Allahbadia, G. N., Allahbadia, S.G., Arora, S., *Hinduism and reproduction in contemporary India*, in Faith and Fertility, op. cit.

[31] Shreemad Bhagvat Purana SB 3.31.1.

[32] See Shrimad Bhagwat 3.31.10, "Thus endowed with the development of consciousness from the seventh month after his conception, the child is tossed downward by the airs that press the embryo during the weeks preceding delivery."

[33] Basu, S., Banerjee, S., 2006, *The quest for manhood: masculine Hinduism and nation in Bengal.* Comparative Studies of South Asia, Africa and the Middle East (2006) 26 (3): 476–490.

It is fascinating to note that in Hindu tradition a woman whose husband was incapable of fathering a child, or who had died, was permitted to have sexual relations with another man in order to bear a child. This can be interpreted as an ancient form of surrogate fatherhood.[34] Hindu scripture also contains a reference to gestational carriers, "Krishna or Shesh gestating as an embryo in the womb of Devki is a part of mine, take it out and transfer it in to the womb of Rohini without any difficulty."[35] There is also a reference to conception and embryonic development occurring outside of the uterus.[36]

In Hinduism the embryo is considered life and must be respected as such, but the use of embryos is permitted for fertility but not for research,[37] and there are circumstances in which it would be permitted to destroy embryos.[38] As such, IVF is permitted.

Hinduism is quite permissive regarding reproductive technology methods, and sources for sperm donation and surrogacy can be found in their literature.

19.6 Judaism[39]

Judaism is based on the teachings of the Torah, the Written Law, given by God to Moses over 3300 years ago, and is interpreted by the Oral Law, comprising a rich literature from the Mishnah, written in the seventh century BCE, and the later Talmud. These interpretations and explanations continue until the present day, with a rich discussion of Talmudic points and their practical application among Torah scholars. These lead to a guide to normative Jewish practice, called halachah, literally the way to go, that encompasses every aspect of a Jew's personal and national life, including each novel development.

In the absence of a central authority to determine halachah, each Rabbi has the authority to guide his congregants according to his understanding and interpretation. However, there are Rabbis who are seen as having a greater authority and weight in making halachic decisions, especially for the wider population; these are called Poskim. Not all Poskim agree with each other, but most observant Orthodox Jews will align themselves with one of them and follow their rulings. Since there are numerous differences of opinion, it is impossible, and counterproductive, to assume that since one couple underwent a particular procedure with Rabbinic approval, this

---

[34] See Kishor op cit., p. 12, for the limitations and specific circumstances in which this is permitted.

[35] Bhagwat Purana 10.2.8.

[36] Kishor, op cit., p. 14.

[37] Sivaraman, M. A. F., Amaris, F., Noor, S. N. M., 2014. Ethics of Embryonic Stem Cell Research According to Buddhist, Hindu, Catholic, and Islamic Religions: Perspective from Malaysia. *Asian Biomedicine* 8(1): 43–52.) and Neaves, W., *The status of the human embryo in various religions*. this shouild not ne in italics *Development*. 2017 Jul 15;144(14):2541–2543.

[38] Kishor op. cit.

[39] See my chapter in Hill and Landau, op cit. For the sources of this section.

will be adopted by other couples. Each couple will consult with their own halachic authority and each may receive a different answer.

Conservative Jews will also follow halachic injunctions, but the interpretations of the Committee on Jewish Law and Standards, the central authority on halacha within Conservative Judaism, may be more liberal and less strict. Reform Jews tend to be less bound by the halacha and see it rather as a cultural and moral directive but not an imperative.

Even those Jews who are not observant of the halacha may be more particular and inclined to do so when having children, since their actions will affect future generations and the legitimacy and acceptance of such children into the community of their offspring.

Judaism sees procreation as a religious act and an obligation; celibacy is not promoted, and a couple should not choose to remain childless. Many communal activities are children-based, and the infertile couple can feel left out and alone. Jewish families can be considerably larger than the general population. There is often great pressure for such couples to have children; even when dealing with secondary infertility, there can be significant stress and a desire to have more children.

Jewish law does not permit masturbation, and many Orthodox men have never masturbated. Menstruation causes a woman to be niddah, ritually impure, and she and her husband cannot have any intimate contact. Uterine bleeding or opening the cervix, e.g., during a hysteroscopy, could possibly render a woman niddah. After becoming niddah, a woman would have to wait a certain number of days before immersing in a mikvah, a ritual bath, and only then could she resume intimate relations with her husband.

These two laws have great impact on fertility diagnosis and treatment. In order to produce a semen sample, a couple would be able to gather semen residue after sexual relations or have relations while wearing a collection condom. This would only be able to be performed when the woman is not niddah. Therefore, the timing of treatment is essential, or, at least, a couple should be instructed to produce and freeze a semen sample during the "pure" period of the menstrual cycle if the treatment is likely to occur during the impure time of the month. In certain, rare, and very specific cases, some Rabbis will permit producing a sample through masturbation, but this would require specific Rabbinic permission.

An Orthodox Jewish woman may want to know whether a particular procedure, e.g., hysterosalpingogram, causes bleeding or opens the cervix. It is essential to give the patient the most exact information possible, prior to and after the procedure. She can then ask her halachic authority as to the ramifications of each procedure.

In vitro fertilization is permitted, but some authorities limit the use of ART to one child; some permit even more, including cases of secondary infertility, even when there are already a number of children. There is a greater debate regarding egg donation and as to the identity of the mother. The accepted opinion is that Jews must be strict, and when either the genetic mother or the birth mother is not Jewish, the child born would need to be converted to Judaism. Some authorities permit the use of donor sperm if the donor is not Jewish to limit the risks of future procreation with a sibling. Embryos are not considered life in Judaism and so can be destroyed if not needed. Surrogacy can also be used in Judaism, but if the surrogate is not Jewish, the baby would need to be converted as such a Jewish surrogate may be preferred. In Judaism it is the mother who confers the religion on the child.

19.7 Buddhism

Buddhism follows the teachings of Buddha and his achievement of enlightenment and triumph over suffering. Buddha means enlightened one in Sanskrit. Although there are three major branches of Buddhism, all Buddhists accept certain common principles: liberation from dukkha, suffering, and the four noble truths—a. the truth of the unsatisfactoriness (dukkha sacca), b. the truth of the cause of the unsatisfactoriness (dukkha-samudāya sacca), c. the truth of the cessation of unsatisfactoriness (dukkha-nirodha sacca), and d. the truth of the way leading to the cessation of unsatisfactoriness (dukkha-nirodha-gamini-paṭipadā sacca). All Buddhists follow the Five Precepts: not taking life, not stealing, not engaging in improper sexual relations, not lying and not consuming intoxicants. Buddhism emphasizes benevolence and non-violence, an interest in helping others, and meditation.

In Buddhism, there is great importance placed on family and respect for parents and children. Since infertility can cause suffering, many sources suggest that IVF is permitted, but there are concerns regarding destroying embryos due to the concern over causing harm or taking life. There does not seem to be a limitation on the use of donor sperm or eggs, and surrogacy can be pursued when necessary and within a strong and loving relationship.[40]

19.8 Ethics and Fertility

Ethics is the study of moral dilemma and moral behavior.[41] Put simply, a normal moral life will contain a clash of morals and principles. The ability to decide which path to follow when values collide gives rise to ethics and determines ethical behavior.

Fertility treatment is also prone to force the practitioner to choose between moral principles; do embryos have rights and should they be preserved at all costs, or can the clinic destroy them if they are not needed for further treatment and become a burden on the storage facility? Should all patients have access to fertility treatment regardless of their age and chances of success, or should fertility clinics limit availability in order to concentrate their efforts on the most potentially successful cases?

---

[40] Ying LY, Har L, Loke A. 2015, *The experience of Chinese couples undergoing* in vitro *fertilization treatment: perception of the treatment process and partner support.* PLoS One. 2015;10:e0139691. https://doi.org/10.1371/journal.pone.0139691

[41] Nagel, Thomas (2006). "Ethics". In Borchert, Donald (ed.). *Encyclopedia of Philosophy* (2 ed.). Macmillan.

Should fertility treatment be offered to people who are related, or does the risk of creating genetically impaired offspring override the desire to have children?[42]

One problem with such ethical dilemmas is the lack of authoritative guidance. Unlike religious imperatives, ethics relies on a personal approach and the generally accepted norms, which tend to change. An ethicist cannot speak with any definitive authority; they are a voice in the deliberations but cannot be "the" voice. Moral ethics are dependent on the approach and perspective of the specific ethicist and can shift and change throughout time.

This makes it challenging to seek and rely on ethical guidance, but all hospitals have an ethics committee, or a similar institutional mechanism, who can be consulted regarding ethical challenges. The committee may be comprised of medical professionals (from different disciplines), ethicists, and even a member of the clergy. They discuss the moral dilemma and present a position statement or ethical guidelines for the medical practitioners and the patients.[43]

In the area of reproductive health, the American Society of Reproductive Medicine (ASRM) has an active Ethics Committee that has published numerous position papers on a wide variety of subjects. These can be accessed on their website,[44] and cover such subjects as family members acting as gamete donors, fertility treatment when partners withhold information from each other, consideration of the gestational carrier, and cross-border reproductive care.

While the Ethics Committee reports are classed as opinions and are not legally binding, they are an excellent source for consideration and a basis for the factors that need to be taken into account when deliberating a moral issue in the fertility laboratory.

19.9 Legislation

In addition to the ethical considerations, there are legal limitations and regulations as to what is permitted to be done. The aim of our legal systems is to protect the rights of the individuals within the society, especially of those who tend to be neglected or mistreated.

As such, the legal system will protect the rights of the unborn or even unconceived child and even the rights of the embryos. As such, most countries will not permit fertility treatment in incestous relations, such as between a father and his daughter, or between two siblings, since the child conceived and born will be disadvantaged and has a high chance of carrying a genetic abnormality. The same may be true for a couple with severe mental disabilities.

---

[42] Serour, G.I., Serour, A.G., 2017. Ethical issues in infertility. *Best Practice & Research Clinical Obstetrics & Gynaecology,* 43:21–31.

[43] Mehta P, Zimba O, Gasparyan AY, Seiil B, Yessirkepov M. Ethics Committees: Structure, Roles, and Issues. *J Korean Med Sci.* 2023 Jun 26;38(25).

[44] https://www.asrm.org/practice-guidance/ethics-opinions/

The recent case in Alabama[45] is a somewhat extreme example of the law protecting embryos, since the judge afforded the same rights of children to frozen embryos. In this case, the law viewed embryos as life, equivalent to any other child, and forbade destroying them, identifying the medical professionals who did so as murderers. This has been contested and has been seen as a threat to the continued operation of fertility facilities.

In the case of third-party treatments, especially gestational carriers, the law can attempt to protect the carrier and determine that she has visitation rights and a claim to motherhood of the child, while other courts of law have protected the rights of the genetic parents and discounted any maternal relationship between the gestational carrier and the child.[46]

Since different states and municipalities have distinct laws, which also tend to change periodically, it is essential to consult with the clinic's legal adviser prior to embarking on a treatment that may raise legal questions. The patients must be informed that the clinic will only proceed with a treatment after receiving legal permission to do so.

There are also financial considerations related both to availability of fertility treatment for those who cannot pay and remuneration for donors.

19.10 Conclusion

My hope is that this brief review expresses the importance of understanding that not all that can be done should be done and may be done. Fertility treatment is a tremendous tool in the hands of the medical practitioner, and it must be used wisely and for the better good. Religion, ethics, and the law all come to determine the definition of the better good.

The informed medical professional is advised to comprehend the wishes and needs of the patient and administer treatment within the religious, ethical, and legal framework that is the most appropriate and applicable.

[45] See Susan Crockin and Francesca Nardi's article, *Alabama Supreme Court Rules Frozen Embryos are "Unborn Children" and admonishes IVF's "Wild West" treatment*, on the ASRM website, https://www.asrm.org/news-and-events/asrm-news/legally-speaking/frozen-embryo-destruction-and%2D%2Dpotential-travel-restrictions-for-surrogacy-arrangements2/

[46] Wilcox, H.M., Cummings, C.L., Pope, T.M., Mercurio, M.R.; Gestational Carrier Pregnancies: Legal and Ethical Considerations for Pediatricians. *Pediatrics*. April 2024;153(4).

The In Vitro Fertilization Protocols: Simple Explanations for Nurses and Patients

20

Michael H. Dahan, Darina Groucha, Shu Qin Wei, Mingju Cao, and Seang Lin Tan

20.1 Introduction

There are many in-vitro fertilization (IVF) protocols, more than can be discussed in any single textbook, and many centers have their own unique protocols. However, there are also several common protocols that are used by many IVF centers. This chapter is divided into two parts. The first section provides short explanations for nurses on how the common IVF protocols are performed. The second section is designed for nurses to explain to patients how they should follow their IVF protocol. Each IVF protocol will be presented individually. We hope that this chapter will aid in both the learning of nurses and help them to teach patients about some of the most common methods of IVF.

M. H. Dahan (✉)
Department of Reproductive Endocrinology and Infertility, McGill University, Montreal, QC, Canada

D. Groucha · S. Q. Wei · M. Cao
OriginElle Fertility Clinic & Women's Health Centre, Montreal, Canada

S. L. Tan
Department of Obstetrics and Gynecology, McGill University, Montreal, Canada

OriginElle Fertility Clinic & Women's Health Centre, Montreal, Canada
e-mail: sltan@orignielle.com

M. Das, M. H. Dahan (eds.), *A Comprehensive Guide to Reproductive Health and Infertility Medicine for Nurses*, https://doi.org/10.1007/978-3-032-24372-0_20

20.2 Nurses Section

20.2.1 GnRH (Gonadotropin Releasing Hormone) Antagonist Protocol [1]

Purpose of Protocol:
- Efficient means of combining ovarian stimulation with ovulation control.

Targeted Population/Indications:

- Most patients are candidates, including high responders, normal responders, and poor responders [1].
- When a short treatment duration is desired

Exclusions:
- Patients who require a flexible treatment schedule
- Patients for whom ovarian stimulation is contraindicated

Materials:
- GnRH Antagonists
- Gonadotropins
- HCG or GnRH agonist trigger

Procedure:
1. On day 1 of menstrual bleeding, the patient notifies the clinic of start of her menstrual cycle. The patient will be scheduled for a baseline ultrasound on day 2–4 to rule out the presence of a potentially ovarian cyst. If there is no cyst present greater than 10 mm in mean diameter, the patient will begin gonadotropins on days 2–4 as per doctor's orders.

   The starting dose of gonadotropins will depend on patient's age, ovarian function, and previous response to gonadotropins (use the dose of HMG/FSH that was effective in a previous cycle). The following may be used as a guide for dosage in women with normal ovarian activity:
   150 IU HMG/FSH <35 years.
   225 IU HMG/FSH 35–38 years.
   300 IU HMG/FSH 39–40 years.
   375 IU HMG/FSH >40 years.

   These doses apply to all presented protocols.

   If polycystic ovaries, use a daily dose that is 75 IU less than would be normally ordered.

   If basal FSH is >10 IU/L or serum AMH or AFC is low, use a higher dose than would be normally ordered. Note, the maximum dose of FSH ordered is 450 IU/day of FSH or 24 mcg daily of rec-FSH-gamma. (As per ESHRE guidelines, the highest dose should not be greater than 300 IU/ daily).

   Use the effective gonadotrophin dose used in a previous cycle as the starting dose in subsequent cycles.

2. Ultrasound scans are scheduled to monitor patient response on day 5–7 of stimulation and every 1–2 days thereafter depending on follicular growth, until the day of trigger. Serum Estradiol (E2) level is checked at the time of ultrasound (up to and including the day of trigger) to further evaluate response.

   Gonadotropin dose may be adjusted based on follicular development and hormonal response. When Estradiol is >13,000 pmol/L or more than 20 follicles are stimulated, a GnRH agonist trigger alone should be used.

   Cycle cancellation may be considered if a patient has fewer than three pre-ovulatory follicles ≥14 mm. In these circumstances, the doctor should counsel the patient and decide individually whether to cancel the cycle.
3. When the patient exhibits a leading follicle >12–14 mm, GnRH antagonist (Orgalutran® Fyremadel® or Cetrotide®) 0.25 mg/day is commenced. Once begun, antagonist continues daily up to and including the day of trigger at 24-hour intervals (Note: on the day of trigger, antagonist should be given before noon) [1].
4. A GnRH antagonist can be initiated at a fixed time point, usually day 5 or 6 of stimulation (without follicular monitoring on that day) and once begun, antagonist continues on a daily basis up to and including the day of trigger at 24-hour intervals (Note: on the day of trigger, antagonist should be given before noon).
5. The trigger should be given as per doctor's orders. Trigger is administered 35–38 hours prior to egg retrieval as per doctor's orders [2].
6. If E2 or the number of follicles suggest high risk of ovarian hyperstimulation syndrome (OHSS), final follicular maturation may be achieved by giving GnRH agonist alone [3].
7. **OHSS Risk Mitigation Protocol**
   - Provide patient education on signs and symptoms of OHSS, as per OHSS Risk Management Handout.
   - Book patient for a follow-up ultrasound 2–4 days after egg collection and OHSS bloodwork post-operation for monitoring as per doctor's orders.

20.2.2 The Progesterone Primed Ovarian Stimulation (PPOS) Protocol [4]

Purpose of Protocol:
- Efficient means of combining ovarian stimulation with ovulation control, with lower cost and avoidance of one injectable medication.

Targeted Population/Indications:
- Most patients are candidates, including high responders, normal responders, and poor responders [4].
- When a short treatment is desired

Exclusions:
- Patients who require a flexible treatment schedule
- Patients for whom stimulation is contraindicated

Materials:

- Medroxyprogesterone acetate (MDPA)10 mg [4]
- Gonadotropins
- HCG or GnRH agonist trigger

Procedure:

1. On day 1 of menstrual bleeding, the patient notifies the clinic of start of her menstrual cycle. The patient will be scheduled for a baseline ultrasound on day 2–4. Ultrasound to rule out the presence of a potentially confounding cyst. If there is no cyst present greater than 10 mm in mean diameter, the patient will begin gonadotropins on days 2–4 as per doctor's orders.
2. Ultrasound scans are scheduled to monitor patient response on day 5–7 of stimulation and every 1–2 days thereafter depending on follicular growth until the day of trigger. Serum estradiol is checked at the time of ultrasound (up to and including the day of trigger) to further evaluate response.

   Gonadotropin dose may be adjusted based on follicular development and hormonal response. When estradiol is >13,000 pmol/L or more than 20 follicles are stimulated, a GnRH agonist trigger alone should be considered.

   Cycle cancellation may be considered if a patient has fewer than two or three preovulatory follicles ≥14 mm. In these circumstances, the doctor should counsel the patient and decide individually whether to cancel the cycle.
3. When the patient exhibits a leading follicle >12–14 mm, MDPA 10 mg daily orally is commenced. Once begun, MDPA continues daily up to and including the day of trigger at 24-hour intervals (Note: on the day of trigger, MDPA should be given before noon).
4. The MDPA can be initiated at a fixed time point, usually day 1 of stimulation or on day 5 or 6 of stimulation (without follicular monitoring on that day). Once begun, MDPA continues daily up to and including the day of trigger at 24-hour intervals (Note: on the day of trigger, MDPA should be given before noon).
5. Trigger should be given as per doctor's orders. Trigger is administered 35–38 hours prior to egg retrieval as per doctor's orders.
6. If E2 or the number of follicles suggest high risk of OHSS, final follicular maturation may be achieved by giving GnRH agonist alone.
7. **OHSS Risk Mitigation Protocol** [5]
   - Provide patient education on signs and symptoms of OHSS, as per OHSS Risk Management Handout.
   - Book patient for a follow-up ultrasound 2–4 days after egg collection and OHSS bloodwork post-operation for monitoring as per doctor's orders.

20.2.3 Low Dose GnRH Agonist Long Protocol with Oral Contraceptive (OC) [6–8]

Purpose of Protocol:

- Efficient, flexible means of achieving downregulation in poor responders, while reducing flare up effect of GnRH agonist.

Targeted Population/Indications:

- Patients with previous long protocol who had poor response relative to AFC
- Low responders, including women with high basal serum FSH, low AFC, or AMH levels.

Exclusions:

- Patients for whom OCs are contraindicated
- Patients with estrogen-sensitive tumors

Materials:

- 1–2 packets of OC
- 2 vials of buserelin acetate or other GNRH agonist
- Gonadotropins
- HCG

Procedure:

1. The patient will begin a low-dose monophasic estrogen OC on day 1–5 of cycle. OC is taken daily (1 tablet/day) and must be continued for a minimum of 14 days but may be extended up to a maximum of 29 days as the patient/clinic schedule requires. The patient should take her last OC on a Monday after taking the requisite minimum 14 days.

   Note: OC is continued without interruption. If more than 21 tablets are required for scheduling, the patient is instructed to begin a new packet on day 22 (and surplus sugar pills are discarded) [6]

   Key Modification:

   - Blood pressure monitoring is required prior to OC initiation.
2. The patient will begin buserelin 200 mcg/day 5 days before stopping OC (i.e. will take both OC and buserelin for 5 days) and continue the same dose for a minimum of 7 days until downregulation (DR) is achieved. Typically, buserelin is started on a Thursday, and the DR ultrasound is scheduled 10–14 days later.
3. At the DR ultrasound, ovaries and uterus are evaluated for evidence of pituitary suppression: absence of ovarian activity (no follicles/cysts) and endometrial thickness < 5 mm. If a follicle/cyst is present, or if the endometrial lining is thick, serum estradiol is evaluated.

   Serum estradiol <150 pmol/L (or 40 pg/mL) is confirmation of suppression.

   If there is a cyst or if lining is >5 mm and serum estradiol is >150 pmol/L, the patient will continue buserelin in the SAME dose (200 mcg/day) and will return 1 week later to reassess suppression. If a cyst/follicle is still present, this should be drained (*Note: cysts > 2.5 cm at the initial DR ultrasound should be drained at that time*).

   Key Modification:

   - Progesterone measurement is added during suppression check to confirm complete downregulation.

4. When suppression is confirmed, gonadotropins are commenced. Buserelin dose is reduced to 50 mcg twice daily (100 mcg/day) (buserelin continues at this dose until and including the day of HCG).

   Ultrasound scans are scheduled to monitor patient response on day 5–8 of stimulation and then every 1–2 days, depending on follicular growth, until and including the day of HCG. Patients with PCO and suspected poor responders (who are not already at the maximum dose) are additionally scheduled for an (early) Day 5 ultrasound.

   Serum estradiol is checked at the time of ultrasound from day 3–8 onward (up to and including the day of HCG) to further evaluate response.

   Cycle cancellation may be considered if a patient has fewer than three pre-ovulatory follicles or too many follicles and there is a risk of OHSS.
5. HCG can be given once three follicles measure (use the average diameter in 3 dimensions) $\geq$18 mm.

   The usual triggering dose of HCG is 250 mcg of recombinant product (or 5000–10,000 IU of urinary product) 35–38 hours before egg retrieval [6].

20.2.4 IVF Long Protocol with Oral Contraceptive [6–8]

This protocol is like the LOW DOSE GnRH AGONIST LONG PROTOCOL—OC, with higher doses of GnRH agonist used. The only modifications as compared with the protocol previously discussed are:

- Patients will begin buserelin (Suprefact®) 500 mcg/day, five days before stopping OC (i.e. will take both OC and buserelin for five days).
- Buserelin will continue at the same dose for a minimum of 7 days until down-regulation (DR) is achieved.
- By convention (for scheduling purposes), patient will begin buserelin on a Friday, and the DR ultrasound is scheduled on Thursday 10–14 days later.

When buserelin is not available or is specifically contraindicated, leuprolide (Lupron®) 500 mcg/day may be substituted (Note: leuprolide is more concentrated than buserelin, and so volumes delivered will be different).

When patients prefer to avoid injections (and are prepared to take an inhaled formulation), nafarelin (Synarel®) may be substituted for buserelin. Nafarelin dose begins at 400 mcg twice daily and decreases to 200 mcg twice daily once suppression has been achieved.

When suppression is confirmed, gonadotropins commence and the buserelin dose is lowered to 200 mcg/day (buserelin continues at this dose until and including the day of HCG); If leuprolide is taken, the dose is reduced to 200 mcg/day.

Modifications to the previously discussed GnRH agonist long protocols may be introduced in that the GnRH agonist may be stopped up to 7 days before trigger with a low risk of premature ovulation.

20.2.5 Microdose Flare Protocol [9, 10]

Purpose of Protocol:

- Ovarian stimulation utilizing the flare-up effect of a GnRH analog and prevention of premature luteinization, combined with gonadotropin ovarian hyperstimulation.

Targeted Population/Indications:

- Patients undergoing IVF who are at risk of poor ovarian response
- Patients with a history of a previous poor ovarian response (less than four follicles recruited and/or peak E2 < 1800 pmol/L)
- Patients with an elevated baseline FSH on days 2–5 (>10 mIU/mL)
- Patients with an AFC < 4 follicles
- Patients >38 years of age with low ovarian reserve

Exclusions:

- Patients for whom OC is contraindicated
- Patients with an estrogen-sensitive tumor

Materials:

- 1–2 packets of OC
- GnRH Analog (Buserelin, Lupron)
- onadotropin
- HCG

Procedure:

1. Patient will begin low-dose monophasic estrogen OC within the first 5 days of menstrual cycle. OC is taken daily (1 tablet/ day) and must be continued for a minimum of 21 days and a maximum of 28 days. Patient will take her last OC on a Saturday after taking the requisite minimum of 21 days. Note: OC is continued without interruption. If more than 21 tablets are required for scheduling, patient is instructed to begin a new packet on day 22 (and surplus pills are discarded).
2. On the third day (Tuesday) after OC discontinuing, patients will have a baseline scan to rule out the presence of a cyst >15 mm.

   If there is no cyst, patients will begin taking the GnRH analog Buserelin 50 mcg twice daily. An alternative to Buserelin is Leuprolide 40 mcg bid (50mcg bid may be taken if dilution permitting 40 mcg is impractical). The GnRH analog is continued at this same dose until and including the day of HCG administration.

   If a cyst is present, the cyst is drained and patient begins GnRH analog as above.
3. On the fifth day (Thursday) after discontinuing the oral contraceptive / the third day of the GnRH analog, gonadotropins are commenced.

The starting dose of gonadotropin depends on the patient's previous response to gonadotropin ovarian stimulation, age, baseline FSH, and AFC.

4. On day 6 (Tuesday) of stimulation with gonadotropin, an ultrasound is scheduled to monitor patient response. The ultrasounds are repeated on day 9 (Friday) and as needed every 1–2 days thereafter, depending on follicular growth, until and including the day of hCG. Serum Estradiol is checked at the time of the ultrasound, until and including the day of hCG.

   The gonadotropin dose will be adjusted based on follicular development and rise of the Estradiol.

   Cycle cancellation may be considered if a patient has fewer than three pre-ovulatory follicles.

5. HCG can be given once the average diameter (in three dimensions) of three follicles measures ≥18 mm. The (usual) triggering dose is 250 mcg recombinant hCG or 5000–10,000 IU urinary hCG.

   HCG is administered 35–38 hours prior to egg retrieval.

20.2.6 Long Day21 Protocol [6–8]

Patient is instructed to call on day 1 of period and register start of cycle with admin team.

Patient starts Buserelin injections 0.5mls daily (OD).

Baseline scan (to check whether suppressed scan) is done with period that follows.

The antral follicle count must be recorded at baseline scan.

The aim of the baseline scan is to confirm that the endometrium is thin (<5 mm) and that there are no functional cysts or dominant follicles (>10 mm) seen in either ovary (see baseline scan algorithm)

(a) If the endometrium is >5 mm or there is a functional cyst or dominant follicle (>10 mm) then blood is to be sent for BHCG and Estradiol.

(i) If the BHCG is positive then stop the Buserelin injections and commence progesterone supplementation to support the potential early pregnancy.

The HCG should then be repeated in 48 hours and if increasing then the patient should be referred to the early pregnancy unit.

(ii) If estradiol is >200 pmol/L and HCG is negative then repeat scan and bloods in 7 days.

If the baseline scan confirms quiescence (endometrium <5 mm and no dominant follicle or functional cyst >10 mm) then FSH stimulation can be commenced at the prescribed dose.

Additionally, the dose of Buserelin is reduced to 0.2mls once daily subcutaneous from the start of FSH and continued at this dose till HCG administration.

The starting dose of FSH should be reviewed at the daily results meeting.

After 5 doses of FSH a blood test should be done for estradiol and this should be between 500 and 1000 pmol/L. Further estradiol monitoring is conducted as outlined below, however, the clinical picture (ultrasound findings, previous history) should always be taken into consideration when altering dose:

(a) If the estradiol is <500 pmol/L, then consider increasing the FSH dose by at least 75iu and repeat estradiol in 48 hours to confirm response to stimulation.
(b) If the estradiol is >1000 pmol/L, then consider reducing the FSH dose by at least 75iu and repeat estradiol in 48 hours.
(c) The aim of estradiol assessment is to monitor response to simulation and confirm the start of ovarian response to stimulation. The repeat estradiol level on day 7 should be double that at day 5 (approx. 1000–2000 pmol/L). If the estradiol is >3000 pmol/L, then reduce the FSH dose by at least 75iu and repeat scan and estradiol level 48 hours later. This doubling should allow for an estradiol level on the day of trigger of approximately 10,000 pmol/L.
(d) The aim should also be to allow at least 7 days of follicular development from that start of confirmed ovarian response (i.e., estradiol >500 pmol/L) before trigger injection is given.
(e) A scan is done on day 7–9 to assess the follicle size and response to stimulation and further scans are arranged as required.

Final Oocyte Maturation Trigger

1. The criteria for triggering final maturation are >3 follicles >18 mm on scan on the day of trigger.
2. If estradiol is >10,000 pmol/L or > 18 follicles on >11 mm are seen on scan, the results must be reviewed by a consultant before a decision is made for trigger and Coasting (withholding of further FSH doses) should be considered.
3. If a decision to coast the patient is made then estradiol levels must be assayed daily until levels fall to <10,000 pmol/L before trigger injection.
4. Egg collection is performed 36–37 hours after trigger.

Luteal Phase Support

Luteal phase support is started on the evening of egg collection, depending on the prescribed preparation and the trigger method as follows:

(i) Progesterone (options as below)

   1. Progesterone 25 mg subcutaneous injections twice daily
   2. Progesterone 25 mg subcutaneous injections once daily and progesterone 400 mg pessaries twice daily
   3. Progesterone IM 100 mg once a day OR
   4. Progesterone pessaries 400 mg twice daily PV/PR

(ii) Estradiol 2 mg tablets twice daily

If pregnancy test is positive then progesterone supplementation is continued till 10 weeks gestation. Estradiol tablets may be discontinued with pregnancy test.

Pregnancy Test

A urine pregnancy test is performed 11 days after a blastocyst embryo transfer

(a) If positive, a pregnancy scan should be booked for 6–8 weeks of pregnancy
(b) If negative, the patient should attend for a serum hCG.
    (i) If this is <2 IU/l, all medications should be stopped. Patients should be advised to expect a bleed within 14 days. If they do not bleed, they should perform a urinary pregnancy test and to contact the fertility unit.
    (ii) If this is 2–5 IU/l on two occasions, 48 hours apart, all medications should be stopped, and a hCG should be repeated in 7 days to confirm it is negative (i.e. <2 IU/l).
    (iii) If this is >5 IU/l but shows a suboptimal rise (<63%) or suboptimal drop (<50%) 48 hours apart, refer to the early pregnancy unit.
    (iv) If this is >5 IU/l and shows an optimal rise then book a pregnancy scan for 7 weeks of pregnancy.
    (v) If the pregnancy test is positive, then medications are continued as follows:

a. b. c. estradiol tablets until pregnancy test
Injectables until 8 + 0 weeks' gestation

Pessaries until 12 + 0 weeks' gestation (if the patient has evidence of bleeding in early pregnancy, then they can continue the progesterone pessaries until 16 + 0 weeks' gestation).

20.2.7 Long Day 21 Depot GnRH Agonist (PROSTAP) Protocol [6–8]

Patient is instructed to call on day 1 of period and register start of cycle with admin team.

Patient attends unit for depot GnRh agonist injection 3.75 mg SC on approximately day 21 (21 days after the first day of period or 7 days before the next expected menstrual cycle, which would be on day 14 in a 21-day cycle).

Baseline scan (suppressed scan) is done with period that follows.

The antral follicle count must be recorded at baseline scan.

The aim of the baseline scan is to confirm that the endometrium is thin (<5 mm) and that there are no functional cysts or dominant follicles (>10 mm) seen in either ovary (see baseline scan algorithm).

a. If the endometrium is >5 mm or there is a functional cyst or dominant follicle (>10 mm) then blood is to be sent for BHCG and estradiol levels.

(i) If the BHCG is positive, then commence progesterone supplementation to support the potential early pregnancy.

The HCG should then be repeated in 48 hours, and if increasing, then the patient should be referred to the early pregnancy unit.

(ii) If estradiol is >200 pmol/L and HCG is negative, then repeat scan and bloods in 7 days.

If the baseline scan confirms quiescence (endometrium <5 mm and no dominant follicle or functional cyst >10 mm) then FSH stimulation can be commenced at the prescribed dose.

The starting dose of FSH should be reviewed at the daily results meeting.

After 5 doses of FSH, a blood test should be done for estradiol, and this should be between 500 and 1000 pmol/L. Further estradiol monitoring is conducted as outlined below; however, the clinical picture (ultrasound findings, previous history) should always be taken into consideration when altering the dose:

(a) If the estradiol is <500 pmol/L, then consider increasing the FSH dose by at least 75iu and repeat estradiol in 48 hours to confirm response to stimulation.
(b) If the estradiol is >1000 pmol/L, then consider reducing the FSH dose by at least 75iu and repeat estradiol in 48 hours.
(c) The aim of estradiol assessment is to monitor response to simulation and confirm the start of ovarian response to stimulation. The repeat estradiol level on day 7 should be double that at day 5 (approx. 1000–2000 pmol/L). If the estradiol is >3000 pmol/L, then reduce the FSH dose by at least 75iu and repeat scan and estradiol level 48 hours later. This doubling should allow for an estradiol level on the day of trigger of approximately 10,000 pmol/L.
(d) The aim should also be to allow at least 7 days of follicular development from that start of confirmed ovarian response (i.e. estradiol >500 pmol/L) before trigger injection is given.
(e) A scan is done on day 7–9 to assess the follicle size and response to stimulation and further scans are arranged as required.

Final oocyte maturation trigger, luteal phase support, and pregnancy tests are the same as in the Long Day 21 Protocol.

20.2.8 Nafarelin Long Day 21 Stimulation Protocol [6–8]

1. Patient is instructed to call on day 1 of period and register start of cycle with the admin team.
2. Patient starts nafarelin 400 mcg taken twice daily as one spray in each nostril in the morning, and one spray to each nostril in the evening (800 mcg/day) from day 21.

3. Baseline scan (suppressed scan) is booked for 2 weeks later.
4. The baseline scan must document the antral follicle count and a blood test performed for FSH, LH, estradiol, and progesterone.

The aim of the baseline scan is to confirm that the endometrium is thin (<5 mm) and that there are no functional cysts or dominant follicles (>10 mm) seen in either ovary.

(a) If the endometrium is >5 mm then a serum B-hCG should be added to the baseline bloods and a scan can be performed the following day.

(i) If the BHCG is positive, it should be managed according to the Pregnancy Test section below.
(ii) If the estradiol level is >200 pmol/l and/or the Progesterone is >2 nmol/L and/or the endometrium is >5 mm, then discuss at the results meeting with the consultant.

5. If the baseline scan confirms quiescence (endometrium <5 mm and no dominant follicle or functional cyst >10 mm) then stimulation can be commenced at the prescribed dose.
6. The dose of nafarelin is unchanged during ovarian stimulation.

The starting dose of stimulation should be reviewed at the results meeting.

After 5 doses of stimulation, a blood test should be done for estradiol, aiming for a level between 500 and 1000 pmol/l. Further estradiol monitoring is conducted as outlined below, however, the clinical picture (ultrasound findings and previous history) should always be taken into consideration when altering dose:

(a) If the estradiol level is <500 pmol/l, then consider increasing the stimulation dose by at least 75iu and repeating the estradiol level in 48 hours to confirm response to stimulation.
(b) If the estradiol level is >1000 pmol/l then consider reducing the stimulation dose by 25iu-75iu with a repeat estradiol level in 48 hours.
(c) The aim of estradiol assessment is to monitor response to simulation and confirm the start of ovarian response to stimulation. The repeat estradiol level on day 7 should be double that at day 5 (approx. 1000–2000 pmol/l). If the estradiol l e v e l is >3000 pmol/l then consider a dose reduction as above with a repeat scan and estradiol level 48 hours later. This doubling should allow for an estradiol level on the day of trigger of approximately 10,000 pmol/l.
(d) The aim is to allow at least 7 days of follicular development from the start of confirmed ovarian response (i.e. estradiol >500 pmol/l) before the trigger injection is given.
(e) A scan is done on days 7–9 to assess the follicle size and response to stimulation and further scans are arranged as required. Send bloods for FSH, LH, estradiol, and progesterone at each scan.

Final oocyte maturation trigger, luteal phase support, and pregnancy test are the same as in the Long Day 21 Protocol.

20.2.9 Frozen Egg/Embryo Transfer Cycle: Natural Cycle [11–13]

Purpose of Protocol:

- To describe patient preparation for frozen embryo replacement for patients who do not require hormonal support

Targeted Population/Indications:

- Patients having a normal ovulatory cycle (28 days–32 days)

Procedure:

1. Confirm that patient is ovulatory with a midluteal serum progesterone test during the menstrual cycle preceding the treatment cycle or using some other test (Note: this is not necessary if the patient has already had a progesterone test suggesting ovulation during the preceding 6 months.) [13].

   If no ovulation is confirmed, physician should revise the medical order and direct patient to follow HRT frozen embryo replacement cycle [11].
2. On day 1 or 2 of cycle, patient will have a baseline ultrasound to identify preexisting cysts and uterine pathology. If ultrasound result is normal, the patient will return for additional ultrasound to track follicular growth on cycle day 8–10 (and every 2–3 days thereafter, if necessary) until the dominant follicle reaches 14 mm.
3. Once the dominant follicle measures 14 mm, the patient is instructed to begin urine LH tests twice daily until a positive result is perceived and to notify the lab when this occurs.
4. The embryo transfer (ET) is scheduled by the lab as follows: (Note: for purposes of scheduling the embryo transfer, day of LH surge is equivalent to the day of HCG). Some centers will add HCG injection on the day of LH surge.

   3 days after LH surge for embryos frozen on day 1 post insemination
   4 days after LH surge for embryos frozen on day 2 post insemination
   5 days after LH surge for embryos frozen on day 3 post insemination (usually)
   7 days after LH surge for embryos frozen on day 5 post insemination
   7 days after LH surge for embryos frozen on day 6 post insemination

Another option is to measure serum progesterone levels daily and time the embryo transfer when the progesterone levels are at least 4.50 ng/ml. Progesterone is the hormone of ovulation and may take up to 4 days to increase after LH surge. In that case, the rise in progesterone would be counted as day 0 with the embryo transfer happening 2–5 days later based on embryo age at the time of freezing.

5. At the time of transfer, cycle cancellation may be considered if:
   - Endometrial thickness is persistently <7 mm
   - Fluid is detected in the endometrial cavity
   - Auterine abnormality is detected

20.2.10 Frozen Egg/Embryo Transfer Cycle: Medicated [14, 15]

Purpose of Protocol:

- To describe patient preparation for frozen embryo replacement for patients who do require hormonal support

This protocol can be combined with Long Day 21 Depot GnRH agonist (PROSTAP) PROTOCOL.

In which the: Patient is instructed to call on day 1 of period and register start of cycle with admin team [15].

Patient attends unit for GnRH agonist injection 3.75 mg SC on approximately day 21 (21 days after the first day of period), or 7 days before the next expected menstrual cycle.

Baseline scan (? suppressed scan) is done with period that follows.

The aim of the baseline scan is to confirm that the endometrium is thin (<5 mm) and that there are no functional cysts or dominant follicles (>10 mm) seen in either ovary (see baseline scan algorithm)

Or this protocol can be combined with GnRH antagonists.

In this case the GnRH antagonist injection is from **Day 2** of cycle and until Day 8 of cycle.

Or can be done without GnRH suppression

Targeted Population/Indications:

- Those desiring ease of timing of the embryo transfer.
- Those who do not ovulate on their own.

1. On day 1 or 2 of cycle, the patient will have a baseline ultrasound scan to identify preexisting cysts and uterine pathology. If the ultrasound result is normal, patient will start taking 6 or more mg daily of estradiol orally or vaginally or an equivalent in patch form, usually 100 mcg patch daily, which is usually changed every 2–3 days. They will return for additional ultrasound to track endometrial growth on cycle days 8–11 of medication.
2. Once the lining reaches an adequate endometrial thickness (usually ≥ 8 mm) progesterone supplementation will be initiated and an embryo transfer will be scheduled after discussion with the embryologists.
3. 2–3 days after progesterone initiation for embryos frozen on day 2 post-insemination

3–4 days after progesterone initiation for embryos frozen on day 3 post-insemination

120–148 hours post progesterone initiation or embryos frozen on days 5–7 post insemination.

The difference in timing will depend on clinic protocols.

20.3 Patient Teaching Section

These guidelines should be modified as per the fertility unit's own guidelines

Antagonist or PPOS
Patient's Guidelines

- Antagonist and PPOS protocols are short protocols that last about 2 weeks. You will be taking medication (pills or/and injections) and coming for ultrasounds and blood tests. You are responsible for booking both ultrasounds and blood tests; medical staff will tell you when these appointments are required.
- You should not start taking any medications before your first ultrasound.
- Please note that day 1 is considered the first day of full menstrual bleeding of your cycle.

Are the following requests completed and signed?
- Serology tests for female and male partners
- IVF consent form

Step	Day	Action
Step 1	Day 1 of your period	**Call clinic** A nurse ensures that you can start your protocol right away or if you must wait, as well as making sure that all of your tests are completed before starting
Step 2	Day 2–4 of your period	**Book an appointment** calling the reception, asking for an "IVF monitoring ultrasound" **for day 2–5**
Step 3	Day 2–4 of your period	**Perform ultrasound #1** Doctor reviews your ultrasound results, and a nurse tells you if and when you can start your medication. You can immediately see a nurse for Step 4
Step 4		**(4.1) Receive calendar and injection teachings** You can have that teaching after the ultrasound #1. Medication, doses, and the dates of ultrasound appointments are written on the calendar **4.2) Book ultrasound #2** The nurse will book your next "IVF monitoring ultrasound scan" appointment, or you may be asked to book this at the reception, before leaving the Clinic
Step 5		**Get medications** Get only the medications you need until next ultrasound
Step 6		**Perform ultrasound #2** The doctor reviews your ultrasound results, and a nurse tells you if you need to get more medication or to repeat another ultrasound. Once the ultrasound results have been reviewed, the doctor decides when you will have the egg collection procedure. A nurse will inform you for the next steps of the treatment
Step 7	Before collection	**Receive collection preparation teaching** 35–38 hours before your egg collection, you are asked to do a trigger injection (Ovidrel, HCG, or Buserelin/Naferelin/Lupron; it is not on your calendar). A nurse tells you when to take it exactly and will give you specific instructions

(continued)

Step	Day	Action
Step 8	Collection day	**Egg collection** Please remember to come at least 1 hour before the time of the collection
Step 9	After collection	**Receive post-egg collection teaching** Start progesterone as directed by the nurse A nurse calls you the day following the **egg** collection to make sure you are fine If a fresh embryo transfer is planned (never in PPOS protocols)
In the case of a fresh embryo transfer		
Step 10	Before transfer	**Receive transfer preparation teaching** Within 48 hours after collection, the embryologist informs you when you will have your transfer based on the number and quality of the embryos. The transfer will take place on day 2–5. The nurse will provide teaching.
Step 11	Transfer day	**Transfer** Please remember to come 30 min before the time of the transfer
Step 12	After transfer	**Receive post-transfer teaching** Your nurse will either ask you to book a pregnancy blood test, or you will be asked to check this at home using a home pregnancy test kit. If you have been asked to come for a pregnancy blood test, ask to book a "pregnancy blood test" at the reception
Step 13	16 days after collection day	**Do a pregnancy test at home using a test kit or a pregnancy blood test**
Step 14	Same or 1 day after pregnancy blood test	**Receive results** Inform the fertility center about your pregnancy test results. If you have had a pregnancy blood test, a nurse calls you to give you the results **Negative results** Stop progesterone Continue all the vitamins Book an appointment with your doctor **Uncertain** Repeat pregnancy blood test in 2 days; continue all medicines **Positive results** Continue progesterone up to 7–12 weeks of pregnancy or as directed by your nurse Stop all vitamins, except folic acid or prenatal vitamins After around 7–16 days from your pregnancy test, book an appointment for "gestational or vitality scan"

We recommend you take 1 month's break between fresh IVF cycles to allow the ovaries resume to normal before being re-stimulated. If you do have frozen embryos remaining from your fresh cycle, however, you can choose to proceed with a frozen embryo transfer cycle when you are ready to do so.

20.4 Low-Dose GnRH Agonist or GnRH Agonist Long Protocol

Patient's Guidelines

- Low-dose agonist and long protocols last about 5 weeks. You will be taking medication (pills and/or injections), coming for ultrasounds and blood tests. You are responsible for booking both ultrasounds and blood tests; medical staff will tell you when to.
- You don't start your treatment with an ultrasound.
- Please, note that day 1 is considered as the first day of full bleeding of your cycle.

Are the following requests completed and signed?
- Serology tests for female and male partners
- IVF consent form

Step	Day	Action
Step 1	Day 1 of your period	**Call the fertility clinic** A nurse ensures that you can start your protocol right away or if you have to wait, as well as making sure that all your tests are completed before starting
Step 2		**Receive calendar and injection teachings** A nurse gives you your calendar, and tells you when you can start taking your **birth control pill (BCP).** Usually, it is fine to **start BCP within first 5 days** of your period, but a nurse has to confirm when
Step 3		**Buy medications and follow the calendar** Carefully note **when you should take the last BCP pill**
Step 4		**Book an appointment** calling the reception, asking for an "IVF monitoring ultrasound" Book on the day the calendar tells you to. It does not matter when your period comes
Step 5		**Perform ultrasound #1** Doctor reviews your ultrasound results, and a nurse tells you if and when you can start your medication
Step 6		**(6.1) Receive calendar and injection teachings** You can have that teaching after the ultrasound #1 or book an appointment one day later. In that case, please book an appointment asking for "nurse teaching" at the reception **(6.2) Book ultrasound #2** Book an ultrasound, asking for an "IVF monitoring ultrasound," before leaving the clinic
Step 7		**Perform ultrasound #2** Doctor reviews your ultrasound results, and a nurse informs you if you need to get more medication and book a repeat ultrasound scan. The doctor reviews the ultrasound scan and decides when you can have your egg collection. The nurse will inform you of the plan once the scan has been reviewed by the doctor

(continued)

Step	Day	Action
Step 8	Before collection	**Receive egg collection preparation teaching** 35–38 hours before your collection, you are asked to do a trigger injection (Ovidrel or HCG; it is not in your calendar). A nurse tells you when to take it exactly
Step 9	Collection day	**Egg collection** Please remember to come 1 hour before the time of the collection
Step 10	After collection	**Receive post-collection teaching** A nurse calls you the following day of the egg collection to enquire how you are
In the event of a fresh embryo transfer		
Step 10	Before transfer	**Receive transfer preparation teaching** Within 48 hours after collection, the embryologist informs you about the embryo's status and possible transfer date (based on number and quality of embryos between day 2 and day 5)
Step 11	Transfer day	**Transfer** Please remember to come 30 min before the time of the transfer
Step 12	After transfer	**Receive post-transfer teaching** Continue taking your progesterone until your "pregnancy test." Your nurse will either ask you to book a pregnancy blood test, or you will be asked to check this at home using a home pregnancy test kit **The nurse will inform you about the date for your pregnancy test on your embryo transfer day. If you have been asked to have a pregnancy blood test, this** will be booked by a nurse on the embryo transfer day
Step 13	16 days after collection day	**Do pregnancy test**
Step 14	Same or 1 day after pregnancy blood test	Inform the fertility center about your pregnancy test results. If you have had a pregnancy blood test, a nurse calls you to give you the results **Negative results** Stop progesterone Continue all the vitamins Book an appointment with your doctor **Uncertain** Repeat pregnancy blood test in 2 days; continue all medicines **Positive results** Continue progesterone up to 7–12 weeks of pregnancy or as directed by the nurse Stop all vitamins, except folic acid or prenatal vitamins After around 7–16 days from your pregnancy test, book an appointment for a "gestational" or "vitality scan"

We recommend that you take 1 month's break between fresh IVF cycles to allow the ovaries resume to normal before being re-stimulated. If you do have frozen embryos remaining from your fresh cycle, however, you can choose to proceed with a frozen embryo transfer cycle when you are ready to do so.

20.5 MicroDose Flare (MDF) with Birth Control Pill (BCP) Patient Guidelines

- MicroDose Flare protocol lasts about 4 weeks. You will be taking medication (pills or/and injections), coming for ultrasounds and blood tests. Please ensure both your ultrasounds and blood tests have been booked; medical staff will tell you the appointment dates and times.
- You don't need to start your treatment with an ultrasound.
- Please, note that day 1 is considered as the first day of full bleeding of your cycle.

Are the following requests completed and signed?
- Serology tests for female and male partners
- IVF consent form

Step	Day	Action
Step 1	Day 1 of your period	**Call the clinic** A nurse ensures that you can start your protocol right away or if you have to wait, as well as makes sure that all of your tests are completed before starting
Step 2		**Get the birth control pill (BCP)**
Step 3		**Follow the calendar** Carefully note **when you should take the last BCP pill**
Step 4		**Book an appointment** by calling the reception, asking for an "IVF monitoring ultrasound" 2 days after stopping BCP Book it on the day the calendar tells you to. It does not matter when your period comes
Step 5		**Perform ultrasound #1** Doctor reviews your ultrasound results, and a nurse informs you if and when you can start your medication
Step 6		**Receive calendar and injection teachings** You can have that teaching after ultrasound #1 or book an appointment 1 day later. In that case, please book an appointment asking for "Nurse Teaching" at the reception
Step 7		**Get medications** Get only the medications you need until next ultrasound. Do not start any medication until a nurse informs you
Step 8		**Book ultrasound #2** Ensure you know the date and time of your next ultrasound scan. If you have been asked to book your next scan at the reception, ensure you do so by asking for an "IVF monitoring ultrasound," before leaving the clinic
Step 9		**Perform ultrasound #2** The doctor reviews your ultrasound results, and a nurse tells you if you need to get more medication or repeat another ultrasound. Once the ultrasound results have been reviewed, the doctor decides when you will have an egg collection. Whatever the ultrasound scan results are, a nurse will inform you about the next steps of the treatment

(continued)

Step	Day	Action
Step 10	Before collection	**Receive collection preparation teaching** 35–38 hours before your egg collection, you are asked to do a trigger injection (Ovidrel or HCG; it is not on your calendar). A nurse will give you instructions on when to take it exactly
Step 11	Collection day	**Collection** Please remember to come 1 hour before the time of the collection
Step 12	After collection	**Receive post-collection teaching** A nurse calls you the day after the egg collection to make sure everything is fine
In the event of a fresh embryo transfer		
Step 13	Before transfer	**Receive transfer preparation teaching** Within 48 hours after collection, the embryologist informs you when you will have your embryo transfer and provides a teaching
Step 14	Transfer day	**Embryo transfer** Please remember to come 30 min before the time of the transfer
Step 12	After transfer	**Receive post-transfer teaching** Continue taking your progesterone until pregnancy test **The nurse will inform you about the date of your pregnancy test on your embryo transfer day. If you have been asked to have a pregnancy blood test, this** will be booked by a nurse on the embryo transfer day
Step 13	16 days after collection day	**Do the pregnancy test**
Step 14	Same or 1 day after pregnancy blood test	Inform the fertility center about your pregnancy test results. If you have had a pregnancy blood test, a nurse calls you to give you the results **Negative results** Stop progesterone Continue all the vitamins Book an appointment with your doctor **Uncertain** Repeat pregnancy blood test in 2 days **Positive results** Continue progesterone up to 7–12 weeks of pregnancy or as directed by the nurse Stop all vitamins, except folic acid and prenatal vitamins After around 7–16 days from your pregnancy test, book an appointment for a “gestational scan” or “vitality scan.”

We recommend you take 1 month’s break between fresh IVF cycles to allow the ovaries to resume normal before being re-stimulated. If you do have frozen embryos remaining from your fresh cycle, however, you can choose to proceed with a frozen embryo transfer cycle when you are ready to do so.

20.6 Frozen Embryo Transfer Cycle (FERC)

Patient's Guidelines

- FERC protocol lasts about 3 weeks.
- You will be taking medication (pills or/and injections), coming for ultrasound scans. You are responsible for booking your ultrasound scan; medical staff will tell you when to.
- You should not start taking any medications before your first ultrasound.
- Please, note that Day 1 is considered the first day of full bleeding of your cycle.

Are the following requests completed and signed?
- Serology tests for female and male partners
- FERC consent form

Step	Day	Action
Step 1	Day 1–4 of your period	**Call the Clinic** A nurse ensures that you can start your protocol right away or if you have to wait, as well as making sure that all of your tests are completed before starting
Step 2	Day 2–4 of your period	**Book an appointment** by calling the reception, asking for an "IVF monitoring ultrasound" **for day 2–4**
Step 3		**Perform ultrasound #1** Doctor reviews your ultrasound results, and a nurse tells you if and when you can start your medication, if needed. You can immediately see a nurse for Step 4
Step 4		**(4.1) Receive calendar and injection teachings** You can have that teaching after the ultrasound #1 or book an appointment one day before it. In that case, please book an appointment asking for "Nurse Teaching" at the reception **(4.2) Book ultrasound #2** Ensure you know the date and time of your next ultrasound scan. If you have been asked to book your next scan at the reception, ensure you do so by asking for an "IVF monitoring ultrasound," before leaving the clinic
Step 5		**Get the estrogen medications if prescribed** You will know the date of the next ultrasound when you receive your calendar
Step 6		**Perform ultrasound #2** The doctor reviews your ultrasound results, and a nurse informs you if you need to get more medication or repeat another ultrasound. The doctor reviews the scan results and decides when you can start new medications. Whatever the ultrasound scan results are, a nurse will inform you about the next steps

(continued)

Step	Day	Action
Step 7 (If Step 4 not done)		**Receive calendar teaching** A nurse tells you when to start your progesterone. The embryologist informs you about the date of your embryo transfer
Step 8	Before transfer	**Receive embryo transfer preparation teaching** The nurse will give you instructions how to take the progesterone medication if prescribed
Step 9	Transfer	**Transfer** Please remember to come 30 min before the time of the transfer
Step 10	After transfer	**Receive post-transfer teaching** Continue taking your estrogen and progesterone if prescribed until your pregnancy test **The nurse will inform you about the date of your pregnancy test on your embryo transfer day. If you have been asked to have a pregnancy blood test, this** will be booked by a nurse on the embryo transfer day
Step 11		**Do pregnancy test** If bleeding, call the clinic, but continue your medications unless told to stop by the IVF center team
Step 14		**Receive results** Inform the fertility center about your pregnancy test results. If you have done a pregnancy blood test, a nurse calls you to give you the results **Negative results** Stop estrogen and progesterone Continue all the vitamins Book an appointment with your doctor **Uncertain** Repeat pregnancy blood test in 2 days; continue all medicines **Positive results** Continue estrogen and progesterone if prescribed up to 7–12 weeks of pregnancy or as directed by the nurse. Stop all vitamins, except folic acid and prenatal vitamins After around 7–16 days from your pregnancy test, book an appointment for “gestational scan,” or “vitality scan”

20.7 Frozen Embryo Replacement Cycle (FERC) Antagonist Protocol

Treatment Plan

Day 1 of Cycle: Please call IVF reception to register for treatment and to book your first scan appointment.

Day 1 of cycle is when you have a proper full bleed before

12:00 hours. Spotting is not counted as a proper full bleed. If you have a proper full bleed after 12:00 hours then the next day will be your Day 1 of the cycle.

We advise patients to use a barrier method of contraception (use of condom) or to abstain from intercourse from day 1 of their cycle and during their treatment.

You may have been advised to attend for a baseline scan; if so, please mention this at the time of your call, and you will be booked in for a baseline ultrasound scan before you start medication.

FERC Antagonist Protocol

You need to start to apply two patches (200 mcg) twice a week or estradiol tablets. 4 mg twice daily (The nurse will advise you when to start the patches or tablets.)

You also need to start the GnRH antagonist injection from **Day 2** of cycle and until

Day 8 of cycle.

After approximately 2 weeks of taking patches, you will have a scan appointment to confirm if you are ready for embryo transfer (E/T).

If you are not ready for E/T, then you will be given another scan appointment.

Start Progesterone Suppositories

If you are ready for embryo transfer, then you will be given instructions on when to commence Progesterone Suppositories (twice a day—one in the morning and one at night, roughly the same time each day).

You MUST continue applying the patches or taking the estradiol tablets until we advise you when to stop taking all your medications.

Day of Embryo Transfer

The number of embryos to thaw and how many are recommended for transfer would have already been discussed with you at Consultation Clinic.

If you decide to change your mind, then please call the IVF reception and ask to speak to the head of the embryologist department.

Information regarding embryo transfer (ET):

- Arrival Time for ET—this will be given to you by your nurse.
- -We advise patients to have a comfortable full bladder when they arrive for E/T, and this helps to visualize the endometrial cavity under ultrasound guidance

- You can eat and drink as normal
- E/T procedure is usually a simple and painless procedure and only takes a few minutes
- You will be able to empty your bladder after E/T (before leaving the IVF Unit)
- Speak to embryologist if you have any queries about your embryos

Post-embryo Transfer Information

Patients will be given an information sheet about what they can do or cannot do after the E/T.

We advise patients to abstain from any heavy lifting and strenuous exercise.

20.7.1 Pregnancy Test at Home

Patients will be given instructions (date and time) regarding urine pregnancy test on the day of embryo transfer.

A pregnancy test kit will be provided to do the test, and patients will be advised to email the results.

Estrogen Patches

The estrogen patch is used to thicken endometrium (lining of womb) before embryo transfer for patients having frozen embryo replacement cycle.

Patients are advised to change patches every other day until we ask them to stop the medication. The patches need to be applied to dry skin below the waist.

Side Effects of Estrogen Patches

Side effects are rare, but patients may have localized skin inflammation. Some patients may also have headaches, nausea and vomiting, increased vaginal discharge, and experience tenderness of the breast.

GnRH Antagonist

The GnRH antagonist blocks the effects of the natural hormone called gonadotropin-releasing hormone (GNRH). GNRH controls the secretion of another hormone called luteinizing hormone (LH), which induces ovulation during menstruation cycle. The antagonist is used to prevent the premature LH surge that might cause a premature release of egg cells.

Side Effects of GNRH Antagonist

Possible side effects of the GnRH antagonist injections are headaches, nausea, vaginal dryness and local irritation, and swelling at the site of injections.

Side effects are rare, but patients may have localized skin inflammation. Some patients may also have headaches, nausea and vomiting, increased vaginal discharge, and experience tenderness of the breast.

Progesterone Suppositories
Patient will be advised when to start progesterone suppositories. It should be inserted vaginally or rectally twice a day roughly the same time (one in the morning and one at night) until we ask patients to stop the medication.

Progesterone is used to keep the lining of the womb thick and to support the growth of the embryo in your womb.

Side Effects of Progesterone Suppositories
Side effects are rare, but patients may have breast tenderness, local inflammation and vaginal discomfort, abdominal swelling, vaginal discharge, constipation, or diarrhea.

Post-embryo Transfer Information
We advise patient to rest on the day of the embryo transfer. Patients will be given an information sheet about what they can do or cannot do after the E/T.

We advise patients to abstain from any heavy lifting and strenuous exercise.

Pregnancy Test at Home
Patients will be given instructions (date and time) regarding Urine Pregnancy Test on the day of embryo transfer. A pregnancy test kit will be provided to do the test, and patients will be advised to email the results to the nursing team.

We hope that this chapter aids in your understanding of the IVF protocols and for patient teaching. The patient teaching sections have been presented individually so they can be photocopied and given out to patients. It is likely that these protocols may vary slightly at your institutions; however, this chapter will still provide a solid basis for patient care.

Conflicts of Interest None of the authors have any conflicts of interest related to this chapter.

References

1. Messinis IE, Messini CI, Anifandis G. Ovarian stimulation protocols in fresh cycles and in elective freeze-all cycles. Syst Biol Reprod Med. 2025;71:307–29.
2. ESHRE Guideline Group on Ovarian Stimulation, Ata B, Bosch E, Broer S, Griesinger G, Grynberg M, Kolibianakis E, Kunicki M, La Marca A, Lainas G, Le Clef N, Massin N, Polyzos NP, Sunkara SK, Timeva T, Töyli M, Urbancsek J, Broekmans F. ESHRE guideline: ovarian stimulation for IVF/ICSI: an update in 2025. Hum Reprod. 2026;41:498–514.
3. Seyhan A, Ata B, Polat M, Son WY, Yarali H, Dahan MH. Severe early ovarian hyperstimulation syndrome following GnRH agonist trigger with the addition of 1500 IU hCG. Hum Reprod. 2013;28:2522–8.
4. Guo YC, Chen PY, Li TT, Jia L, Sun P, Zhu WS, Deng CC, Fang C, Liang XY. Different progestin-primed ovarian stimulation protocols in infertile women undergoing in vitro fertilization/intracytoplasmic sperm injection: an analysis of 1188 cycles. Arch Gynecol Obstet. 2019;299:1201–12.
5. Melado L, Ata B, Kalafat E, Del Gallego R, Bayram A, ElKhatib I, Lawrenz B, Fatemi H. Outcomes of GnRH agonist trigger in dydrogesterone-based PPOS versus GnRH antagonist cycles: a retrospective parallel cohort in freeze-all IVF treatment. Eur J Obstet Gynecol Reprod Biol. 2026;322:115101.
6. Awadalla SG, Friedman CI, Chin NW, Dodds W, Park JM, Kim MH. Follicular stimulation for in vitro fertilization using pituitary suppression and human menopausal gonadotropins. Fertil Steril. 1987;48:811–5.
7. Droesch K, Muasher SJ, Brzyski RG, Jones GS, Simonetti S, Liu HC, Rosenwaks Z. Value of suppression with a gonadotropin-releasing hormone agonist prior to gonadotropin stimulation for in vitro fertilization. Fertil Steril. 1989;51:292–7.
8. Kalaitzopoulos DR, Voros C, Blockeel C. Back to the future! Is there still a role for the GnRH agonist protocol in ovarian stimulation? Reprod Biomed Online. 2026;53:105733.
9. Schoolcraft W, Schlenker T, Gee M, Stevens J, Wagley L. Improved controlled ovarian hyperstimulation in poor responder in vitro fertilization patients with a microdose follicle-stimulating hormone flare, growth hormone protocol. Fertil Steril. 1997;67:93–7.
10. Surrey ES, Bower J, Hill DM, Ramsey J, Surrey MW. Clinical and endocrine effects of a microdose GnRH agonist flare regimen administered to poor responders who are undergoing in vitro fertilization. Fertil Steril. 1998;69:419–24.
11. Labrosse J, Haab E, Entezami F, Massin N. Outcomes of frozen embryo transfers from a large monocentric cohort (2982 cycles): towards a preferential use of cycles with a corpus luteum for endometrial preparation. Front Endocrinol (Lausanne). 2026;17:180860.
12. Marques LM, Van Muylder A, Brijs M, Lawrenz B, Fatemi HM, Luyten J. Cost-effectiveness of single euploid frozen embryo transfer in a true natural versus a hormonal replacement cycle. Fertil Steril. 2025;124(5 Pt 2):1032–41.

13. Edades J, Kalafat E, Ata B, Del Gallego R, Fatemi H, Lawrenz B. Assessment of interindividual follicular size variation at ovulation in natural-cycle frozen embryo transfer. Ultrasound Obstet Gynecol. 2025;65:125–7.
14. Li X, Shi W, Gao Y, Shi J, Li N, Bai H. Is duration of estrogen supplementation associated with clinical outcomes in frozen-thawed autologous single-blastocyst transfer cycles? J Assist Reprod Genet. 2022;39:1087–94.
15. al-Shawaf T, Yang D, al-Magid Y, Seaton A, Iketubosin F, Craft I. Ultrasonic monitoring during replacement of frozen/thawed embryos in natural and hormone replacement cycles. Hum Reprod. 1993;8:2068–74.

21 Nursing Leadership

Caitlin R. Hebert

21.1 Introduction

The field of reproductive endocrinology and infertility (REI) has grown substantially since 1978. The total number of children born via in vitro fertilization (IVF) is expected to approach 10 million worldwide [1]. These numbers would not be possible without the important contributions of the nurses who care for these patients and support fertility clinics across the world. While modern fertility case management practices vary widely across roles and regions, nursing staff have the most frequent and intimate involvement with the care of patients [2]. In this book, we have discussed how fertility nurses coordinate among interdisciplinary teams to help patients accomplish the goal of completing fertility cycles. As new nurses become experienced in this field, they may begin to wonder what it means to be nurse leaders in this field.

The nurse leader does not necessarily have to hold official titles such as nurse manager, charge nurse, or nurse executive. To become leaders in the REI field, all nurses need is to gain relevant experience, excel as team players, and have a strong desire to lead. Common characteristics of a strong REI nurse include strong communication skills, critical thinking, flexibility, and empathy. The same skills utilized in patient care are what also make nurses excellent leaders, whether in the designated leadership position or as peers in the unit.

In this chapter, we explore the multifaceted role of the nurse leader in the REI clinic, focusing on three areas: quality management, education and training, and career development. Nurse leaders play an important role in ensuring high standards of care, and this chapter examines how their leadership impacts quality

C. R. Hebert (✉)
Shady Grove Fertility, Rockville, MD, USA
e-mail: caitlin.hebert@sgfertility.com

M. Das, M. H. Dahan (eds.), *A Comprehensive Guide to Reproductive Health and Infertility Medicine for Nurses*, https://doi.org/10.1007/978-3-032-24372-0_21

management in fertility units and clinics. Given the specialized nature of REI nursing, effective education and training are essential responsibilities for nurse leaders, who ensure that their teams are prepared to provide exceptional care. The chapter concludes by discussing how nurse leaders can advance their own professional growth and career development.

21.2 Quality Management in the Fertility Unit

Over the last fifty years, there have been many theories and much research on how leadership impacts quality management [3]. What do we mean by quality management in the fertility unit, and how do nurses, as leaders, contribute to quality management? In general, quality management involves systems or organizations to set a standard of care that leads to excellence, including key issues of patient safety, clinical effectiveness, patient experience, and regulatory compliance [4]. Given that nurses are involved in multiple components of care, the nurse coordinator carries a heavy burden of responsibility and additionally serves as a second set of eyes for elements for which they are not responsible.

Assisted reproductive technology (ART) is still a relatively new field. However, there has been a strong focus on quality management, particularly in the form of key performance indicators (KPIs) within the ART space. KPIs are seen as a valid way to check that the healthcare provided is high in quality and operates within acceptable limits. With respect to ART, there has been research on best practices across multiple disciplines, including effective treatments during stimulation, air quality standards in the laboratory, and limiting the number of embryos transferred. The commitments to quality management have increased ART success rates substantially since its inception. Throughout the world, ART has been regulated by many nations. Examples of this include the US, requirements of cycle outcome reporting to national entities such as the Centers for Disease Control (CDC) or, in the United Kingdom, inspections carried out by the Human Fertilization & Embryology Authority (HFEA). In both US clinics and UK clinics, nurses are frequently the individuals gathering delivery outcomes for reporting to their respective collection agencies and are the ones who help ensure appropriate protocols and documentation are completed to pass regulatory inspections.

At the beginning of the patient's journey, nurses are responsible for setting the stage for patient safety and patient experience by reviewing the process in detail and confirming that patients have provided fully informed consent. Conveying both the strictness of aspects of care in combination with the unpredictable nature of a personalized response to treatment is essential for patients preparing for their treatment cycles. Nurses play crucial roles in consent, education, and compliance.

Nursing teams are frequently the primary educators of patients related to medication administration. The accuracy of the prescribed therapies must be strictly adhered to maximize clinical success. The safety of medication management requires comprehensive education, including about usage (mixing, administering, handling, and storing), side effect education, medication interactions, and adverse reactions. Nurses' ability to provide comprehensive education can have profound impacts on patients. The stringent aspects of trigger shots (typically given within a tightly prescribed window), which constitute an essential part of successful ART cycles [5], are discussed in Chap. 9. If the nurse has not adequately educated the patient on proper administration or provided the appropriate window for triggering, there is a chance that the patient will not experience final oocyte maturation or ovulation prior to egg retrieval. Both outcomes not only compromise the clinical success of patients but also contribute to a negative patient experience.

Research suggests that ART procedures are relatively safe [6]; however, there are complications that can occur as a result of controlled ovarian hyperstimulation, oocyte retrieval and early pregnancy challenges. ART complications, as discussed in Chap. 14, and early pregnancy problems are frequently identified through nurse and patient communication. The nurse leaders on the unit look not only to help other nurses triage patients who are experiencing complications appropriately, but also to help address patterns within the practice. Research suggests that specialized nurses with high levels of expertise are able to identify, prevent adverse events and minimize patient suffering [7]. Nursing leaders on the unit are promoters of a culture of continuous improvement.

Case Scenario:

You are the senior nurse on your clinic's fertility unit. A nurse with less than six months of experience comes to you because a patient is unhappy with the requirement to complete a series of infectious disease bloodwork tests prior to starting treatment. The patient requested that their concerns be escalated to a senior nurse.

Context: The new nurse reported that a previous nurse had allowed the patient to proceed with REI treatment without completing this requirement.

Approach: You call the patient back to review the rationale for blood testing. Some of these tests are required by law, and others are required by national standards of care. You also counsel the patient that some tests are important to rule out problems that could reduce their chance of conception or increase the risk to mother or baby.

Outcome: The patient verbalizes the understanding of the rationale and states that they will obtain the bloodwork drawn prior to the start of the treatment cycle.

Discussion Questions:

- How can nursing leaders on the unit handle situations where patients are dissatisfied with requirements while upholding ethical, clinical, and legal compliance?
- What strategies can be utilized to mentor peers when managing patient interactions and expectations?
- How would you address the new nurses' report of prior deviation from the protocol as a leader on the unit?

21.3 Education and Training

Unlike many other nursing specialties, the majority of nurses moving into the REI field do not come into the field with strong reproductive health and infertility foundational knowledge. Research suggests that the nursing education received prior to obtaining licensure includes limited evidence of sexual and reproductive healthcare content [8]. There is a strong learning curve for new nurses, not only in terms of clinical information but also because many nurses come from the bedside, they must also learn best practices of case management.

There have been efforts from organizations such as ASRM (Association for Reproductive Medicine) and ESHRE (European Society of Human Reproduction and Embryology) to create education content that can be utilized to support the transition of nurses. ASRM offers a foundational course called "Nurses in REI Communication, Knowledge, and Skills" as well as a subsequent course for the more experienced REI nurse called the Nurse Certificate Course in Reproductive Endocrinology and Infertility. ESHRE offers a certification for nurses and midwives that is available to those nurses practicing in REI with a minimum educational level of a bachelor's degree or equivalent. With the understanding that certification promotes a commitment to lifelong learning, increases competency and allows nurses to establish a sense of pride in their work [9], the NPG (Nurses' Professional Group) of ASRM has worked with NCC (National Certification Corporation) to reinstate a national certification to be available for American and Canadian nurses. Even with these courses available, the majority of nurses report that the type of training they receive as an REI care coordinator is "observational on the job" [10]. This leaves the responsibility of training new nurses to the experienced nursing leaders in the unit.

An additional challenge in the education and training of reproductive health and infertility nurses is the many differences in what nurses and midwives in the field are responsible for in different countries and clinics [11]. Without established baseline expectations of the nurse's role, it is difficult for national or international educational programs to provide comprehensive knowledge to successfully establish new nurses in the role. Furthermore, without clear metrics for success (similar to the KPIs established for the embryology lab), it can be very difficult for nursing leaders to communicate what success looks like for those unfamiliar with the clinical role, i.e., stakeholders who may be in roles that control their staffing, evaluations, and compensation.

Case Scenario:
A new nurse has joined your busy private practice, and another senior nurse has been tasked with precepting the new nurse employee. The new nurse reported that they feel overwhelmed by the complexity of the unit's procedures and that when she goes to work with the senior nurse tasked to precept her, she is told that they do not have time to review the information.

Context: This senior nurse is excellent at providing comprehensive care, but they also have the largest and most complex patient load on the unit.

Approach: You go to your nursing supervisor and offer to precept the new hire since you feel you have the capacity to take on this responsibility. They approve the transition to the new hire under your guidance.

Outcome: The new hire reported that they feel more confident in caring for patients; however, their senior nurse colleague reported feeling undermined that leadership took away the training responsibility from them.

Discussion Questions:

- What steps could you take to ensure that the senior nurse feels supported along with the new hire?
- What strategies can be used to ensure that preceptors have the time and resources to effectively mentor new nurses?
- How can mentorship or training responsibilities be shared across teams to build a sustainable training model in your clinic?

21.4 Career Development

There are many facets of career development, including continuing education, taking on new titles or responsibilities, and committing to lifelong learning.

Improving the quality of nursing care, improving safety, and decreasing healthcare costs are all extrinsic and important positive impacts that promote career development in nurses providing care to patients and organizations [12]. For clinics, there is value in prioritizing career development because it creates a more versatile, resilient, and effective workforce. For the nurse leader, career development may also reap rewards of personal satisfaction, respect from colleagues, and increased salaries.

Both ESHRE and ASRM (professional organizations) host conferences with content created for and by nurses, including symposia, postgraduates, round tables and venues for nurses to share their research. Conferences are a great way for nurse leaders to get to know others in the field, learn about best practices, and develop specific skills.

As the nurse leader takes on more responsibility or cases with greater complexity, they are also taking on additional learning opportunities. As the nurse leader takes stock of their long-term goals, they should not only look at what their previous experiences show that they have strength in but also seek to find places where they find their joy.

Since nurse leaders frequently participate in some facet of training, their passion may involve the education and training of new nurses. They may choose to pursue additional education, including master's or doctorate degrees in nursing education. REI nurse leaders may also want to pursue leadership roles within their practice or continue education on the business side. Nurses who like working within EMRs (electronic medical records) may want to consider informatics (a specialty that combines nursing science with computer science and information science). There are also careers in industry (such as pharmaceutical companies) or academia and research. Additionally, some nurses have decided to pursue advanced clinical practice (DNP); with this degree, more nurses are working at the top of their licensures within clinics, helping with patient consultation and procedures. Whatever path the nurse in REI decides to pursue, the skills cultivated in their case management will set them up for success.

Case Scenario:

Thomas is an experienced nurse at your fertility practice who would like to transition into a greater leadership role. In the past three years, he has precepted new nurses, was a superuser for the EMR, and has helped lead the lunch time journal club. He has come to you for advice.

Context: Thomas has a bachelor's degree but is unsure if he would like to do any additional education at this time.

Approach: You have Thomas spend time thinking about what of his previous activities made him feel the most fulfilled by or that he felt the most affinity for. You recommend that he investigate what types of leadership development opportunities are available at your practice to support him. You encourage him to look at conferences and to discuss how he feels after completing some of these activities.

Outcome: Thomas is able to attend a conference through which he was able to talk to a nurse who recently became the team lead in their clinic. He comes back and discusses with his supervisor about taking on the additional responsibilities and value that he can add to this role. His manager agreed, and he was promoted to a nursing team lead position.

Discussion Questions:

- What sorts of barriers might nurses face in pursuing leadership roles, and how can they be addressed?
- How can reflecting on past experiences help identify what career development path you might want to follow?
- How can practices create pathways for leadership growth without requiring additional formal education, or how can they make formal education more affordable?

21.5 Conclusion

As discussed, leadership is not confined to formal titles; it is reflected in nurses' ability to inspire their peers, support their patients, and drive improvements within their clinic. REI nurse case managers are uniquely positioned to influence patient outcomes and organizational success and develop the next generation of nurse coordinators in the field. The continued success of ART depends on the development and dedication of nursing professionals. As you reflect on your journey in this field, consider how you will set new benchmarks of excellence in your clinic, your peers, and yourself.

References

1. Centers for Disease Control and Prevention. 2018 Assisted Reproductive Technology National Summary Report US Dept of Health and Human Services; 2021.
2. Hariton E, Alvero R, Hill MJ, Mersereau JE, Perman S, Sable D, et al. Meeting the demand for fertility services: the present and future of reproductive endocrinology and infertility in the United States. Fertil Steril. 2023;120(4):755–66.
3. Hirtz PD, Murray SL, Riordan CA. The effects of leadership on quality. Eng Manag J. 2007 Mar;19(1):22–7.
4. Bhattacharya S, Hamilton M. Reproductive medicine for the MRCOG. Cambridge University Press; 2021. p. 157–8.
5. Maghraby H, Saleh H, Fourtia IL, Rasheed S, Elmahdy M, Abdelbadie AS, et al. The dilemma of the trigger timing in IVF: a review. Middle East Fertil Soc J. 2024;29(1).
6. Wang J, Sauer MV. In vitro fertilization (IVF): a review of 3 decades of clinical innovation and technological advancement. Ther Clin Risk Manag. 2006;2(4):355–64.
7. Glarcher M, Vaismoradi M. A systematic integrative review of specialized nurses' role to establish a culture of patient safety: a modeling perspective. J Adv Nurs. 2024.
8. Cappiello J, Coplon L, Carpenter H. Systematic review of sexual and reproductive health care content in nursing curricula. J Obstetr Gynecol Neonat Nurs. 2017;46(5):e157–67. Available from: https://www.jognn.org/article/S0884-2175(17)30272-1/fulltext
9. Garrison E, Schulz C, Nelson C, Lindquist C. Specialty certification. Nursing Manage (Springhouse). 2018;49(5):42–7.
10. Vlasic J, Stevenson E, Landrum M, Gedzyk-Nieman S, Wood J. Reproductive endocrinology and infertility nurse online orientation program evaluation: a quality improvement initiative. F&S Reports [Internet]. 2023;4(4):390–5. Available from: https://pubmed.ncbi.nlm.nih.gov/38204951/
11. Somers S, Cotton H, Kendrew H, Pomper J, Pinborg A, Jorgensen IR, et al. Empowering nurses and midwives: the evidence-base for the nurses and midwives certification Programme of ESHRE. Hum Reprod. 2024;39:2171.
12. Vázquez-Calatayud M, Errasti-Ibarrondo B, Choperena A. Nurses' continuing professional development: a systematic literature review. Nurse Educ Pract [Internet]. 2021;50(1):102963. Available from: https://www.sciencedirect.com/science/article/pii/S1471595320310490

How to Use the Fertility Medications, What Are Their Indications, and How to Deal with Complications

22

Michael H. Dahan and Seang Lin Tan

22.1 Introduction

The first human menopausal gonadotropin preparations were registered in the 1950s [18]. Recombinant human follicle-stimulating hormone (FSH) to treat infertility was first brought to market in 1995 [11], which was followed by recombinant luteinizing hormone (LH) in the early 2000s. These are the medicines used to stimulate follicles to grow for IVF and for other indications. Nurses will deal with many questions related to the administration of and complications related to the use of these medicines. In this chapter, we will present an introduction to these medicines and the other medicines we use in fertility care, how they are administered, and how to troubleshoot complications related to their use. There are four major producers of these medicines: Ferring, IBSA, Merck, and Organon. Many other companies also manufacture generic versions of these medications, which are known as biosimilars and are sold as both menopausal gonadotropins and recombinant human FSH.

22.2 Indications

In adult women, gonadotropins (FSH alone or with LH or LH activity) are indicated for:

M. H. Dahan (✉)
Department of Reproductive Endocrinology and Infertility, McGill University, Montreal, QC, Canada

S. L. Tan
Department of Obstetrics and Gynecology, McGill University, Montreal, Canada

OriginElle Fertility Clinic & Women' Health Centre, Montreal, Canada
e-mail: sltan@orignielle.com

M. Das, M. H. Dahan (eds.), *A Comprehensive Guide to Reproductive Health and Infertility Medicine for Nurses*, https://doi.org/10.1007/978-3-032-24372-0_22

1. anovulation (including polyendocrine metabolic ovarian syndrome) in women who have been unresponsive to treatment withclomiphene citrate or letrozole (or other oral ovulation induction medicines)
2. for ovulation inductions with or without intra-uterine insemination,
3. stimulation of multifollicular development in women undergoing superovulation for assisted reproductivetechnologies (ART) such as in vitro fertilization (IVF), gamete intra-fallopian transfer and zygote intra-fallopiantransfer, and
4. in association with a luteinizing hormone (LH) preparation for the stimulation of follicular development in women with severe LH and FSH deficiency [11, 12].

FSH or hMG (human menopausal gonadotropins) are also indicated for use in adult men for the stimulation of spermatogenesis in those who have congenital or acquired hypogonadotrophic hypogonadism. For this indication, FSH must be administered with concomitant human chorionic gonadotropin (hCG) therapy. This is not required when hMG is used. hCG provides LH activity in this case, since both LH and FSH are needed when both are lacking.

The active component of recombinant FSH mimics the action of endogenous FSH (FSH produced by the brain), which is secreted by the pituitary gland under the pulsatile stimulus of gonadotropin-releasing hormone (GnRH). In women, FSH induces follicular growth by regulating follicle recruitment in the ovary, and subsequent oocyte selection and the synthesis of steroid hormones [20, 21], thus preparing the reproductive tract for fertilization, implantation, and pregnancy [4]. In men, FSH mediates testicular development and spermatogenesis [4].

For women undergoing ovarian stimulation for multiple follicle development before ART, a dose of 150 to 225 IU/day of FSH is normally recommended, starting on Days 2 or 3 of the menstrual cycle. The first day of full flow is day one. However, in clinical practice, the starting dose is typically individualized based on specific baseline characteristics that are known to predict how a patient will respond to treatment. These include markers of ovarian reserve, age, body weight, and ovarian response to a previous cycle of ovarian stimulation. Accordingly, if a low ovarian response (hypo-response) is anticipated, the starting dose may be increased in a stepwise manner but should not exceed 450 IU/day. Alternatively, if an excessive ovarian response (hyper-response) is expected, the starting dose may be decreased to lower than 150 IU/day. During ovarian stimulation, ovarian response should be monitored carefully using ultrasound and hormonal monitoring [3], with adjustment to the starting dose after 3–7 days in increments of 75–150 IU/day [11, 12, 15], at the discretion of the treating physician [14, 19].

For men with hypogonadotropic hypogonadism, FSH should be given at a dose of 150 IU three times a week, concomitantly with hCG, for a minimum of 4 months. If, after this period, the patient has not responded, the combination treatment may be continued; current clinical experience indicates that treatment for up to 18 months may be necessary to achieve spermatogenesis [11, 12] in some men.

Human chorionic gonadotropin (hCG) is indicated for adult women undergoing multi-follicular development prior to egg collection and is administered to trigger final follicular maturation and stimulate development of the corpus luteum after ovarian stimulation. It is also indicated to trigger ovulation and corpus luteum development in anovulatory or oligo-ovulatory women following ovarian stimulation [9] with or without intrauterine insemination. The dose used is much higher than that found in hMG, 5000–10,000 units trigger ovulation, as compared to 75–300 units of hCG in hMG.

During ovarian stimulation, it is vital that ovulation is precisely timed, so that the oocyte retrieval process can be performed at the optimum time to retrieve the maximum number of mature oocytes. Otherwise, the patient will ovulate, and the eggs will be lost in the belly cavity. In natural cycles, a mid-cycle increase in the levels of luteinizing hormone (LH surge) indicates that ovulation will occur within 24–36 hours. In women undergoing ovarian stimulation, it can be difficult to predict when the LH surge will occur, and it may happen before many of the follicles are fully mature.

To ensure the precise coordination of ovulation and mature oocyte retrieval, women undergoing ovarian stimulation are given drugs (gonadotropin-releasing hormone [GnRH] antagonists, agonists, or progesterones) that prevent this rise [6, 16]. Because the LH surge has been prevented, ovulation needs to be induced in women treated with GnRH antagonists, agonists, or progesterones using preparations that stimulate LH release from the patient's brain or hCG. LH and hCG bind to the same receptor in the pituitary gland, although the two molecules have different binding affinity (strength of attachment and duration of action) [2, 13, 17]. This LH or hCG trigger ensures timed final follicular maturation and ovulation that can be synchronized with the oocyte retrieval procedure [5, 17]. Trigger normally occurs 33–38 hours before egg collection. The eggs detach from the follicle wall 32–33 hours after the trigger and ovulation will occur at about 40 hours, at which time the eggs will be lost.

hCG is administered 24–48 hours after the last administration of any gonadotropin preparation used for ovarian stimulation or when the lead follicle is at least 18 mm in mean diameter after oral medications for ovulation induction, once optimal stimulation of follicular growth has been achieved. This is done for intrauterine insemination or intercourse since the sperm live for up to 4 days in the women's reproductive tract and the egg lives for about 24 hours after ovulation, given a significant time overlap for fertilization to occur.

Another option is to administer a single injection of GNRH agonist to trigger ovulation in IVF cycle, not in intercourse or insemination cycles. This can be done in the GNRH antagonist cycle and the progesterone primed ovarian stimulation cycles, and it will induce an LH surge from the patient's pituitary gland. This can be done to prevent ovarian hyperstimulation syndrome, which usually requires an injection of hCG to occur in a woman with many follicles stimulated. This type of trigger cannot be used in women with hypothalamic pituitary dysfunction or women being treated with GnRH agonist IVF protocols.

Gonadotropin-releasing hormone (GnRH) antagonist binds to the GnRH receptor in the anterior pituitary, providing immediate and reversible inhibition of the natural LH surge that precedes ovulation [6, 16]. This ensures that optimal stimulation of follicular growth can be achieved and oocyte retrieval timed precisely.

GnRH antagonists can be administered as either a fixed or a flexible protocol. In the fixed protocol, the GnRH antagonist is typically started on Day 5 or 6 of ovarian stimulation and should continue throughout the gonadotropin treatment period, including the day of ovulation induction. However, the starting day of the GnRH antagonist is dependent on ovarian response and can be delayed in the absence of follicular growth [7–10]. In the flexible protocol, the GnRH antagonist is started when the largest ovarian follicle has reached a specific size, usually between 12 and 14 mm, and/or when serum estradiol reaches a specific threshold [1]. Estradiol produced by the ovary can act as the messenger to the brain to release LH and trigger ovulation.

In both the fixed and the flexible protocols, the GnRH antagonist should be administered once daily, at 24 h intervals, either in the morning or the evening, via subcutaneous injection in the lower abdominal wall [7–10]. The timing of injection should not vary more than 1-hour from the 24-hour window, although this will not result in spontaneous ovulation in many cases. Occasionally if patients ovulate pre-egg collection on a single daily dose of GnRH antagonist, 12-hour interval dosing should be considered, particularly if the patient is obese. However, verification of proper use of the medicine should be verified.

Another option to prevent spontaneous ovulation in an IVF cycle is to provide the patient with progesterone. This is usually done as oral medication, once daily. This has the benefit of being a pill instead of an injection; it is inexpensive when compared to other medication such as GnRH antagonists and can be started as a fixed or flexible protocol. The progesterone can start with stimulation day 1 or 5–6 or when the lead follicle is 12–14 mm in mean diameter. In this protocol, a fresh embryo transfer cannot be undertaken, since the prolonged use of the progesterone will make the uterine lining out of phase with the embryo preventing implantation.

A third option to prevent ovulation is the daily GnRH agonist. It can be used for the downregulation and prevention of premature LH surges. Treatment can be started in the early follicular phase (day 2 or 3 of the menstrual cycle) or in the mid-luteal phase (day 21–23 of the menstrual cycle or 5–7 days before expected start of menses). It is with that subsequent menses that the ovarian stimulation starts. Controlled ovarian stimulation with gonadotropins should be started after approximately 2–4 weeks of GnRH agonist treatment. When a suitable number of follicles have reached an appropriate size, treatment with the GnRH agonist and gonadotropin (FSH or hMG) is stopped and a single injection of hCG is administered to induce the final follicular maturation.

Progesterone supplementation is needed during the luteal phase of an ART procedure, which helps to prepare the lining of the uterus to receive the fertilized oocyte. Daily application of the progesterone should be continued for a total of 5 to 10 weeks if there is laboratory evidence of pregnancy, although this may vary according to clinical judgment. Progesterone is provided both in IVF patients and women who used FSH medications for ovulation induction with or without intrauterine insemination, the lack of which reduces pregnancy rates.

22.3 Known Contraindications to the Use of FSH and hMG

Known contraindications include the following: hypersensitivity to the active substance or to any of the excipients; malignant tumors of the ovary, breast, uterus, pituitary, or hypothalamus; abnormal (not menstrual) vaginal bleeding without a known/diagnosed cause due to the possibility of cancer; the presence of uncontrolled non-gonadal endocrinopathies (e.g., thyroid, adrenal, or pituitary disorders); primary ovarian failure as these medicines will not work; and ovarian cysts or enlarged ovaries. Unless a surrogate is used or the patient is awaiting surgery, other contraindications are fibroid tumors of the uterus incompatible with pregnancy or malformations of the reproductive organs incompatible with pregnancy.

22.4 Complications of Ovarian Stimulation and IVF Caused by These Medicines

Care should be taken in women with the following risk factors for OHSS: a history of ovarian hyperstimulation syndrome (OHSS), a previous COS cycle that resulted in more than 30 follicles ≥11 mm measured by ultrasound examination, basal antral follicle count >20, and polyendocrine metabolic ovarian syndrome (PMOS).

- **Ovarian Hyperstimulation Syndrome (OHSS):**
  - Nurses should be vigilant for signs of OHSS, a possible side effect characterized by rapid weight gain, abdominal pain, nausea, diarrhea, and enlarged ovaries. Patients at risks of developing OHSS should avoid hCG administration or should avoid further hCG injections if already occurring, to prevent further complications, and the condition should be closely managed under medical supervision. Please refer to local policy and/or protocols.
- **Venous Thromboembolism (VTE) Risk:** Nurses should be aware of the increased risk of venous thromboembolism (VTE) in patients undergoing fertility treatments, particularly those involving ovarian stimulation. Women with recognized risk factors for VTE, such as a personal or family history of thromboembolic events, obesity (BMI > 30 kg/m^2), or thrombophilia, may be at heightened risk of developing blood clots during or following treatment with gonadotropins. It is essential for nurses to assess the patient's history thoroughly and collaborate closely with the fertility specialist to mitigate this risk. Monitoring for signs of VTE, including unexplained leg pain, swelling, and shortness of breath, is crucial. In high-risk patients, preventive measures, such as anticoagulant therapy, may be considered. Patient education on recognizing VTE symptoms and seeking immediate medical attention is also a critical component of care.
- **Multiple Pregnancies.**
- Women undergoing ovulation induction with or without intrauterine insemination with FSH or hMG have an increased risk of multiple pregnancies (primarily

twins). Nurses should inform patients of this risk and ensure regular monitoring to minimize it.

Fertility medications are administered through various routes, including intramuscular or subcutaneous injection, and commonly require several administrations over a number of days. Prefilled multi-dose injectors to deliver these medications are now widely available from most of the major companies. The most essential characteristics of injector pens are the devices having a multi-use, ready-to-use construction which does not require mixing, dose confirmation, and having a dose counter with digits.

22.5 Instructions for Use

What to do before you start using the injector pens.

1. Getting the pen ready for injection, including:
   - Checking the reservoir is not cracked and the solution is clear.
   - Verifying that the dose display is set to zero.
2. Attaching the single-use needle before each injection.
3. Setting the dose:
   - The dose-setting knob should be turned clockwise for some pens, bidirectionally for others, until the prescribed dose shows in the dose-display window.
   - If the knob is turned past the prescribed dose, the dose-setting knob can be turned counterclockwise until the correct dose is displayed.
4. Injecting the dose as indicated by a healthcare professional into the upper thigh or abdomen:
   - Before injection, patients should double-check that the correct dose is shown in the dose-display window and adjust if necessary.
   - The needle should be inserted into a raised section of skin at the designated injection site at a 90-degree angle to the skin and, with the needle in the skin, the injection button should be depressed for at least 5 seconds to ensure the full dose is injected.
5. After injecting:
   - The dose window should show zero to indicate that the full dose has been administered.
   - If the dose window does not show zero, the pen is empty and the full dose has not been administered.
   - In this event, the number shown by the dose display is the missing amount that will have to be injected using a new pen injector; the dose indicated on the empty pen injector is the exact dose that should be dialled on the new pen to complete the daily dose.

For injectable medicines, after inserting the needle and pressing down the injection button (until the number "0" lines up with the dose indicator) in the case of pens, the patient should wait at least 5 seconds before releasing the injection button or removing the needle form under the skin. After this time, the needle should be slowly removed from the injection site.

22.5.1 How to Inject Fertility Medications

Hands should be washed thoroughly with soap and water. The most convenient site for injection is the abdomen a few inches from the navel or the upper thigh. The injection site should be cleaned with a disinfectant to remove any surface bacteria. Let the area dry for at least a minute. With the syringe held upward, remove the needle cover if present. Pinch a large area of skin around the clean area with the forefinger and thumb. For comfort, rotate the injection site daily. The needle should be inserted at the base of the pinched-up skin at an angle of 45–90 degrees to the skin surface. With the needle inserted in the correct position, pull back on the plunger slightly if not using a pen or injector to ensure there is no blood return into the syringe. The patient will encounter some resistance in doing so. If the patient sees blood, the needle may have hit a vein or artery. If this happens, draw back slightly and reposition the needle without removing it for injection. If the needle is completely removed, a new, sterile, prefilled syringe should be used. Cover the injection site with a swab containing disinfectant and hold pressure. The site should stop bleeding in 1–2 minutes. Once the needle is correctly placed, depress the plunger slowly and steadily so the solution is correctly injected, and the skin is not damaged. Pull the plunger out quickly after waiting 5 seconds under the skin and apply pressure to the site with a swab containing disinfectant. Dispose of the syringe or needle cap in an appropriate sharps container.

22.6 Troubleshooting the Medications

Q What should I do when I cannot push the injection button to deliver the dose?

A This means the pen is empty and unable to provide the desired dose.

Q What do I do if there is not enough medicine remaining in the pen for my prescribed dose?

A If the dose display shows a number higher than "0" after injection, this indicates that the pen is empty and that the complete dose has not been given. If this happens, the number shown in the dose display indicates the missing amount that needs to be injected using a new pen to complete the dose.

Q What do I do if I dialled the wrong dose?

A To adjust the dialled dose, the injection button can be turned either clockwise or counterclockwise. Some pens only can be dialled in one direction. Once the correct dose is indicated in the display window, you can proceed with the injection.

Q How does storage outside the recommended storage conditions influence the stability of the product?

A A product should not be stored outside the recommended storage conditions (please refer to the product information).

Q What should I do if there are any air bubbles in the syringe?

A To remove the air bubbles, hold the syringe with the needle pointing upward and gently flick the syringe until all the air collects at the top. Push the plunger until the air bubbles are gone.

Q What should I do if the syringe shows visible signs of deterioration or if the liquid contains particles or is not clear?

A Do not use the product if you notice these signs.

Q What if the product has been exposed to a higher or lower temperature than recommended, such as by leaving it in a car?

A Do not use the product and obtain new product.

Q My patient is very anxious about needles and injection site pain.

A echniques such as cooling the injection site with an ice pack beforehand and bringing medicine out of the fridge 30 minutes before injection so it is at room temperature can be helpful.

Q What if my patient has difficulty inserting the vaginal progesterone with the applicator?

A The applicator with the insert can be placed into the vagina while the patient is standing, sitting, or lying on her back with knees bent.

Q What if my patient misses a dose of vaginal progesterone?

A A missed dose can be taken as soon as the patient remembers but should not be more than the daily dose prescribed.[5]

Q How should the multi-use applicator for certain vaginal progesterone (where available) be cleaned between uses?

A The applicator should be rinsed thoroughly in warm running water and wiped dry with a soft tissue.[5]

22.7 For Gonadotropin Powder that Needs Reconstituting

Q What if the powder does not dissolve when the solvent is added?

A If the powder is not dissolving once the solvent has been added, roll the vial gently between your hands until the solution is clear. Shaking should be avoided. The solution should not be administered if it contains particles or is not clear.

Q How many hMG or FSH or LH vials can I mix at a time?

A Mostly, multiple powder vials can be dissolved with one ampoule/vial of solvent. Please check your local label for specific guidance.

Q How far in advance can hMG or FSH or LH be reconstituted?

A These medicines must only be reconstituted immediately before first use. Where available, multidose formulations can be stored for a maximum of 28 days at not more than 25 ° C after reconstitution.

Important to note is that:

The injection site should be varied to prevent lipoatrophy.
Medicinal products must not be used after the expiry date.

22.8 Adverse Reactions

The most frequently reported adverse drug reactions (ADR) during treatment with FSH-containing products in clinical trials, in order of seriousness, are ovarian hyperstimulation syndrome (OHSS), headache, abdominal pain, abdominal distension, and injection site pain.

Vaginal progesterone can cause vaginal irritation and even non-uterine vaginal bleeding. Other forms of progesterone luteal support can be attempted. The patient should be reassured that the bleeding is not likely to affect the pregnancy; however, an evaluation by the physician should be undertaken. Intramuscular injections of progesterone in oil for luteal phase support commonly cause redness and a rash at the injection sight which if localized and without shortness of breath are more likely reactionary than allergic in origin. The pain that commonly accompanies these injections are minimized by rotating injections in opposite sides of the gluteus maximus, a large muscle, and using ice packs before and after the injections. Other muscles should not be used for injection of intra-muscular progesterone. Care should be taken to avoid injection in the sciatic nerve, which also is located close to this muscle, by injecting in the upper one-third of the muscle. Inflammation and sterile abscesses are also known to occur, and if swelling occurs, the patient should be referred to the doctor. Use of progesterone injections in water or oral luteal support progesterone can help avoid these complications. Only a single oral progesterone, that is effective for luteal support is on the market and it is not available in many countries. Most progesterone is metabolized rapidly by the liver preventing oral administration for luteal support in fertility care. The marketed oral product is an exception.

22.9 Specific Companies' Fertility Medications

Note that some of these products may not be approved for use/available in your country, and there may be slight differences in prescribing information (PI) in different countries. So, please check with your local pharmaceutical representative for details.

Key safety data may vary from country to country. Please refer to your local product label.

We at first present the trade name since this is likely how these products will be called in your fertility centers and you will need to be familiar with this name. This is followed by the generic name.

22.10 Products by the Ferring Pharmaceuticals

22.10.1 Menopur®

Menopur® which is the brand name of menotropin is highly purified human menopausal gonadotropin (HP-hMG) containing human follicle-stimulating hormone (FSH) bioactivity and human luteinizing hormone (LH) bioactivity in a 1:1 ratio. LH bioactivity is mainly derived from hCG (human chorionic gonadotropin). It is available in two forms.

22.10.2 Powder and Solvent for Solution for Injection

Appearance of powder: white to off-white lyophilized cake. Appearance of solvent: clear colorless solution. Available in 75 IU and 150 IU single-dose presentations and 600 IU and 1200 IU multidose presentations. The multidose formulation can be used to give more than one dose of menotropin. The powder must be reconstituted with the solvent provided in the package prior to use. The powder should only be dissolved immediately before use. The exact prescribed dose of reconstituted solution should be drawn up from the vial using one of the disposable syringes provided for injection and the dose should be administered immediately. There is a primming step. After reconstitution, the solution may be stored for a maximum of 28 days at not more than 25 °C. The un-reconstituted powder is stable for 3 years.

22.10.3 Solution for Injection in Prefilled Pen

· The prefilled pen is a disposable, dial-a-dose pen that can be used to give more than 1 dose of menotropin. The pen can be dialed to give doses from 6.25 IU to 450 IU of menotropin in marked increments of 6.25 IU. *Normal a*ppearance of solution is clear. It is available in 600 IU/0.96 ml and 1200 IU/1.92 ml presentations.

Menotropin 75 IU and 150 IU formulations: Do not store above 25 ° C. Do not freeze. Store in the original container to protect from light.

Menotropin 600 IU and 1200 IU formulations: Prior to reconstitution, store in a refrigerator at 2 ° C—8 ° C. Do not freeze. One reconstituted always store with the pen cap on to prevent degradation from light.

22.10.4 Rekovelle®

Rekovelle® is recombinant FSH delta.

Available forms.

FSH delta 12 micrograms/0.36 mL solution for injection in prefilled pen: one prefilled multidose pen delivers 12 micrograms follitropin delta in 0.36 mL solution.

FSH delta 36 micrograms/1.08 mL solution for injection in prefilled pen: one prefilled multidose pen delivers 36 micrograms follitropin delta in 1.08 mL solution.

FSH delta 72 micrograms/2.16 mL solution for injection in prefilled pen: one prefilled multidose pen delivers 72 micrograms follitropin delta in 2.16 mL solution.

One mL of solution contains 33.3 micrograms of follitropin delta.

FSH delta is dosed very differently than other FSH medications used in fertility care. This is due to the fact that equivalent daily doses in IUs with follitropin delta and other recombinant FSHs (determined using the Steelman Pohley rat bioassay) resulted in a higher ovarian response with follitropin delta. As the rat bioassay might not fully reflect the potency of the FSH in follitropin delta in humans, FSH delta is dosed in micrograms and not IUs.

For the first treatment cycle, the individual daily dose will be determined based on the FSH delta dosing algorithm (described in the label) which is based on the woman's serum anti-Müllerian hormone (AMH) concentration and her body weight. For women with AMH <15 pmol/L, the daily dose is 12 micrograms, irrespective of body weight. For women with AMH ≥15 pmol/L, the daily dose decreases from 0.19 to 0.10 micrograms/kg by increasing AMH concentration. The maximum daily dose for the first treatment cycle is 12 micrograms. For subsequent treatment cycles, the daily dose of FSH delta should be maintained or modified according to the patient's ovarian response in the previous cycle. The maximum daily dose for subsequent treatment cycles is 24 micrograms.

The pen can be dialed to give doses from 0.33 micrograms to 20 micrograms of FSH delta in marked increments of 0.33 micrograms. Before using the pen for the first time, the air and any bubbles should be removed from the cartridge (priming) to receive the correct dose. The dose can be corrected either up or down without loss of medicine by turning the dose knob in either direction until the correct dose lines up with the dose indicator.

The FSH delta prefilled pen only needs to be primed before the first use.

Chorapur®/Brevactid® is human chorionic gonadotropin. Human chorionic gonadotropin (hCG) is a glycoprotein comprising an alpha subunit that is common to luteinizing hormone (LH) and follicle-stimulating hormone (FSH), and a beta subunit that is unique to hCG. hCG is obtained from the urine of pregnant women, in this case. The amount of hCG is indicated in units of the biological action.

Powder: The powder for solution for injection is supplied in colorless, type 1 glass vials with rubber stopper closed with a cap. Solvent: The solvent for solution for injection is supplied in colorless, type 1 glass ampoules.

The shelf life is 3 years. For immediate, single use following reconstitution. It cannot be saved for future later injections.

22.10.4.1 hCG 5000 IU

In assisted reproductive technology programs such as in vitro fertilization (IVF), hCG 5000 IU is administered to trigger final follicular maturation and luteinization after stimulation of follicular growth.

It can be used to treat delayed puberty in boys with concomitant hypogonadotropic hypogonadism. Diagnosis should be made after assessment of the function of the testes in patients with hypogonadotropic hypogonadism before a stimulation treatment. Differential diagnosis includes cryptorchism and anorchism.

22.10.4.2 hCG 1500 IU

In case of hypogonadotropic hypogonadism, one vial of hCG1500 IU twice a week (corresponding to 3000 IU chorionic gonadotropin per week) in combination with hMG or FSH over a period of several months is recommended. The treatment should be continued for at least 3 months before any improvement in spermatogenesis can be expected. During this treatment, testosterone replacement therapy should be suspended, and testosterone levels should be monitored at intervals. It may be necessary to increase the hCG dose to achieve normal testosterone levels. If the response to general hCG therapy is not sufficient, additional administration of hMG or FSH may be necessary. Once an improvement has been achieved under combination therapy, it may in some cases be maintained by hCG alone.

22.10.5 Pediatric Population

Therapy of undescended testes should be completed by the end of the first year of life. The following dosage is recommended in young infants: 250 IU/dose (0.17 ml of the 1500 IU vial) twice a week for 5 weeks.

Gonapeptyl®/Decapeptyl® is the brand name of triptorelin acetate, which is a gonadotropin-releasing hormone (GnRH) agonist and is a synthetic decapeptide analogue of natural GnRH. Chronic administration of a GnRH agonist results in inhibition of pituitary LH and FSH secretion. Triptorelin-induced downregulation of the pituitary can prevent the LH surge and thereby prevent premature ovulation and/or follicle luteinization. The pituitary suppression effects were found to last 6 days from the end of treatment. It is provided as a clear colorless solution. This medication is injected as 0.1 mg/ml and is intended for subcutaneous injection once daily. For the downregulation and prevention of premature LH surges, treatment can be started in the early follicular phase (day 2 or 3 of the menstrual cycle) or in the mid-luteal phase (day 21–23 of the menstrual cycle or 5–7 days before expected start of menses). Controlled ovarian stimulation with gonadotropins should be started after approximately 2–4 weeks of GnRH agonist treatment. When a suitable number of follicles have reached an appropriate size, treatment with the GnRH agonist and gonadotropin is stopped and a single injection of hCG is administered to induce the final follicular maturation.

The most frequent adverse events are headache, vaginal bleeding/spotting, abdominal pain, injection site inflammation, and nausea. Ovarian cysts have been reported to occur during the initial phase of treatment with this medicine. They will reabsorb with time but may negatively influence an ovarian stimulation cycle.

Triptorelin is intended for subcutaneous injection once daily into the lower abdominal wall. Following the first administration, it is advised that the patient be kept under medical supervision for 30 minutes to ensure there is no allergic/

pseudo-allergic reaction to the injection. Facilities for treatment for such reactions should be immediately available. The following injections may be self-administered if the patient is made aware of the signs and symptoms that may indicate hypersensitivity, the consequences of such a reaction, and the need for immediate medical intervention. The injection site should be varied to prevent lipoatrophy.

Lutinus®/Endometrin® is the brand name of progesterone used for luteal support in fertility care. Each vaginal tablet contains 100 mg of progesterone. The dose is 100 mg administered vaginally two or three times daily starting at oocyte retrieval and continuing for up to 10 weeks total duration (or 12 weeks of gestation). It has a three-year shelf life at room temperature. This medicine is to be placed directly into the vagina by the applicator provided.

1. Unwrap the applicator.
2. Put one tablet in the space provided at the end of the applicator. The tablet should fit securely and not fall out.
3. The applicator with the tablet may be inserted into the vagina while you are standing, sitting, or when lying on your back with your knees bent. Gently insert the thin end of the applicator well into the vagina.
4. Push the plunger to release the tablet.

Remove the applicator and rinse it thoroughly in warm running water, wipe dry with a soft tissue, and keep the applicator for subsequent use.

Store in the original container. This medicinal product does not require any special storage conditions.

22.11 Products by the IBSA Group Pharmaceuticals

Meriofert® (menotrophin) is a human menopausal gonadotropin used in controlled ovarian stimulation (COS). It contains a combination of follicle-stimulating hormone (FSH) and luteinizing hormone (LH) activity, which helps in the recruitment and maturation of multiple ovarian follicles. The HMG contained in this menotrophin is extracted from the urine of post-menopausal women. Human chorionic gonadotrophin (hCG), extracted from the urine of pregnant women, is added to contribute to the total LH activity.

Available products

- IBSA's menotrophin prefilled syringe (PFS) 900 IU (multi-dose vial)—for subcutaneous administration only.
- IBSA's menotrophin 150 IU (single-use vial)— for subcutaneous or intramuscular administration.
- IBSA's menotrophin 75 IU (single-use vial)—for subcutaneous or intramuscular administration.

Indications:

1. Ovulation Induction:
2. IBSA's menotrophin prefilled syringes 900 IU/ 150 IU single vial and 75 IU single vial are used to induce ovulation or multi-folliculogenesis in women.

Complications

The most relevant adverse drug reaction in clinical trials with IBSA's menotrophin was dose related, ovarian hyperstimulation (OHSS).

The most frequent adverse reactions with IBSA's menotrophin were headache and abdominal distension, nausea, fatigue, dizziness, and pain at the injection site.

22.11.1 IBSA's Menotrophin 75 IU and 150 IU

Reconstitution of IBSA's menotrophin should be carried out under aseptic conditions using only the solvent provided. The solution must be prepared immediately before injection to ensure its integrity. Prior to reconstitution, a clean preparation area should be established, and hands should be thoroughly washed. To prevent the formation of foam, the vial should be gently rolled between the hands rather than shaken. Once reconstituted, the solution should be clear and colorless; any solution exhibiting particles or discoloration must not be used.

22.11.2 Transporting IBSA's Menotrophin 900 IU

No cool bag is required to transport the product home. However, store it in the refrigerator (2–8 °C) as soon as possible, ideally within a few hours. Short periods at room temperature (15–25 °C) do not affect efficacy or safety.

22.11.3 Storing Outside the Fridge

If IBSA's menotrophin 900 IU is left outside the fridge for a few days before reconstitution, do not use it. It must be stored in the fridge at 2–8 °C to maintain safety and efficacy.

22.11.4 Reconstitution Timing

IBSA's menotrophin 75 IU and 150 IU should be reconstituted immediately before use with the solvent provided. In contrast, IBSA's menotrophin multidose (900 IU) can be reconstituted and stored for use within 28 days. To prevent painful injections and minimize leakage from the injection site, IBSA's menotrophin should be slowly administered subcutaneously. The subcutaneous injection site should be alternated to prevent lipoatrophy. Any unused solution should be discarded.

Please note that the IBSA's menotrophin may be known under different names in different areas. Other names include Lifecell®, Meriofert®, Merional®, Fostimon®, Meriofert spuit®, or Mensinorm®.

22.11.5 Lubion® (Progesterone) Prefilled Syringe

Lubion® is a subcutaneous progesterone injection that can be injected intramuscularly as well and is indicated for luteal phase support in assisted reproductive technology (ART) treatments. It is injected once daily. It is the only subcutaneous progesterone currently available for luteal phase support. This form of progesterone is water-based which minimizes pain and decreased the risks of inflammation at the injection site and potentially abscess formation. Subcutaneous administration requires once-daily injections of 25 mg.

22.11.6 Nature and Contents of Container

Single-Use Vial:

IBSA's injectable progesterone is provided in a colorless glass vial, designed for single use. Each vial is sealed with a bromobutyl rubber stopper and secured with an aluminum seal and a "flip-off" cap. The medication is available in pack sizes containing 1, 7, or 14 vials, though not all these sizes may be available in every market.

Prefilled Syringe

Siliconized colorless glass syringe with a staked stainless-steel needle, closed at one end by a needle shield and at the other end by a siliconized bromobutyl plunger stopper.

There are two formulations: single-use-vial solution for injection and solution for injection in prefilled syringe.

- Each vial and prefilled syringe contains progesterone 25 mg solution for injection.

22.11.7 Dosage and Administration

IBSA's injectable progesterone is intended for intramuscular or subcutaneous administration.

Administer 25 mg once daily starting from the day of oocyte retrieval, typically continuing until 7–12 weeks of confirmed pregnancy.

22.11.8 Administration Methods

- Intramuscular (IM) injection (only applicable for the solution for injection formulation):
  - Select an area in the femoral quadriceps (right or left thigh).
  - Clean the area with a swab.
  - Administer the injection deeply at a 90° angle.
  - Inject slowly to minimize tissue damage.
- Subcutaneous (SC) Injection (applicable to both formulations):
  - Choose the front of the thigh or lower abdomen.
  - Swab the area, pinch the skin, and insert the needle at a 45° to 90° angle.
  - Inject slowly to reduce tissue damage.

1. Commonly Reported Adverse Events:
   - Injection site reactions: Pain, swelling, pruritus (itching), and hematomas at the site of injection. Nurses should monitor and manage these reactions by ensuring proper injection technique and providing post-injection care.
   - Breast and vulvovaginal disorders: Patients frequently reported breast tenderness, breast pain, vaginal discharge, vulvovaginal pruritus, and vulvovaginal discomfort. These symptoms, while common, should be noted, and patients should be reassured.
   - Gastrointestinal symptoms: Patients may experience nausea, vomiting, abdominal pain, and constipation. Symptomatic relief can be offered to alleviate discomfort.
   - Mood alterations and sleep disturbances: Mood changes, including depression, and sleep disorders like insomnia were noted. Nurses should closely monitor patients with a history of mental health disorders.
   - Neurological effects: Headaches, dizziness, and somnolence (drowsiness) were reported. Patients should be advised to avoid operating heavy machinery or driving if they experience these symptoms.
2. Less Common Adverse Events:
   - Skin and Subcutaneous Reactions: Some patients may experience skin issues such as rash, urticaria (hives), or pruritus.
   - Weight gain: A minority of patients reported an increase in body weight during treatment. Regular weight monitoring can help identify significant changes.
   - Fluid Retention: As progesterone may cause fluid retention, conditions such as epilepsy, migraine, or cardiac/renal dysfunction can be exacerbated. Nurses should monitor fluid balance and report any concerning symptoms.

3. Serious Adverse Events:
   - Hepatic disorders: While rare, some patients may develop jaundice or other liver-related issues. Patients with preexisting liver conditions should be closely monitored.

- Precautions with Medical Conditions:
  - Patients with hepatic or renal dysfunction should be carefully monitored, as accumulation of cyclodextrins can occur, especially in cases of moderate to severe renal dysfunction on IBSA's injectable progesterone.
  - Progesterone can cause fluid retention, so extra caution is advised for patients with conditions influenced by fluid retention such as epilepsy, migraine, asthma, or cardiac/renal dysfunction.
  - Diabetic patients need to be observed as progesterone can reduce insulin sensitivity and affect glucose tolerance.
- Risks for Older Adults and Smokers: In patients over 35 years, smokers, or those with risk factors for atherosclerosis, there is an increased risk of retinal vascular lesions and other complications like transient ischemic attacks or sudden severe headaches. Use should be terminated if such symptoms occur.
- Depression: Patients with a history of depression should be closely observed, as progesterone can exacerbate symptoms. Discontinuation should be considered if symptoms worsen.

22.11.9 Special Precautions for Storage

22.11.9.1 Storage Conditions for IBSA's Injectable Progesterone

Proper storage of medication is essential to ensure its efficacy and safety during IVF treatments. Nurses should be aware of the following guidelines for the storage of IBSA's injectable progesterone:

- Temperature Requirements: IBSA's injectable progesterone must be stored at a temperature below 25 °C. It is crucial to ensure that the medication is kept in a controlled environment and not exposed to excessive heat.
- Do Not Refrigerate or Freeze: Refrigeration or freezing can damage the solution. Make sure that IBSA's injectable progesterone is stored at room temperature and that patients are advised to avoid placing it in refrigerators or freezers at home.
- Protection from Light: The medication should remain in its original packaging to protect it from light exposure, which could degrade the solution's potency.
- Single-Use Vial: Once opened, the solution must be used immediately. Any leftover product should be discarded and must not be stored for future use.
- Prefilled syringe: Store in the original package in order to protect from light.

IBSA's injectable progesterone is known by many brand names including Alterpure®, Prolutex®, Progedex®, Pleyris®, Inprosub®, Lubion®, and Progiron®.

Fostimon® is a urofollitropin collected form the urine of menopausal women, which is a purified form of follicle-stimulating hormone (FSH). IBSA's purified urinary FSH is a hormone naturally produced by the pituitary gland and plays a critical role in the regulation of reproduction. IBSA's purified urinary FSH works by mimicking the natural FSH hormone, which encourages the growth and maturation of ovarian follicles, increasing the chances of ovulation or producing multiple eggs in women undergoing fertility treatments.

22.11.10 Formulations

- IBSA's purified urinary FSH 75 IU, powder, and solvent for solution for injection.
- IBSA's purified urinary FSH 150 IU, powder, and solvent for solution for injection.

IBSA's purified urinary FSH is administered via subcutaneous or intramuscular injection. It is crucial to alternate injection sites to avoid lipoatrophy. Administer the injection slowly to reduce discomfort and minimize leakage.

The powder should be reconstituted immediately prior to use with the solvent provided.

IBSA's purified urinary FSH is also known by other names including Fostimonkit®, Fostipur®, and Altermon®.

Zivafert® is human chorionic gonadotropin (hCG) and is used to trigger final oocyte maturation and ovulation in women undergoing ART procedures. It comes in a prefilled syringe containing 5000 IU of human chorionic gonadotropin (hCG), which is derived from human urine. It comes in a powder form that must be reconstituted for injection. A single dose of 5000 IU (one vial) or 10,000 IU (two vials) is typically administered 24–48 hours after follicular stimulation and 34–38 hours prior to IVF egg collection.

After reconstituting the powder with the provided solvent, the solution should be administered intramuscularly or subcutaneously. Any unused solution should be discarded.

Do not store above 25 °C.

Keep the vial and solvent in the prefilled syringe in the original package to protect the.

medicine from the light.

22.11.11 Nature and Contents of Container

1 pack contains: Powder in a vial (type I glass), sealed with a rubber closure and held in place with a flip-off cap.

1 ml of solvent in a prefilled syringe (type I glass), one long needle for the reconstitution and for the intramuscular injection and one short needle for the subcutaneous injection.

Multipack containing two packs of five vials + five prefilled syringes of solvent, as described above.

Not all pack sizes may be marketed.

IBSA hCG may also be known by other names in different markets including Dinaron®, Zivafert®, Choriomon®, Gonasi®, and Gonadotrophine Chorionique®.

22.12 Products by Merck®, Darmstadt, Germany

22.12.1 Gonal-*f*®

Gonal-*f*® is a medicine that contains the active component follitropin. Follitropin alfa is produced using recombinant DNA technology [8, 11].

Follitropin alfa is supplied in a vial containing either 1050 IU/1.75 mL or 75 IU powder and solvent and solution for injection, or as a prefilled, multidose injector (Follitropin Pen Injector 2.0), available in four dosing presentations (150 IU, 300 IU, 450 IU, and 900 IU). The required dose is dialed before each injection, with a maximum individual dose of 150 IU for the 150 IU presentation, 300 IU for the 300 IU presentation, and 450 IU for the 450 IU and 900 IU presentations. Each pen can deliver multiple injections, and users can dial the required dose in small increments of 12.5 IU (0.92 μg).

22.12.2 Pergoveris®

Pergoveris® is a medicine that contains the active substances follitropin alfa and lutropin alfa, in a fixed 2:1 ratio. Both components are produced using recombinant DNA technology and are free of urine-derived proteins (Lunenfeld 2004).

This medicine is supplied in a vial containing 150 IU follitropin alfa and 75 IU lutropin alfa or as a prefilled pen containing 300 IU/150 IU, 450 IU/225 IU, or 900 IU/450 IU follitropin alfa/lutropin alfa, respectively, where the higher number refers to the amount of follitropin alfa contained in each pen [7–10]. Each prefilled pen can deliver multiple doses of this medicine.

22.12.3 Luveris®

Luveris® is a medicine that contains the active substance lutropin alfa (recombinant human luteinizing hormone [r-hLH]; Merck KGaA, Darmstadt, Germany). Lutropin alfa, produced using recombinant DNA technology is free of urine-derived proteins and other contaminants. Lutropin alfa is available as a powder and solvent that are made up into a solution for injection [11, 12]. Lutropin alfa is indicated, in combination with a FSH preparation, for the treatment of adult women with infertility to stimulate the development of the follicles in the ovary.

22.12.4 Ovitrelle® or Ovidrel® (Different Names Based on Location)

Ovitrelle® is a medicine that contains the active ingredient human choriogonadotropin alfa (recombinant human chorionic gonadotropin [r-hCG]; Merck KGaA, Darmstadt, Germany). The r-hCG is produced using recombinant DNA technology. r-hCG contains 250 μg r-hCG (equivalent to approximately 6500 IU) in a 0.5 mL solution for injection in a prefilled syringe or a prefilled, single-dose, single-use pen injector [7–10].

22.12.5 Cetrotide®

Cetrotide® is a class of drug known as a gonadotropin releasing hormone (GnRH) antagonist. This GnRH antagonist contains the active ingredient Cetrorelix. It is supplied as a vial containing 0.25 mg GnRH antagonist and a solvent for solution for injection; after reconstitution with the solvent, each mL of the solution contains 0.25 mg GnRH antagonist.

22.12.6 Crinone®

Crinone® is an 8% vaginal progesterone gel, supplied as a 90 mg/g vaginal gel in a specially designed sealed applicator. Each applicator delivers 1.125 g of gel containing 90 mg of progesterone. 8% vaginal progesterone gel should be applied every day; the starting day is decided based on clinician judgment and is usually within a few days after the oocyte retrieval. It can be used once or twice daily with most studies showing similar live birth rates, although rates of vaginal bleeding in pregnancy are higher with once daily dosing.

22.13 The Organon & Co.® Products

22.13.1 Corifollitropin Alfa Is Marketed as Elonva®

22.13.1.1 Molecule Information

Corifollitropin alfa is designed as a sustained follicle stimulant with the same pharmacodynamic profile as (rec)FSH, but with a markedly prolonged duration of FSH activity, thus differentiating it from other rFSH products. The long duration of FSH activity was achieved by adding the carboxy-terminal peptide of the β-subunit of human chorionic gonadotropin (hCG) to the β-chain of human FSH. Corifollitropin alfa does not display any intrinsic LH/hCG activity. The half-life of CFA is approximately 70 h compared to 33 h for rFSH.

22.13.1.2 How to Use

Corifollitropin alfa is available in two different doses: (1) 100 microgram solution for injection—each prefilled syringe contains 100 microgram of corifollitropin alfa in 0.5 mL solution for injection and (2) 150 microgram solution for injection—each prefilled syringe contains 150 microgram of corifollitropin alfa in 0.5 mL solution for injection. In the treatment of women of reproductive age, the dose of corifollitropin alfa is based on weight and age. A single 100-microgram dose is recommended in women who weigh less than or equal to 60 kilograms and who are 36 years of age or younger. A single 150-microgram dose is recommended in women who weigh more than 60 kilograms, regardless of age, or who weigh 50 kilograms or more and who are older than 36 years of age. Women older than 36 years of age who weighed less than 50 kilograms were not studied.

Due to corifollitropin alfa's ability to initiate and sustain multiple follicular growth for an entire week, a single subcutaneous injection of the recommended dose of corifollitropin alfa may replace the first seven injections of any daily (rec) FSH preparation in a COS treatment cycle. Corifollitropin alfa is indicated for controlled ovarian stimulation (COS) for the development of multiple follicles in women participating in IVF.

Corifollitropin alfa is also indicated for the treatment of adolescent males (14 years and older) with hypogonadotropic hypogonadism, in combination with human chorionic gonadotropin (hCG).

Corifollitropin alfa should be administered as a single subcutaneous injection, preferably in the abdominal wall, typically during the early follicular phase of the menstrual cycle. On stimulation day 5 or 6, the concurrent determination of serum estradiol levels may be useful. Stimulation day 8: Seven days after the injection with corifollitropin alfa on stimulation day 1, COS treatment may be continued with daily injections of (recombinant) follicle-stimulating hormone [(rec)FSH] until the criterion for triggering final oocyte maturation has been reached. The daily dose of (rec)FSH may depend on the ovarian response. In normal responders, a daily dose of 150 IU (rec)FSH is advised, but doses as high as 300–450 IU have been used. Administration of (rec)FSH on the day of human chorionic gonadotropin (hCG) administration can be omitted, depending on the ovarian response. In general, adequate follicular development is achieved on average by the ninth day of treatment (range 6 to 18 days). As soon as adequate numbers of mature follicles are observed, a single injection of triggering medications is administered the same day or the day thereafter to induce final oocyte maturation. In case of an excessive ovarian response (>18 Follicles), a GnRH agonist can be given followed by vitrification of all oocytes or embryos to reduce the risk for developing ovarian hyperstimulation syndrome (OHSS). Subcutaneous injection of corifollitropin alfa may be carried out by the woman herself or her partner, provided that proper instructions are given by the physician.

22.13.2 Puregon®/Follistim®: The Brand Name of Follitropin Beta

Follitropin beta is a gonadotropin medication. Follitropin beta contains a recombinant FSH (rFSH). This is produced by recombinant DNA technology, using a Chinese hamster ovary cell line transfected with human FSH subunit genes. The primary amino acid sequence is identical to that of natural human FSH.

22.13.2.1 Indications

Follitropin beta is indicated for the induction of ovulation (OI) in anovulatory infertile women in whom the cause of infertility is not due to primary ovarian failure. It is also indicated for normal ovulatory women undergoing controlled ovarian stimulation as part of in vitro fertilization (IVF) or intracytoplasmic sperm injection (ICSI) cycle.

In men, follitropin beta is indicated for the induction of spermatogenesis with primary and secondary hypogonadotropic hypogonadism (HH) in whom the cause of infertility is not due to primary testicular failure.

22.13.2.2 Dosage Forms and Strengths

Follistim AQ® Cartridge is a clear and colorless solution available as:

Injection: 300 international units per 0.36 mL in a single-patient-use cartridge.

Injection: 600 international units per 0.72 mL in a single-patient-use cartridge.

Injection: 900 international units per 1.08 mL in a single-patient-use cartridge.

Medication storage: Store unused cartridge refrigerated at 2 °C to 8 °C (36 °F to 46 °F) until the expiration date, or at room temperature at up to 25 °C (77 °F) for 3 months or until expiration date, whichever occurs first. After first use, store at 2 °C to 25 °C (36 °F to 77 °F) and discard after 28 days. Store in the original carton to protect from light. Do not freeze. Do not add any other medicines into the follitropin beta cartridge.

22.13.3 Use

Gently pull off the outer needle shield, leaving the inner needle shield in place, and set aside. Use an alcohol pad to clean about a 2-inch area of skin where the needle will enter. Do not discard the outer needle shield. Carefully remove the inner needle shield and discard. Do not touch the needle or let it touch any surface while uncapped. Hold the follitropin beta pen with the needle pointing upward. Tap the cartridge holder gently with the finger to force air bubbles to the top of the needle. Dial the dosage knob until a click is heard. With the needle pointing upward, push in the injection button. Look for a droplet of medicine at the needle tip. If a droplet is not seen, repeat the steps above; otherwise, the patient might not receive the correct dose. If the patient has already used the follitropin beta pen (injection) and they need to give themselves another dose, attach a new Pen Needle and look for a droplet forming at the tip of the needle. If they do not see a droplet, repeat the previous 2 steps. For doses of 50 International Units (IU) up to 450 IU, turn the dosage knob until the correct dosage aligns with the dosage markers on each side of the dosage window. If they dial past your dose, they should not turn the dosage knob backward (they will not damage the pen, but medicine will be lost). Instead, the patient should continue turning until you pass the 450 IU mark, as far as it will turn. The dosage knob must move freely. They should push the injection button in as far as it will go. The patient should start dialing from "0" upward until they reach the correct dosage. The patient should never try to correct a dose-dialing mistake while the needle is in their skin. This may result in an incorrect dose. If the prescribed dose exceeds the deliverable dose of the follitropin beta pen or exceeds the amount remaining in the cartridge, the patient will need to give themselves more than one injection.

The most common adverse reactions (≥2%) in women undergoing ovulation induction are ovarian hyperstimulation syndrome, ovarian cyst, abdominal discomfort, abdominal pain, and lower abdominal pain.

The most common adverse reactions (≥2%) in women undergoing controlled ovarian stimulation as part of an IVF or ICSI cycle are pelvic discomfort, headache, ovarian hyperstimulation syndrome, pelvic pain, nausea, and fatigue.

The most common (≥2%) adverse reactions in men undergoing induction of spermatogenesis are headache, acne, injection site reaction, injection site pain, gynecomastia (breast enlargement), rash, and dermoid cyst.

22.13.4 Orgalutran®: The Brand Name of Ganirelix Acetate

22.13.4.1 Background

Ganirelix acetate is a gonadotropin-releasing hormone (GnRH) antagonist. This injectable medication blocks the GnRH receptor by competitively binding to the receptor in the pituitary gland preventing the release of FSH and LH. This action is immediate rather than the few days required to suppress the pituitary with GnRH agonists. Ganirelix acetate is supplied as a colorless, odorless, sterile, ready-to-use solution intended for SQ use. It is packaged as a single dose, prefilled syringe indicated for the inhibition of premature LH surges in women undergoing controlled ovarian hyperstimulation.

22.13.4.2 How It Is Supplied

Ganirelix acetate injection is supplied in a carton containing one of the following:

1. Disposable, ready-to-use, single-dose, prefilled, 1-ml glass syringe containing 250 mcg/0.5 mL aqueous solution closed with a rubber piston that does not contain latex. Each ganirelix acetate sterile, prefilled syringe is affixed with a 27 gauge x ½ inch needle closed by a needle shield of dry natural rubber/latex that comes into contact with the product.
2. Disposable, ready-to-use, single-dose, prefilled 1-ml glass syringe containing 250 mcg/0.5 mL aqueous solution closed with a plunger stopper. Each ganirelix acetate sterile, prefilled syringe is affixed with a 27 gauge × ½ inch staked needle closed by a rigid needle shield (RNS) not made with natural rubber latex (2).

When removing the prefilled syringe from the packaging, the patient may notice air bubbles in the syringe. This is expected and removal is not needed.

22.13.4.3 Storage

Ganirelix acetate injection should be stored at 77 °F (25 °C); excursions permitted to 59–86 °F (15–30 °C) and should be protected from direct light (2).

22.13.5 Pregnyl®: Brand Name of Chorionic Gonadotropin for Injection

It is indicated for induction of ovulation. It is supplied as a sterile, dried powder for intramuscular injection after reconstitution. Each multiple-dose vial is only for use in one patient and contains 10,000 USP units of chorionic gonadotropin with dibasic sodium phosphate (4.4 mg) and monobasic sodium phosphate (5 mg). If required, pH is adjusted with sodium hydroxide and/or phosphoric acid by Organon®. Each package also contains a 10-mL vial of solvent containing water for injection with 0.56% sodium chloride and 0.9% benzyl alcohol (preservative). Only 1 ml of solvent should be mixed in the powder dissolved and then re-aspirated and injected into the patient.

In conclusion, this chapter provides you with a broad overview of how to use and manage fertility medications. Although biosimilar products were not discussed, they will be used in a similar manner to these medications presented in this chapter. This information is invaluable for nurses who will perform the bulk of teaching related to these medicines.

Acknowledgments We wish to acknowledge the teams from Ferring®, IBSA®, Merck®, and Organon® without whose contributions this chapter would not have been possible.

Conflicts of Interests MHD has received speaker's stipends from Merck and Ferring. He has received a research grant from Merck and has been an expert for Merck, Ferring, and Organon (under previous company names). SLT has no conflicts of interest to declare.

References

1. Al-Inany H, Aboulghar MA, Mansour RT, Serour GI. Optimizing GnRH antagonist administration: meta-analysis of fixed versus flexible protocol. Reprod Biomed Online. 2005;10(5):567–70.
2. Almeida BE, Oliveira JE, Carvalho CM, Dalmora SL, Bartolini P, Ribela MT. Analysis of human luteinizing hormone and human chorionic gonadotropin preparations of different origins by reversed-phase high-performance liquid chromatography. J Pharm Biomed Anal. 2010;53(1):90–7.
3. Bosch E, Broer S, Griesinger G, Grynberg M, Humaidan P, Kolibianakis E, Kunicki M, La Marca A, Lainas G, Le Clef N, Massin N, Mastenbroek S, Polyzos N, Sunkara SK, Timeva T, Töyli M, Urbancsek J, Vermeulen N, Broekmans F. ESHRE guideline: ovarian stimulation for IVF/ICSI(†). Hum Reprod Open. 2020;2020(2):hoaa009.

4. Casarini L, Crépieux P. Molecular mechanisms of action of FSH. Front Endocrinol (Lausanne). 2019;10:305.
5. Dallagiovanna C, Mensi L, Di Gesaro L, La Vecchia I, Reschini M. satisfaction and usability of the recombinant chorionic gonadotropin prefilled pen: a survey in Italy. Drugs Context. 2022;11
6. Depalo R, Jayakrishan K, Garruti G, Totaro I, Panzarino M, Giorgino F, Selvaggi LE. GnRH agonist versus GnRH antagonist in in vitro fertilization and embryo transfer (IVF/ET). Reprod Biol Endocrinol. 2012;10:26.
7. EMA. Cetrotide: summary of product characteristics; 2023a. Retrieved October, 2024, from https://www.ema.europa.eu/en/documents/product-information/cetrotide-epar-product-information_en.pdf
8. EMA. GONAL-f: summary of product characteristics; 2023b. 11 October 2023, from https://www.ema.europa.eu/en/documents/product-information/gonal-f-epar-product-information_en.pdf
9. EMA. Ovitrelle: summary of product characteristics; 2023c. Retrieved October, 2024, from https://www.ema.europa.eu/en/medicines/human/EPAR/ovitrelle
10. EMA. Pergoveris: summary or product characteristics; 2023d. Retrieved October, 2024, from https://www.ema.europa.eu/en/documents/product-information/pergoveris-epar-product-information_en.pdf
11. EMA. Gonal-f: summary of product characteristics; 2024a. from https://www.ema.europa.eu/en/documents/product-information/gonal-f-epar-product-information_en.pdf
12. EMA. Luveris: summary of product characteristics; 2024b. Retrieved October, 2024, from https://www.ema.europa.eu/en/documents/product-information/luveris-epar-product-information_en.pdf
13. Ezcurra D, Humaidan P. A review of luteinising hormone and human chorionic gonadotropin when used in assisted reproductive technology. Reprod Biol Endocrinol. 2014;12:95.
14. Fatemi H, Bilger W, Denis D, Griesinger G, La Marca A, Longobardi S, Mahony M, Yin X, D'Hooghe T. Dose adjustment of follicle-stimulating hormone (FSH) during ovarian stimulation as part of medically-assisted reproduction in clinical studies: a systematic review covering 10 years (2007-2017). Reprod Biol Endocrinol. 2021;19(1):68.
15. FDA. Gonal-f: summary of product charaacteristics; 2020. From https://www.accessdata.fda.gov/drugsatfda_docs/label/2020/020378s045,s067,s075lbl.pdf
16. La Marca A, Sunkara SK. Individualization of controlled ovarian stimulation in IVF using ovarian reserve markers: from theory to practice. Hum Reprod Update. 2014;20(1):124–40.
17. Leão Rde B, Esteves SC. Gonadotropin therapy in assisted reproduction: an evolutionary perspective from biologics to biotech. Clinics (Sao Paulo). 2014;69(4):279–93.
18. Lunenfeld B, Bilger W, Longobardi S, Alam V, D'Hooghe T, Sunkara SK. The development of gonadotropins for clinical use in the treatment of infertility. Front Endocrinol (Lausanne). 2019;10:429.
19. Mahony MC, Hayward B, Mottla GL, Richter KS, Beall S, Ball GD, D'Hooghe T. Recombinant human follicle-stimulating hormone alfa dose adjustment in US clinical practice: an observational, retrospective analysis of a real-world electronic medical records database. Front Endocrinol (Lausanne). 2021;12:742089.
20. Marques P, Lages ADS, Skorupskaite K, et al. Physiology of GnRH and gonadotrophin secretion. In: Feingold KR, Adler RA, Ahmed SF, Anawalt B, Blackman MR, et al., editors. Endotext. South Dartmouth (MA): MDText.com; 2024.
21. McGee EA, Hsueh AJ. Initial and cyclic recruitment of ovarian follicles. Endocr Rev. 2000;21(2):200–14.

GPSR Compliance

The European Union's (EU) General Product Safety Regulation (GPSR) is a set of rules that requires consumer products to be safe and our obligations to ensure this.

If you have any concerns about our products, you can contact us on ProductSafety@springernature.com

In case Publisher is established outside the EU, the EU authorized representative is:

Springer Nature Customer Service Center GmbH
Europaplatz 3
69115 Heidelberg, Germany

Batch number: 10927743

Printed by Printforce, the Netherlands